IDEAL BODY

The New Science of Cosmetic Surgery

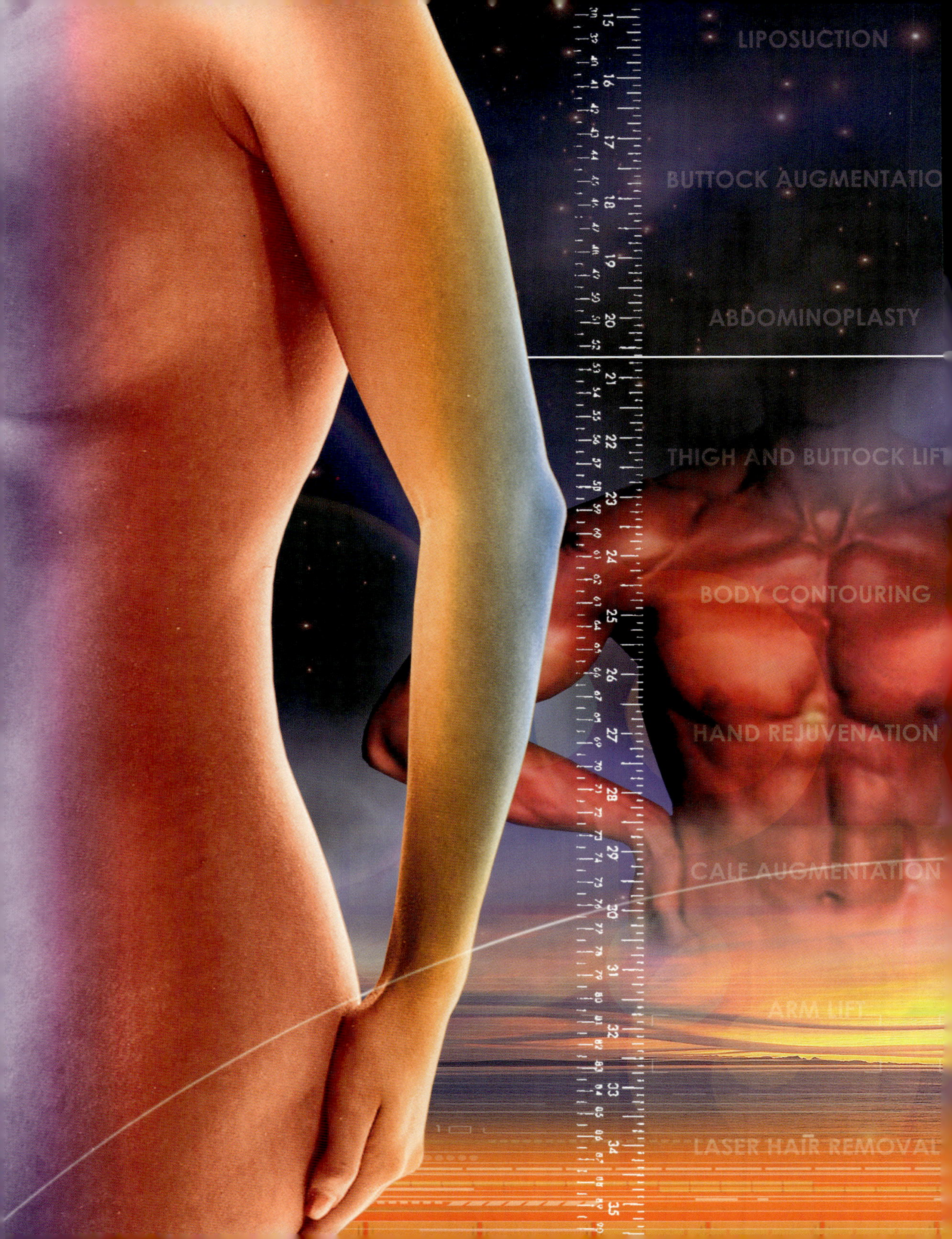
LIPOSUCTION
BUTTOCK AUGMENTATIO
ABDOMINOPLASTY
THIGH AND BUTTOCK LIF
BODY CONTOURING
HAND REJUVENATION
CALF AUGMENTATION
ARM LIFT
LASER HAIR REMOVAL

IDEAL BODY

The New Science of Cosmetic Surgery

BY

Eric Swanson, MD, FRCS(C), FACS

IDEAL LOOK

Published in the United States by:

Ideal Look LLC
11413 Ash
Leawood, KS 66211

For ordering information, contact:
ideallook.info

Ideal Look™ Series:

Ideal Face	ISBN 978-0-578-03663-2
Ideal Facelift	ISBN 978-0-578-03664-9
Ideal Body	ISBN 978-0-578-03665-6
Ideal Breast	ISBN 978-0-578-03666-3

Library of Congress Control Number:
2009911801

Library of Congress Cataloging-in-Publication Data is available.

Gwendolyn Godfrey, Illustrator
Scott Rule, Graphic Designer

Printed in the United States of America
November 2009

5 4 3 2 1

Dedication

The *Ideal Look* series is dedicated to my wife, Cindy, who has worked closely with me since I decided to specialize in cosmetic surgery. Behind many plastic surgeons, there is a trusted assistant who is their biggest fan and also their most discerning critic, and Cindy is mine. Many of my treatments have been influenced by Cindy's input, which is in turn derived from spending countless hours talking to patients and getting their feedback. There have been many times when this work seemed too large and too diverse to complete. What started as one volume has become four, yet this work still serves as an introduction and cannot be considered comprehensive. No doubt many of the techniques discussed here will be modified and some changed completely within a few years of publication.

A big thanks goes to my patients, who have placed their trust in me to make them look better and younger. Given the importance of appearance, there is hardly a more sincere gesture of trust, and it is one that I do not take lightly. Most of what I know has been learned from my patients. I am grateful for their willingness to share their experiences and photographs.

Acknowledgments

I would like to acknowledge the talented assistance of several individuals: Lindsey Wordekemper, B.S.N., for collecting the data and putting it on ever-expanding spreadsheets; Jane Thompson, Ph.D., for the biostatistical analyses that helped make sense of the voluminous clinical data; Gwendolyn Godfrey, for medical illustrations and cover art; and Scott Rule for layout and design.

Table of Contents

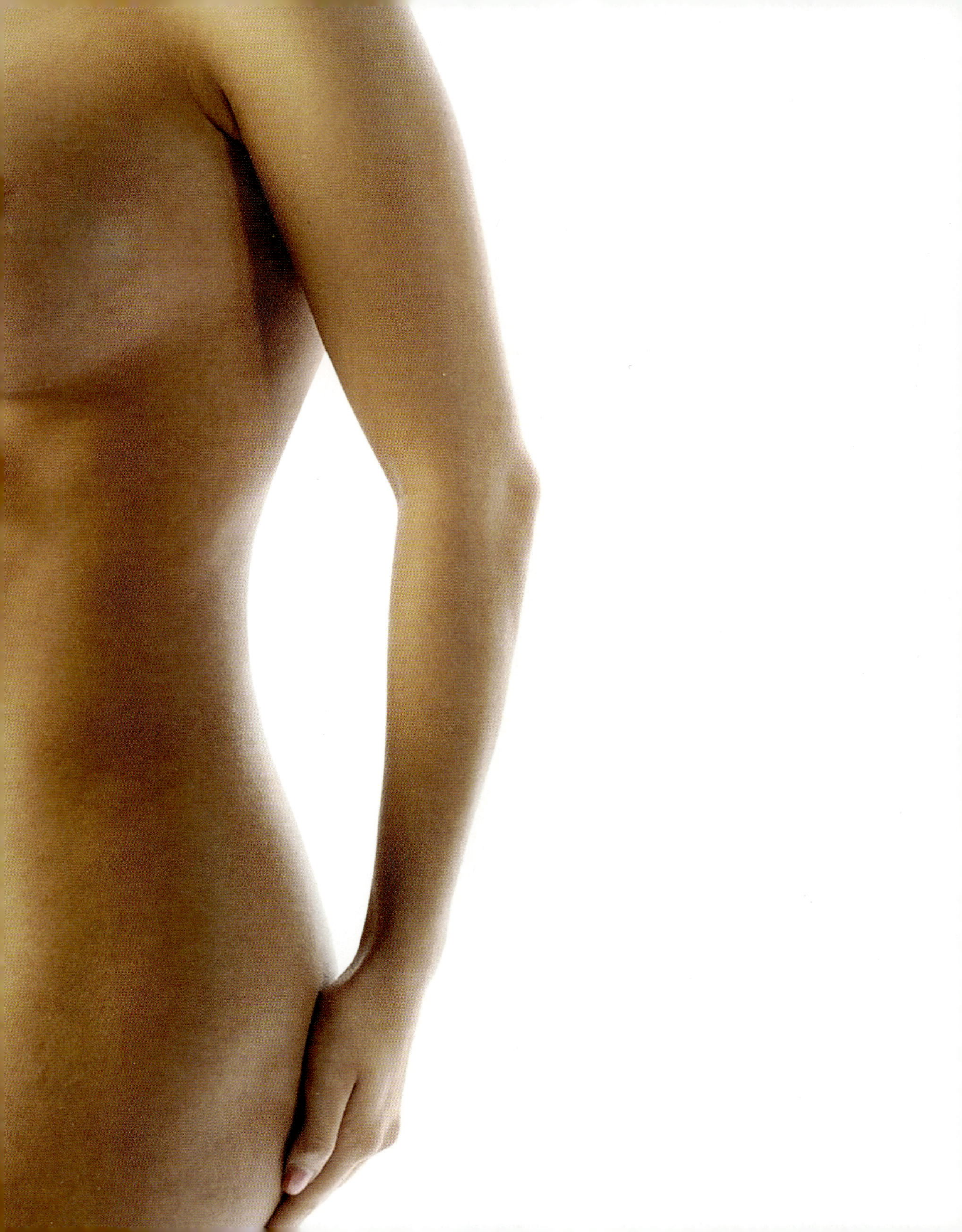

Foreword – Science and the Ideal Body

*"It is by the real that we exist;
it is by the ideal that we live."*
~Victor Hugo

Like the face, there is no denying the importance of the appearance of our bodies. Having an ideal weight is a great start to looking good, feeling good, and living longer. Obesity is a huge problem in the United States today, with one-third of adults obese, and another third overweight. It doesn't have to be this way. In France, only 9% of adults are obese; in Japan, only 3%.

What is obese? Obesity is defined as a body mass index of 30 or more. This index (BMI for short) relates weight to height. Obese people are aware of the prejudice they encounter socially and in the workplace because of their weight. Their thinner counterparts may interpret their obesity as a lack of self-discipline and self-esteem, so there is plenty of motivation to lose weight. Plastic surgeons are seeing more patients who have successfully lost weight, either through dieting or surgery. Out-patient, laparascopic "Lap-Band" surgery is now available as an effective and safe surgical option. However, after losing weight, patients find there is still work to be done. They need plastic surgery to deal with the stretched out skin. Corrective operations including tummy tucks, thigh lifts, and the combination treatment—a "lower body lift"—have gained popularity.

Out of the blue, liposuction became the most commonly performed plastic surgical procedure.

Body disproportion is also very common, but it is not the same as obesity. The medical name for this problem is "lipodystrophy." The affected areas are typically the lower body in women, including the thighs ("saddlebags"), and the tummy and flanks ("love handles") in men. No amount of dieting or exercising can correct this disproportion, which is caused by a genetic maldistribution of fat cells. It is remarkable to consider that prior to the 1980s there was no good medical treatment for this problem, despite its relatively low-tech solution.

Liposuction offered the first reliable means to reshape patients, correcting their disproportion for the rest of their lives. Women who struggled to fit pants over their thighs and then found them loose in the waist could finally be rid of this nuisance. They could start wearing flattering, form-fitting clothing. Out of the blue, liposuction became the most commonly performed plastic surgical procedure. One patient of mine who was subject to ridicule as a teenager told me, "I wish I'd done this when I was 19. It would have changed my life." The problem is not trivial.

Another problem, excess breast tissue in men, can have profound psychological ramifications. A few hours of surgery and this blight on self-confidence and masculinity is gone.

However, as in other areas of the cosmetic surgery business, such a common problem attracts those who seek to profit from the public's emotional vulnerability. A recent example is the dramatic rise and fall of LipoDissolve, a series of injections that was marketed to melt away fat. This company was started by two gynecologists who gathered investors and sank millions of dollars into advertising, opening clinics in several states that were staffed by sales consultants, whose job it was to sign people up and collect large deposits in advance. This business was started despite a lack of research regarding the effectiveness and safety of the procedure, and without even FDA approval of the injected substances. The marketers took aim at liposuction with billboards that read, "It doesn't suck!" featuring eye-catching buff models (See page 31). Even some plastic surgeons hopped on board the LipoDissolve bandwagon. Others scratched their heads, wondering if they were crazy not to get on board with them. Their rationality was challenged by the hype. But they were not crazy after all. As it turned out, LipoDissolve did not live up to its promises and soon went out of business.

The challenge today is skin tone (tightness). Ultrasound is used to stimulate skin contraction by heating the subcutaneous tissues. However, it is difficult to study the degree of skin contraction, and this phenomenon has not been subjected to rigorous scientific evaluation. Claims of skin contraction, including mine, remain unquantified.

Cellulite, the unsightly skin dimpling that patients sometimes compare to hail damage, remains an unsolved problem.

Cellulite, the unsightly skin dimpling that patients sometimes compare to hail damage, remains an unsolved problem. Tabloids show photographs of cellulite on celebrities, who must be mortified to see them (no doubt wondering, Where was that body double when I needed her?). It is easy to understand the pressure to do something, *anything* that might help. Patients are disappointed to learn that plastic surgeons today do not have much to offer. We can effectively treat bulges and body disproportion, but we are still in the dark as to how to smooth skin dimpling. To fill this treatment vacuum, the marketplace is full of diets, creams, and machines that are supposed to help, but there is no scientific validation.

Endermologie® (LPG Systems, Nice, Fr.) is a massage system that combines rollers and suction. It can be a pleasant massage experience and patients report a temporary benefit in cellulite, but treatments must be continued on a regular basis to maintain results.

VelaShape™, an upgrade of the VelaSmooth™ system (Syneron Inc., Irvine, Ca.) is a machine that uses a combination of four modalities—radiofrequency energy, infrared light, rollers, and suction—in a shotgun effort to smooth cellulite. The manufacturer also claims this treatment can reduce the circumference of the abdomen, buttocks, and thighs. Extraordinary claims; disappointing results.

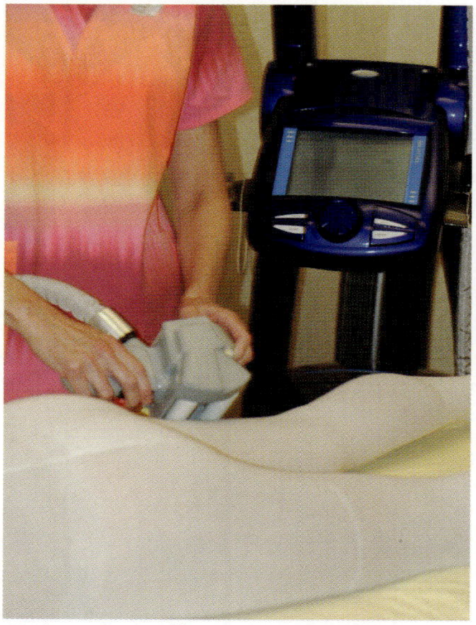

Endermologie offers a massage system to help smooth cellulite.

So what is the science of liposuction? Liposuction has been subjected to scientific study by pioneers in the field of ultrasonic liposuction. In 2002, our center launched its own intensive multipart investigation to answer basic questions and test liposuction's validity as a treatment. We examined weight changes, changes in cholesterol and triglycerides, levels of circulating anesthetic agents, hemoglobin, liver enzymes, electrolytes, and fasting blood sugar. We were fortunate to have volunteers who submitted to MRIs before and after surgery to allow quantification of changes in the thickness of the fat layer.

Patients often ask about the recovery period and when they will get back to normal activities after surgery. They deserve realistic information so that they have the right expectations. There is no better source for this information than patients themselves. After surgery, our patients submitted to detailed surveys administered by our nurses to assess their outcomes. These surveys included questions about the recovery period, result ratings on a scale of 1 to 10 (always of interest to the surgeon), and the psychological effects. This kind of detailed, in-person data-gathering in consecutive patients ensured high response rates and reliability, essential to evidence-based medicine. The findings are relevant to anyone considering body contouring surgery, and are contained in this volume—*Ideal Body*.

CHAPTER ONE

Liposuction

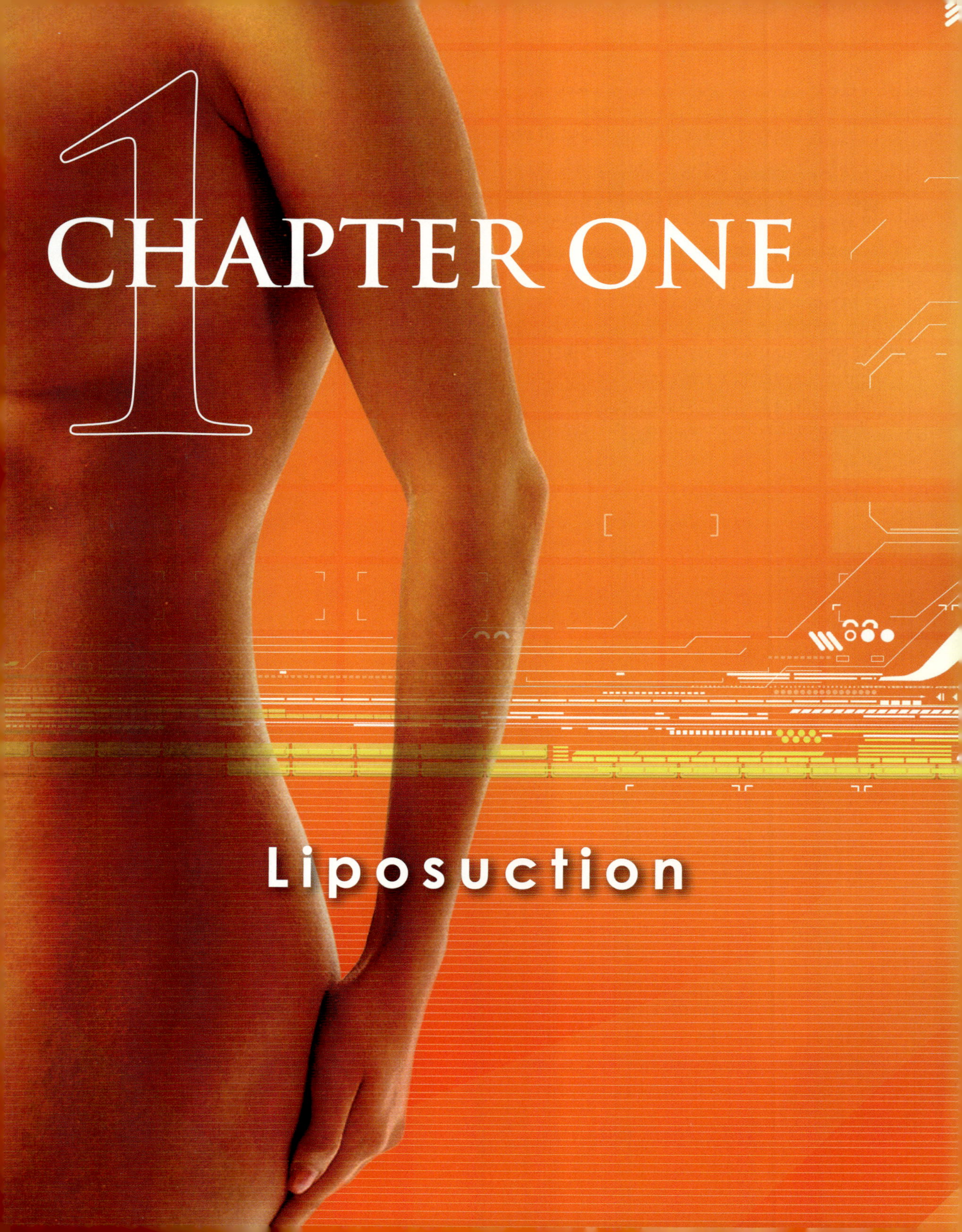

The Ideal Body

What is the ideal body? In centuries past, a full-figured female form has been the standard in most cultures, a sign of health and nutrition. You won't find any "six-packs" or well-toned biceps on Greek statues of women. In the last several decades, some testosterone has been mixed in to the notion of the ideal female body, giving way in the late 20th century to a sinewy, lean look, but with full breasts and rounded buttocks. This combination is unusual in nature. Few women are naturally endowed with an enviable lean physique and full breasts (and round buttocks for that matter). Similarly, few men are endowed with the physique of Michelangelo's David. David did not have love handles!

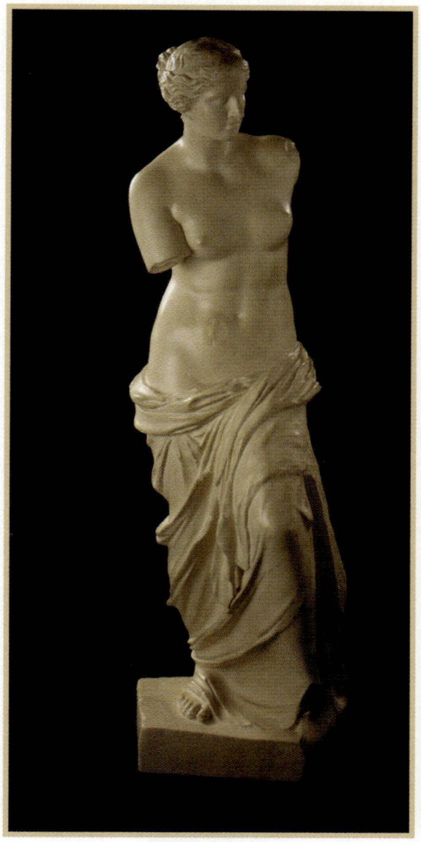

Venus de Milo

Healthy premenopausal women have waist-to-hip ratios of 0.67 to 0.80. This means that their waist circumference is seven- to eight-tenths as large as their hips. A healthy man's waist-to-hip ratio is between 0.85 and 0.95. Moderate weight gain does not alter these basic female and male shapes.

Men have an innate preference for female bodies with narrow waists and full hips, which signal high fertility, high estrogen, and low testosterone. Interestingly, this preference for feminine waist-to-hip ratios is not limited to Caucasian males, but is true for women and other cultures and races as well.

The 1950s bombshell and early *Playboy* centerfold, Jayne Mansfield, reportedly had measurements of 40-21-35, giving her a waist-to-hip ratio of 0.60. (She also said her IQ was 163, but the public was more interested in her other measurements.) Cartoon characters and virtual images of females like Jessica Rabbit (*Who Framed Roger Rabbit*, 1988), and Lara Croft (*Lara Croft* movies starring Angelina Jolie, 2001, 2003, and video games) typically have exaggerated proportions. Barbie™ (1959-) has measurements of 36-18-33, with a 0.54 waist-to-hip ratio (at least before "breaking up" with Ken in 2004, so tragic).

In centuries past, a full-figured female form has been the standard in most cultures, a sign of health and nutrition.

During the 20th century, Miss Americas (1923-87) and *Playboy* centerfolds (1955-65, 1976-90) alike had waist-to-hip ratios that ranged from 0.68 to 0.72. The average Miss America measurements in 1940 were 34-24.5-35; in 1987, they were a slightly bustier and trimmer 35-23.5-34.5. Of course, these measurements took place before and after the introduction of breast implants in the early 1960s and liposuction in the 1980s, enhancements that no doubt influenced later measurements. By the end of the 20th century, the average fashion model was four inches taller than the average woman, but maintained an hourglass 0.70 waist-to-hip ratio, combining a tall, lean body with curves. These measurements counter the notion that the aesthetic ideal has become sleeker and less curvaceous in recent years—sleeker yes, less curvaceous no. These models seem to have their cake and eat it too (or perhaps I should say their tofu)!

The Miss Americas of the 1960s averaged five feet six inches tall and weighed 120 pounds. Twenty years later they had gained two inches in height but remained the same weight. *Playboy* playmates also gained an inch in height and dropped several pounds in weight during the same period. Even the Columbia Pictures logo, the torch-bearing woman, was slimmed in 1992. Who knows if the Statue of Liberty is next?

How do these ideals compare to reality? Today, 64% of American adults are overweight, defined as having a body mass index of 25 or greater, and 31% are obese, having a body mass of 30 or greater. Only one state, Colorado, can claim less than a 20% obesity rate. Alarmingly, six states have rates higher than 30%. The proportion of overweight children (ages 6-19) has jumped from about 5% to 17% in the last 30 years, an indication that this problem is unlikely to get much better in the near future.

Fat Cells and Body Weight

Any discussion of liposuction needs to start with an understanding of fat cells and body weight. An excellent resource on this topic of interest to almost everyone is Robert Pool's scholarly review, *Fat. Fighting the Obesity Epidemic*.

For the nonobese, body fat distribution and number of fat cells is determined genetically. Nonobese people form fat cells only up to age two, and then again from age 10 to 18 as a consequence of puberty—we talk about teenagers "filling out." By contrast, obese children continue to form fat cells up to the age of 24, ending up with more fat cells in adulthood than their leaner friends.

Unlike neurons or cardiac muscle cells, fat cells do not consume much energy.

An adult female who weighs 160 pounds has about 40 pounds of fat. Her lean body mass is 120 pounds. At 200 pounds, she has about 70 pounds of fat, but her lean body mass increases only about 10 pounds (accounting for the extra weight of connective tissue, muscle and blood vessels to support the fat). You might think that a much heavier person would have proportionately larger energy requirements caused by the extra metabolic load of the additional fat cells, but this additional fatty tissue adds little to the body's energy requirements. Unlike neurons or cardiac muscle cells, fat cells do not consume much energy.

Until studies were done in the 1960s by Dr. Jules Hirsch and co-workers, it was unknown whether obese people had an excess number of fat cells or their fat cells simply got bigger or both. Research showed that, as a person's weight increases from ideal body weight to obesity, the number of fat cells remains the same. Each fat cell swells to accommodate more fat-storing triglycerides. But this cellular expansion has a limit. A fat cell can expand to about four times its original size before it needs to divide to store more fat. This works out to about a 60 pound weight gain in the average adult, corresponding to a body mass index well over 30. Within a range of about 60 pounds over ideal weight, fat cell numbers stay the same. Any changes are purely due to an increase or decrease in the size of individual fat cells. An average fat cell is about one-tenth of a millimeter in diameter, about the width of a human hair. In obese people the fat cell may be twice as big, and in lean people half as big.

Body Mass Index

Body Mass Index: Weight (kg) / height $(m)^2$

Underweight	< 18.5
Average weight	18.5-24.99
Overweight	≥ 25
Obese	≥ 30

So what happens if an obese person loses a lot of weight? Does the number of fat cells drop too? The answer is yes, but only with great difficulty. Researchers found that in extremely obese patients who underwent successful bariatric surgery, lost massive amounts of weight, and maintained the weight loss, fat cell *size* dropped sharply. However, reduction in cell *number* was not as impressive; only about a sixth of the fat cells seemed to disappear. Like a benevolent employer, the body does not want to let go of the extra fat cells after they have been recruited.

Like a benevolent employer, the body does not want to let go of the extra fat cells after they have been recruited.

You might wonder, as I have, what causes an obese patient's weight to level out. If extra fat adds little to the body's energy requirements, what stops obese people from gaining weight indefinitely? The answer requires an understanding of homeostasis and metabolic rate.

Homeostatic Set Point

Nonobese people probably think the main problem in obesity is simply that obese people eat too much. We might imagine that they have an entrenched low self-esteem and poor willpower. Obese people do not get much sympathy.

We all might be a little more sympathetic once we understand that the underlying problem is not that they are eating too much. That is secondary. The primary problem in obese people is a change in homeostasis—the "set point" for their weight. The set point is the weight that the body considers normal. In obesity, this equilibrium may become reset at a much higher weight than normal. If their weight creeps up *above* this point, their metabolic rate increases to burn calories, they tend to lose their hunger, and their weight drifts back to this set point. If their weight drops *below* this set point, their brain receives hunger signals, their metabolic rate drops to conserve energy (despite the abundance of energy-stuffed fat cells), and they eat more. We are all slaves to this set point. Nonobese people are fortunate to have a normal set point. An analogy might be resetting the home thermostat to 100°F and finding that this feels most comfortable and that normal room temperature feels too cold.

In the obese person whose weight drops below this elevated set point, the body wrongly reacts as if it is starving and needs to conserve fuel. This explains why a 350 pound woman may consume fewer calories each day than her normal-weight friend and still not lose weight. So when an obese patient claims to be consuming only 2,000 calories a day and not losing weight, she may not be kidding. Doctors need to know this so they are not inclined to think that the patient is being dishonest or making excuses for failing to lose weight.

How does the brain know when to feel hungry and when to feel satiated? Part of the answer involves the hormone leptin, which is produced by fat cells. This hormone takes part in a feedback loop with the hypothalamus of the brain. People born without the gene for this hormone, an exceedingly rare condition, always feel hungry and become severely obese (and may be successfully treated with injections of this hormone). The problem is that obese people already have high levels of circulating leptin, so this strategy would not work for them. The fat cells are doing their job—sending a signal that they have enough energy now, thank you—but the brain isn't "listening." It seems the receptors in the brain become insensitive to this hormone, just the way the body can become insensitive to insulin in conditions of obesity. The brain is still in the hunter-gatherer mode, a long period in our evolution during which starvation was the constant threat to life, not obesity. The brain hasn't evolved to deal with conditions of such an abundant energy supply.

The fat cells are doing their job—sending a signal that they have enough energy now, thank you—but the brain isn't "listening."

In nonobese people, this homeostatic mechanism is very finely tuned, so that their body weight changes little in the course of a year, despite large swings in the number of calories in and calories out. However, there is a general trend upward, with the average American man or woman gaining about 20 pounds between the age of 25 and 55 (a finding that probably does not surprise most of us).

Studies in volunteers have shown that nonobese people who gain weight intentionally tend to lose it quickly, and the weight gain is entirely due to fat cell expansion. Their normal set point remains close to their ideal body weight. This normal set point explains how a nonobese movie star can gain weight for a role (Renee Zellweger in the movie *Bridget Jones Diary*, for example) and then lose it quickly.

However, obese people feel hungry when their weight is below this set point, *even if this set point is 350 pounds*. This fact explains why people who have successfully dropped hundreds of pounds without surgery are so few and far between, and almost maniacal in their efforts to stay thin. They must exert tremendous willpower to stay thin because they often feel hungry. They may have even developed some obsessive behavior in an effort to keep the weight off, such as jogging six miles a day or counting every calorie. Unfortunately, this artificially raised set point does not change easily in people who have been obese.

As it turns out, weight control is not just a simple matter of calories in and calories out. Change in homeostatic set point partially explains why obesity is so hard to cure, and why billions of dollars are spent each year on weight loss programs with such unimpressive results. We are all aware of celebrities who have fought weight issues (Oprah Winfrey), or even written books about weight control (Dr. Phil), but don't seem to succeed despite all the personal and professional incentives.

There are rare cases of genetic mutations causing obesity (Prader-Willi syndrome), but in these patients the obesity is extreme, and there are other obvious physical abnormalities. A review of increasing obesity rates in the United States shows that genetic predisposition cannot be the major cause of obesity. Easy access to high-fat foods, our sedentary culture, and the fact that only 22% of American adults exercise regularly are no doubt major contributing factors.

Unfortunately, although its benefits are undeniable, exercise may be overrated for weight control. Recent studies suggest that proper diet is much more important because the calories burned by exercise are so modest compared with the calories consumed in a single serving of french fries, for example, or a muffin. Furthermore, exercise tends to increase hunger, creating a vicious cycle. Any increased consumption negates the caloric benefit of the exercise. The calculation of how much exercise is needed to work off an Almond Joy bar is discouraging.

Research shows that childhood obesity is particularly insidious. Once those extra fat cells are deposited, it is very difficult for people to drop back to ideal body weight. One study found that 75% of children who were obese at age 10-14 were obese at age 25. Parents who teach their children poor eating habits are doing them a disservice that may last a lifetime.

The take-home message? Avoid childhood obesity and avoid gaining so much weight as an adult that your body produces more fat cells, raising the homeostatic set point for body weight. Once that happens, you are going to have a hard time losing weight and keeping it off.

Avoid childhood obesity and avoid gaining so much weight as an adult that your body produces more fat cells, raising the homeostatic set point for body weight.

Body Shape is Hereditary

It comes as no surprise to most of us that our body shape resembles other family members. Women sometimes refer to an "apple shape" or "pear shape" to describe their (nonideal) proportions. (In fact, there is no fruit that women prefer to resemble.)

Men sometimes remark, "Even when I was in boot camp, I had these love handles." With weight gain and loss, these fat cells enlarge and shrink along with fat cells in other areas of the body, but they never go away.

When we gain weight, our existing fat cells swell, and when we lose weight, they shrink. *But their number and distribution remain the same.* This fact explains why we find that our dimensions are reduced after weight loss, and increased after weight gain, but our body proportions stay about the same. Women with a "pear" shape (also unfavorably compared to a bowling pin) may find that they can drop from a size eight to a size six, but their jeans are still tight on their thighs and loose at the waist. No amount of exercise and fat burning can overcome genetics. Consequently, even professional athletes, bodybuilders (See P.K., Patient Photographs), personal trainers, and aerobics instructors have liposuction.

Body Shape and Pregnancy

Pregnancy does not alter body fat proportions. The tummy is stretched out, of course, and the body swells during pregnancy, but there is no net gain or loss of fat cells. This fact explains why, after losing their extra weight after pregnancy, women find that their body shape is unchanged. The abdominal skin and muscles have been stretched, so the skin tone is not as tight as it was before pregnancy, and there is likely to be some degree of abdominal "pouch" due to stretching of the muscles (which allows the abdomen to bulge forward), but even in the tummy, there is no fat that was not there before.

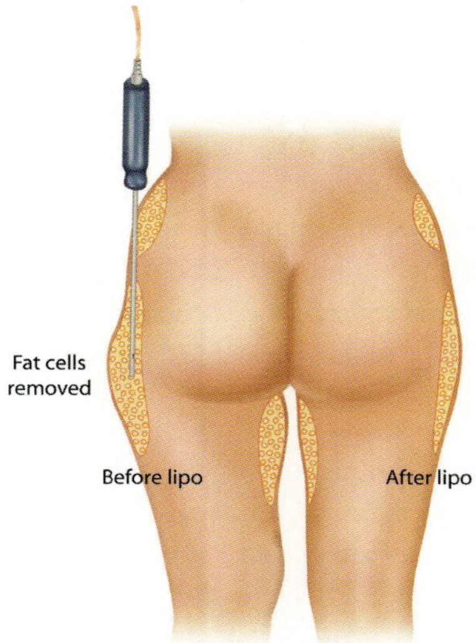

Liposuction permanently removes fat cells from affected areas.

Weight Changes after Liposuction

Patients sometimes remark, "I heard that if you have liposuction on the hips and thighs, when you gain weight you'll gain it in other places like your face and your arms." This rumor is untrue. Any weight gain after liposuction is *evenly* distributed all over the body—it does not return specifically to the treated areas, or accumulate instead in untreated areas (See Illustration, next page). Think of it this way: fat cells in other areas of the body are unaware that their fat cell neighbors in the love handles have "left the building." And even if they did have this information, they do not have the capability of multiplying to compensate. All they can due is swell or shrink, in response to the circulating caloric balance.

Like an expandable suitcase, fat cell size is determined simply by how many calories are delivered to it versus how many are consumed. The fat cell swells if the body consumes more calories than it burns, or shrinks if the body burns more calories than it takes in.

So how does a rumor like this get started? One possible explanation is that people rely on how they fit their clothes as a guide to know when to cut back on calories. After liposuction, they fit their clothes more loosely because fat cells in these areas have departed. By not being attentive to diet and exercise, their weight may creep up until their clothes fit like they did before liposuction. The remaining fat cells in these treated areas swell with the weight gain until their jeans fit the same again. Only now they are fuller in other parts of the body that were not reduced with liposuction, such as the face and arms. In these untreated areas, the fat cells have swelled with no compensatory reduction in numbers.

These patients see me in follow-up and say, "Doctor, I'm disappointed. I really didn't notice much of a difference after liposuction." Before any further discussion, they are asked to step on the scales. Invariably they weigh more, sometimes 10 pounds more, than they did at the time of liposuction. Of course they should weigh less, not more, because the fat that was removed at surgery weighed several pounds, sometimes as much as 10 pounds. Patients are often surprised to learn of this weight gain.

These patients have gained weight after surgery and this superimposed weight gain compromises their reduction from liposuction. In fact, if they had not had liposuction, they would likely not be able to fit into their pants. They ask me how they could have gained this weight. Likely they gained weight because

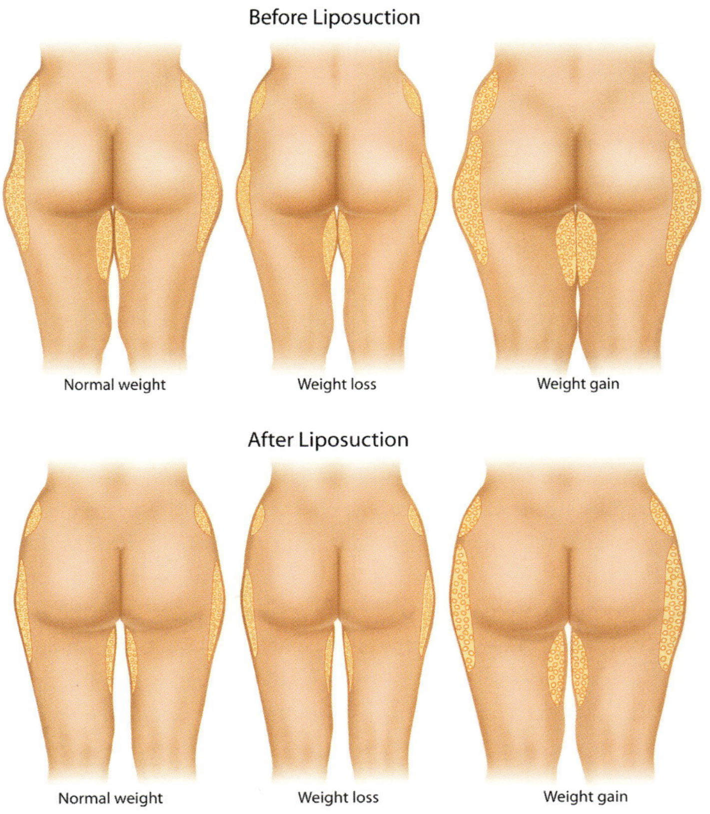

(Above) Weight gain before and (below) after liposuction. After liposuction, the treated areas contain fewer fat cells, making them trimmer at any given weight.

they were less active after surgery, but continued eating the same way. Same calories, less exercise equals weight gain. Plus their usual "alarm"—fitting clothes—did not alert them to cut back.

Fortunately, the outcome can still be a favorable one. She (or he) has not wasted her time and money having liposuction. Because the number of fat cells is fixed, there is no permanent harm done by temporary swelling of the fat cells. The benefits of liposuction can still be realized. But the patient needs to return to full activity and proper diet. When her weight returns to normal (the same as it was at the time of surgery, or less, to account for the fat removed by liposuction), she will appreciate the difference produced by liposuction, unaffected by any weight fluctuation. If she is able to reduce her weight below her preoperative weight (if she started above ideal body weight), the fat cells will be in their shrinking mode, working to her advantage (See Illustration, bottom row middle). The result just gets better and better.

I usually take photographs at least three months after liposuction. This allows enough time for the swelling to go down fully. Ideally, the patient's weight at the time of this follow-up visit is the same as it was on the day of surgery or even a little less, accounting for the weight of fat removed by liposuction. Fat weighs about two pounds per liter, so if a patient had three liters (3,000 cc) of fat removed by liposuction, she should weigh six pounds less when the swelling has gone down. Therefore, to appreciate the results of liposuction without any compromise from postoperative weight gain, this patient should weigh six pounds less than on the day of surgery.

Our studies showed that three months after liposuction, patients lost an average of 2.2 pounds overall. Patients with liposuction volumes over 3,000 cc lost an average of 5.2 pounds. While seemingly modest, these findings were statistically highly significant. Of course, this weight loss represents pure fat removed from specific areas of excess; it cannot be compared with an overall weight loss of the same amount. Removal of this volume of fat from specific problem areas gives the illusion of a larger amount of weight loss. Patients who remain the same weight, or even *gain* weight, often look much trimmer in their "after" photos. Many of the patients featured in the Patient Photographs section had weight losses of several pounds but appear to have lost many more (one dramatic example is T.M., Patient Photographs).

We know from our studies that liposuction can lower circulating triglycerides. This effect is particularly pronounced in patients with liposuction volumes over three liters. A lower level of circulating triglycerides can only be helpful. Whether liposuction has any effect on the homeostatic set point and metabolic rate is unknown.

A Permanent Improvement in Body Proportions

Because adults have a fixed number of fat cells, the only effective and safe way to remove these fat cells is by liposuction (mesotherapy, an alternative treatment, is discussed later). Liposuction works. It provides a permanent correction of body disproportions.

Another popular misconception about liposuction is that benefits may be negated by future weight gain. The patient may say, "If I gain weight, the fat will just come back and I will have wasted my time and money having liposuction." Certainly, if any benefit realized by liposuction were lost the next time the patient put on five pounds, there would be no point in having liposuction in the first place. But the results are still there at the higher weight. The patient will always fit her clothes better, regardless of how much she weighs, for the rest of her life because there are fewer fat cells in the treated areas. And when she loses the five pounds, her shape will shrink to what it was right after liposuction. In fact, it is impossible to lose the benefit of liposuction, barring extreme weight gain. Not to worry—no woman has ever told me she missed her old pear shape, and no man has told me he regretted losing his love handles.

No woman has ever told me she missed her old pear shape, and no man has told me he regretted losing his love handles.

Patients sometimes look at me with a degree of skepticism when I explain that the result is permanent, but they need only look at long-term results for confirmation (See H.E. and T.M., Patient Photographs). They understand the concept once they know that fat cell numbers are genetically determined and do not change with weight gain or loss. The only way to change fat cell distribution is by physically removing them using liposuction (or adding by fat injection). *Liposuction permanently improves body proportions.* This capability is the reason liposuction has been the most popular cosmetic operation for the last couple of decades.

Most patients are attentive to diet and exercise after surgery and lose rather than gain weight. After correction of their body disproportions, they may experience a psychological benefit and find they are more motivated to maintain their improved body form.

Fluid Management

Using the "tumescent" technique, fluids are injected into the tissues before liposuction is performed. The original tumescent technique involved giving so much fluid, as much as 10 liters, that the tissues became tightly distended. The "superwet" technique is a modified form of tumescent liposuction, in which fluids are infused in approximately a 1:1 ratio with the volume suctioned off by liposuction (the "aspirate"). This ratio represents an ideal balance between what is infused and what is removed, providing the liquid medium needed to facilitate ultrasonic liposuction, but avoiding over- or underhydration of the patient.

During surgery, the anesthetist gives "maintenance" fluids through the I.V.. The surgeon adds fluids by injecting the tissues with the infusion solution, and then subtracts fluids by performing liposuction. The surgeon and anesthetist work together to ensure that the patient's state of hydration is just right. If too much fluid is given, there may be a backup of fluid in the patient. Fluid may even start to accumulate in the lungs. This would take quite a large volume of fluid because healthy kidneys are very efficient in removing fluids from the circulation (as any college fraternity brother will attest). However, if too little replacement fluid is given during surgery, the patient's blood pressure may drop, along with perfusion of vital organs. Both extremes are obviously best avoided. Like any team, the more experience the surgeon and anesthetist have working together, the better.

Obese Patients

We know that liposuction is the only viable means to reduce the number of fat cells (except perhaps for extreme weight loss after bariatric surgery, as mentioned earlier). Might liposuction be a useful treatment for obesity? Although liposuction has been used to treat obesity, it is now recognized that this is not the best application of liposuction. In very obese patients, the volume of fat and fluid removed may be much larger—over five liters—making fluid management more difficult and increasing the risk. This is called "large volume liposuction." Furthermore, the difference in body contours is proportionately less, making the procedure less worthwhile. Also, these patients have not developed good eating habits and exercise regimens, so that they may be more likely to gain weight after surgery, particularly if they are even less active than they were before surgery.

"Beer Belly"

Only weight loss by dieting can reduce a "beer belly."

Patients with a "beer belly" are not candidates for liposuction. These patients have a very protuberant abdomen, but minimal subcutaneous fat. There is not much surface fat to grab. Almost all the fat is inside the abdomen ("intraperitoneal"), wrapped around the organs and therefore inaccessible to liposuction. These people are understandably disappointed to hear that liposuction is not an option, but are sorted out early in the consultation. They are glad to be told candidly that they are not good candidates, so they do not waste their time and money having a procedure that is unlikely to help much. I recommend professional weight loss counseling. Only weight loss by dieting can reduce a "beer belly." There is no substitute.

Touchup Liposuction

It is not unusual for patients to return after liposuction, asking for additional treatment of problem areas. This is called touchup liposuction. These patients tend to be pleased with their overall result, but wonder if more might be accomplished with another treatment. About 20% of my patients return for a touchup liposuction. A touchup liposuction is not regarded as a sign of treatment failure, but as "fine-tuning."

Returning for a touchup does not mean the patient was undertreated at the first operation. Patients understand there is a limit to what can be safely removed at one operation. If the surgeon is too aggressive, there is more tissue trauma, jeopardizing skin contraction. With overtreatment there is likely to be greater blood loss and more postoperative pain and swelling.

Rather than trying to do too much, it is preferable to come back later, if necessary, to re-treat areas. This approach reduces the risk of complications and optimizes the skin response. I tell patients with major body disproportion to plan on another liposuction procedure later on. But I also reassure them that I will do as much as I can in one operation, knowing that the reality is they may or may not have another opportunity. My job is to be as aggressive as I can in removing fat (patients frequently tell me before surgery, "Now don't hold back, doc"), without sacrificing safety, raising the risk of skin irregularities, or compromising skin recoil by causing excessive tissue trauma.

There is always less fat removed at a touchup. The recovery is faster than it was after the first liposuction, even when the same areas are treated. Bruising and swelling usually resolve more quickly, and there is less discomfort. Whenever possible, the same incisions are used for access, so there are no additional scars. Patient satisfaction is high.

How It's Done

Advances in Liposuction

Advances in liposuction include the evolution of instruments, energy source, wetting solutions used to pretreat the areas, and anesthesia.

Instrument	Energy	Solution	Results
Liposuction (1982) Large-bore, sharp cannulae	Physical	None	Small volumes Spot treatments Skin irregularities Significant blood loss
Tumescent technique (1990) Finer-caliber, blunt cannulae	Physical	Saline Lidocaine Epinephrine	Larger volumes Multiple areas Smoother borders Less blood loss

Ultrasonic liposuction (1995)			
Ultrasonic generator	Ultrasound Physical	Saline Lidocaine Epinephrine	Selective fat removal Less tissue trauma Better skin contraction (?)

A Short History of Liposuction

Liposuction was introduced by an Italian gynecologist, Dr. Giorgio Fischer, in 1974. In 1977, a French plastic surgeon, Dr. Yves-Gerard Illouz, refined the technique for cosmetic applications by pre-injecting tissues with fluid and using a safer blunt cannula (metal tube with a hole at the end). A long time coming, liposuction was a huge step forward in body contouring surgery when the technique burst on the scene after a presentation by Dr. Illouz in 1982. Previously, there was no good treatment for fat bulges. One might wonder why it did not occur to anybody to try it decades earlier. After all, the concept is pretty simple and "low-tech." In fact, it was tried in the early 1920s by another pioneering French surgeon, but there was one particularly bad outcome in a French model, who ended up with an amputation, that quickly cooled enthusiasm for it.

One might wonder why it did not occur to anybody to try it decades earlier. After all, the concept is pretty simple and "low-tech."

In 1990 an American dermatologist, Dr. Jeffrey Klein, described the tumescent technique. This modification represented another big step forward. He injected the tissues with a large volume of saline solution before performing liposuction. This saline solution contained the hormone epinephrine, to reduce blood loss, and lidocaine, a local anesthetic. The local anesthetic allowed the procedure to be performed using local anesthesia alone, in the doctor's office, making this popular technique available to nonsurgeons.

The fluid injected into the tissues served to hydrate the patient during surgery, so that little or no extra I.V. fluid administration was needed (also avoiding the need for an anesthetist). The infusion of fluid filled up the tissues, making them "tumesce." This tissue injection facilitated liposuction by enlarging the fat layer, helping to make the contours smoother because it was easier for the operator to avoid suctioning too close to the skin or overtreating areas, which might cause irregularities.

The epinephrine contained in this fluid greatly reduced blood loss, enabling the operator to treat multiple areas at one time and remove greater quantities of fat. The operator was no longer limited to spot treatments. All of the affected areas could now be treated simultaneously. Patients could be treated at one setting instead of returning for multiple procedures, expanding the capabilities and popularity of this new technique. Liposuction quickly became the most common plastic surgery operation performed in the United States, a distinction held for most of the last two decades, although liposuction was recently edged to second place by breast augmentation.

Ultrasonic Liposuction

Ultrasonic liposuction, also called ultrasonic-assisted liposuction, was developed by an Italian plastic surgeon, Dr. Michele Zocchi, in 1988. Ultrasonic liposuction was used extensively in Europe and South America for several years before being introduced to the United States in 1995.

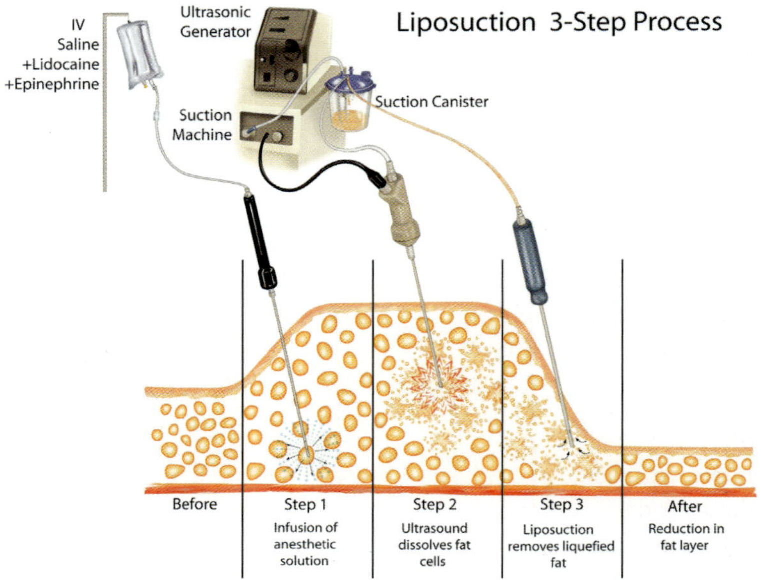

Ultrasonic energy has been used in many areas of medicine since the 1970s. One of its first applications was in eye surgery, to selectively dissolve cataracts. Ultrasound was subsequently used to remove tumors in neurosurgery. The same principle was applied to fat removal.

An ultrasonic probe produces a high frequency sound wave that causes fat cells to dissolve. The technique was introduced in combination with tumescent (or more precisely superwet) liposuction. This was a perfect matching of techniques because ultrasonic energy propagates best in a liquid environment and the fluid absorbs the heat energy generated by ultrasound.

With the introduction of ultrasonic assistance, liposuction evolved from two steps to three—the tissues are first injected with fluid, the ultrasonic probe is introduced to dissolve fat cells, and the liquefied fat is then suctioned out (See Illustration).

The infusion solution (also called wetting solution), which had not even been used in the early days of "dry liposuction," now serves multiple purposes—local anesthesia, reduced blood loss, fluid replacement, and a liquid medium for ultrasound.

Ultrasonic liposuction does not replace tumescent liposuction but rather complements it. It improves results in fibrous areas that are difficult to treat with traditional liposuction—the upper abdomen, flanks, back, and male breasts. The fat is liquefied before its removal, so that the resulting contours are smooth. Because ultrasonic energy is used to break up the fat cells, less physical force is required from the plastic surgeon. With less physical force, one might expect better preservation of the connective tissue under the skin, along with nerves and blood vessels. Less tissue trauma may mean less bruising of the tissues, less discomfort, and a shorter recovery time. An added advantage of ultrasonic liposuction may be improved skin tone and appearance, due to improved preservation of the underlying connective tissue. With selective defatting under the skin, the skin's capacity to contract is optimized. Nevertheless, it is important to recognize that these are largely theoretical benefits that have not been clinically proven in a published randomized study comparing ultrasonic with traditional liposuction.

Another favorable observation has been the rarity of infection after ultrasonic liposuction. Dr. Zocchi attributes this finding to the conversion of some of the water molecules into peroxide molecules as they are exposed to ultrasonic energy. Ultrasonic assistance may also reduce the risk of a rare complication called fat embolism syndrome (See Complications).

Patients (and even surgeons!) may be forgiven for confusing "tumescent," "ultrasonic," "laser," "Vaser®," "power-assisted, or PAL," and recently, "Water-Jet-assisted, or WAL," all words or acronyms to describe different modifications of liposuction. Stated simply, patients want the modern, up-to-date kind of liposuction that works better, but is kinder and gentler than the old-fashioned technique. They especially would like to avoid the technique they saw on television, featuring a surgeon apparently pummeling a patient with a long metal instrument!

Usually multiple sites are treated using small incisions to correct body contour disproportions. In women, the lower body is usually affected, consisting of the abdomen, hips, flanks, back, buttocks, thighs, and knees. In men, the problem areas are typically the abdomen, flanks, and breasts. Each of these areas is treated at the same operation, removing more fat in some areas and less in others to produce optimal body contours and results that look good from all angles. Spot treatments are obsolete, except for touchups. People are three-dimensional and deserve to be treated in a 3-D fashion. This is what is meant by "lower body liposuction"—circumferential treatment from the rib cage to the knees. Other commonly treated areas are the arms, calves, and under the chin ("submental lipectomy"). The knowledge of how much to remove and how much to leave behind comes only with experience.

Selectivity for Fat Cells

In the past, surgeons have relied on physical energy alone to dislodge fat cells. The surgeon literally pummeled the fat with a blunt instrument (cannula). The flimsy fat cells were dislodged from their attachments and suctioned away. This technique was effective, but nonselective. Other tissues were traumatized too.

The important tissues are preserved intact; the nerves, blood vessels, and connective tissue stay behind, like the branches of a tree that has lost its leaves.

Surgeons prefer selective techniques because there is less "collateral damage" to other tissues. This principle is familiar, also applied to medical laser treatments that target skin pigments, such as laser treatment of birthmarks, and laser hair removal. In the case of ultrasonic liposuction, a cell type is targeted—the lowly fat cell, which is like a flimsy balloon full of Jell-O. If a fat cell is exposed to high frequency sound waves, microbubbles are generated from pressure changes, called cavitation. The fragile cell membrane cannot contain these bubbles and gives way, releasing its liquid fat contents ("emulsification"), which are then suctioned out of the body. The important tissues are preserved intact; the nerves, blood vessels, and connective tissue stay behind, like the branches of a tree that has lost its leaves. No question, these tissues have been traumatized, but not as much as they would have been without the benefit of ultrasound.

Skin Tone

The most important advantage of ultrasonic liposuction may be improved skin contraction. Every woman wishes to preserve her skin tone as much as possible, so any advantage the surgeon can provide in this regard is very much appreciated.

The main component of connective tissue is collagen, the body's most abundant protein. It turns out that if you heat up collagen just the right amount, it contracts. Surgeons observe this effect when using the laser on facial skin; the skin visibly contracts. It is possible that a similar shrinking process is going on under the skin during ultrasonic liposuction. Surgeons have noticed improved skin contraction after ultrasonic treatment. However, this effect has not been scientifically validated.

In some patients, I perform ultrasonic liposuction primarily for the *skin-tightening* effect, not so much for fat removal. This is the opposite of liposuction's original purpose—to eliminate fat, but possibly at the expense of loose skin. Now we are, in effect, asking liposuction to do something more than remove fat, a task that's not really part of its job description. The benefit in skin tone is usually modest and influenced greatly by the patient's inherent skin quality and elasticity. I tell patients not to expect an improvement in skin tone; any tightening is a welcome bonus.

In the early days of liposuction (circa 1983, the year I graduated from medical school), surgeons advised their patients: "Yes, I can reduce your bulges, but at the expense of loose skin. You may need additional surgery later on to tighten loose skin, and these procedures leave long scars." So it was with understandable apprehension that women chose liposuction. That they chose it at all is a testament to their dissatisfaction with their body shape. In fact, early on, plastic surgeons recommended not performing liposuction on patients over 50 because of concern about their skin response. How times have changed!

Certainly, if secondary skin excision can be avoided, so much the better. With tumescent (superwet) and ultrasonic techniques, skin tone is usually no worse after surgery than it was before, and can be better. Some patients, whom I thought would need a tummy tuck later on, seemed to do remarkably well with liposuction alone, the skin showing much better ability to contract than expected (See T.N. and B.D., Patient Photographs). Even some older patients, for whom I would have recommended arm lifts (brachioplasties) in the past (See S.D., Liposuction of Arms), have done well enough with liposuction alone. With ultrasonic liposuction, excisional procedures, such as tummy tucks or arm lifts, with their long scars, may sometimes be avoided or at least deferred. And if the skin does not respond well, no bridges have been burnt; patients can always return later for the excisional surgery (i.e., cutting out tissue) if it is needed.

Skin that has already been severely stretched by pregnancy or weight gain is still best treated with a tummy tuck.

However, there are limits to skin recoil. Skin that has already been severely stretched by pregnancy or weight gain is still best treated with a tummy tuck, particularly if loose skin is the main concern. Liposuction alone will not suffice. This is a judgment call that is made by the patient and surgeon, considering factors such as the patient's goals, the significance of the scars, downtime, and expense.

Less Trauma

In the past, before I started using ultrasonic assistance, I would be exhausted after a day doing liposuction. I recall plastic surgeons sometimes calling this their "liposuction workout." Not anymore. After pretreating an area with ultrasound, the "mop up" liposuction is physically much less demanding. Of course, I do not object to a personal workout if that's what it takes to give my patient the best result, but if I can deliver a better result with less physical trauma to the patient, so much the better! Less trauma to the tissues should mean an easier and less painful recovery. It's a win-win situation—less trauma, better result. One plastic surgeon is fond of reminding surgeons at meetings, "Remember, we [plastic surgeons] enjoy surgery much more than our patients." Anything we can do to lessen the trauma and reduce discomfort is appreciated by our patients.

How Does Ultrasound Work?

Ultrasonic waves are produced by transforming electrical energy that comes out of the wall outlet into high-frequency sound energy, 20,000 cycles per second, which is too high to be perceived by the human ear. This happens in the ultrasonic generator.

This energy is transmitted to the handpiece, which transforms it into mechanical vibrations. The titanium rod connected to the handpiece actually moves back and forth invisibly at an almost unimaginable 20,000 times a second! This vibration causes little bubbles to form in the fat cells, destabilizing them. The flimsy cell membranes disintegrate, releasing the liquefied fat. Fortunately, this disintegration does not happen in denser tissue types such as connective tissue, nerves, or blood vessels. The treatment is selective for fat cells.

The flimsy cell membranes disintegrate, releasing the liquefied fat. Fortunately, this disintegration does not happen in denser tissue types such as connective tissue, nerves, or blood vessels. The treatment is selective for fat cells.

Some of the energy converts to heat, warming the tissues in contact with the probe. For this reason, the surgeon keeps the probe moving when ultrasound is applied. Otherwise, a localized heat buildup might cause a burn. Ultrasound is always used in a liquid medium (remember, sound travels better in water), maximizing the effect of ultrasound to dissolve fat cells, and minimizing the risk of overheating the tissues. The incision is protected with a plastic sleeve, so it is not burned. The skin incision is made a little longer than the diameter of the liposuction cannula, to accommodate this plastic protector.

With the introduction of ultrasound, a two-step process (injection, then suction) becomes a three-step process (injection, then ultrasound, then suction). The advantages of the tumescent technique are maintained. Added to these are the advantages of ultrasonic assistance.

Ultrasound – Pros and Cons

Advantages of Ultrasound

- Less trauma to the tissues
- More effective fat removal in fibrous areas
- In theory, better skin contraction

Disadvantages of Ultrasound

- Expense of equipment
- Possibility of burning the skin
- Slightly longer incisions

How do the advantages compare with the disadvantages? Well, expense should not even be on the list. Any surgeon who does an appreciable volume of liposuction can afford to invest in ultrasonic equipment. The added time is insignificant. In fact, the ultrasound treatment compensates for the extra time by making the mop up liposuction part of the procedure easier, less tiring, and shorter. I find that ultrasonic assistance adds very little surgical time. And burns? In over 2,500 cases, I have experienced two small burns (See C.M., Complications), both of which were easily revised and of no lasting consequence to the patients. Finally, it does not really matter that the incision is eight millimeters long rather than six millimeters long, particularly if the incisions are minimized and strategically placed in well-concealed locations and natural creases.

However, I caution patients that the tools always take a back seat to the technical prowess of the surgeon. There are some skilled surgeons practicing without ultrasound who can achieve excellent results, and there are less-skilled plastic surgeons using ultrasonic liposuction with mediocre outcomes due to inexpert technique. It has been said that the most important part of a stethoscope is the part between the earpieces. Similarly, the hand holding the liposuction instrument is more important than the tool itself. Of course, the right hands and the right instrument make for an ideal combination.

The hand holding the liposuction instrument is more important than the tool itself.

Similar to laser skin resurfacing, the ultrasonic technique came on the scene with much fanfare. This burst of popularity of a new technique is the "zealot stage." Then came troubling reports of complications such as burns and fluid collections under the skin ("seromas"). Similar to complications after laser skin resurfacing, these problems resulted from overtreatment. Burns may be avoided with proper skin protection and by always moving the cannula when in use, like ironing clothing. Seromas are very rare after liposuction if treatment areas are not subjected to excessive trauma, and can be avoided almost entirely by using conservative (short) ultrasound times.

Overtreatment causes the development of a potential ("dead") space under the skin that fills with fluid caused by inflammation from excessive tissue trauma. Experienced surgeons know that it is preferable to come back another day and re-treat an area rather than overtreat it and risk problems.

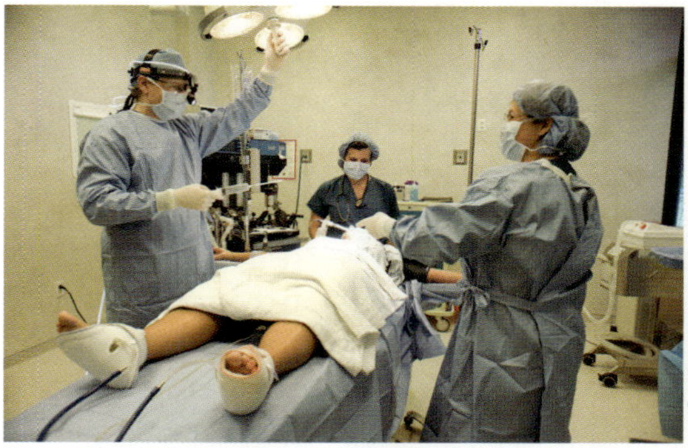

Operating Room in Ambulatory Surgery Center

Concerned about complications, some plastic surgeons reverted to traditional liposuction, without ultrasonic assistance. However, with the prudent use of this tool, by limiting ultrasound times to a few minutes per area, the advantages may be realized without additional risks. Moderation is the key. *Using the optimal ultrasound times is like prescribing the correct dose of medication.*

Ambulatory Surgery Center

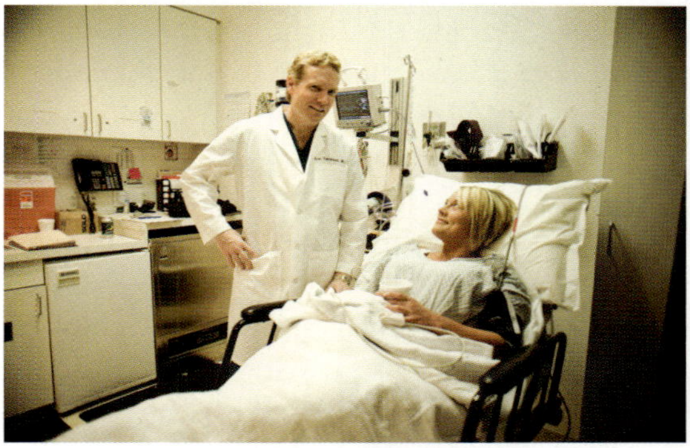

Waking up in the Recovery Room

Improvements in anesthesia have shortened patient recovery times, allowing surgery to be performed safely in an out-patient setting. Benefits include greater convenience, easier scheduling, greater consistency in medical personnel, cost containment, and avoidance of hospital-acquired ("nosocomial") infections. As a safety measure, the American Society of Plastic Surgeons mandates that its members use only accredited out-patient facilities or licensed ambulatory surgery centers.

I perform liposuction in a state-licensed ambulatory surgery center, under an unconscious intravenous anesthetic. The surgery takes one to two hours, depending on the number of areas treated. Patients are asleep for surgery and awaken in the Recovery Room (also called the Post Anesthesia Care Unit or "PACU") afterward. Because local anesthetic solution is injected into the tissues, patients require less I.V. medication and usually recover quickly after surgery, with minimal discomfort. Patients go home the same day. Touchups are done either under a brief intravenous sedation or local anesthesia alone if the treatment area is small. I do have a preference for intravenous sedation, even for touchups, because our surgical facility is conveniently located on-site and I.V. sedation offers optimal patient comfort.

"Laser" Liposuction

It is easy for patients to confuse ultrasonic liposuction with laser liposuction. Adding to the confusion is the term "Vaser®" liposuction (which is simply a type of ultrasonic liposuction). Both "ultrasonic" and "laser" sound high-tech. Both involve pre-injection of the treatment areas with fluid before the dissolved fat is suctioned away. However, beyond this similarity they are quite different. Ultrasonic liposuction uses a high frequency sound wave to selectively disrupt fat cells. Laser systems (for example: Smartlipo™, Cynosure Inc., Westford, Ma.) use a low-energy laser light beam to break up fat cells. Laser systems are costly and add a price increment to surgery because a nonreusable tip is needed for each patient. Importantly, laser use in liposuction does not selectively target fat cells, which is the principle advantage of ultrasonic assistance. Studies have failed to show a definite advantage for liposuction devices that incorporate a laser. Investigators found greater cellular damage to the fat cells and greater release of triglycerides from laser treatments (versus liposuction without laser pretreatment) and no improvement in skin retraction. The word "laser" has marketing appeal in medicine, and investigators caution against "putting commerce before research."

The latest marketing scheme is external laser treatment that is being sold as a noninvasive way to lose fat "without the dangers of surgery" (See Illustration). At least when used internally in combination with traditional liposuction, there is a scientific basis for laser disruption of fat cells (the question being whether this provides any benefit over regular liposuction), but certainly this does not mean that laser light applied *externally* to the skin surface without liposuction has any effect on fat cells. You might as well shine a laser pointer on your skin. This important distinction is not disclosed by the purveyors of this contraption that looks like something out of the *Matrix* movies. Even on a theoretical level, it is not plausible that low-power diode laser energy can penetrate the skin and emulsify fat (and that's probably a good thing). No wonder the treatment is painless, and no wonder it's unproven to have any benefit. Admittedly, "myzerona.com" is a catchy name, recalling a popular 1970s song, just right for baby boomers. But it's all hype.

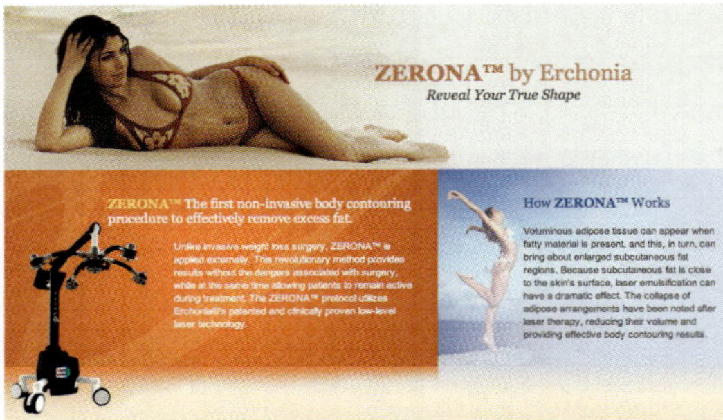

Zerona™ claims to be the first non-invasive body contouring procedure to effectively remove excess fat.

While laser resurfacing of skin turned out to be a winning application of laser technology, fat removal appears to be a better served by ultrasonic technology.

LipoDissolve: Does it Work?

LipoDissolve, a type of mesotherapy, makes use of an injection of chemicals (one is phosphatidylcholine) under the skin to dissolve fat. It is not new, having been used for decades in Europe. Recently, it was marketed in the United States by two St. Louis-based gynecologists who hired sales consultants to sell it as an alternative to liposuction. After all, the sales pitch went, who wants surgery if there is a nonsurgical alternative?

The problem is that there are no controlled scientific studies showing LipoDissolve to be safe and effective. Unlike Botox® Cosmetic, which was used for treating eye conditions before being FDA-approved for cosmetic uses (its safety being proven and FDA approval obtained for other medical uses), the FDA has still not approved LipoDissolve or phosphatidylcholine for *any* purpose. The American Society for Aesthetic Plastic Surgery recommends against its members using LipoDissolve until it has been properly evaluated.

Although nonsurgical and often performed by nonsurgeons, LipoDissolve is not without risks, including skin indentations, pigmentation changes, and infections, which can be resistant to antibiotics. Unfortunately, plastic surgeons are now seeing unhappy patients who complain about painful injections, hard knots at the injection sites, and disappointment with the results. LipoDissolve is sometimes recommended to patients who would benefit much more from liposuction and tummy tucks.

According to Dr. Rod Rohrich, the editor of the *Journal of Plastic and Reconstructive Surgery*: "It is mind-boggling to think that a physician would inject patients—or that patients would allow physicians to inject them—with unknown, unproved substances based on hearsay and unsubstantiated clinical findings." And it is "inconceivable" that plastic surgeons would embrace such a treatment.

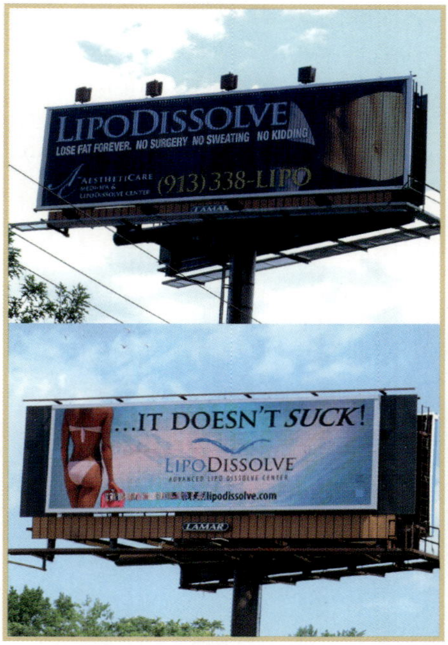

Billboards advertising LipoDissolve. LipoDissolve was marketed heavily, but the results did not live up to the hype.

Liposuction, on the other hand, has been shown to be safe, effective, and is FDA-approved. Ultrasonic liposuction selectively targets fat cells. The liquefied fat is then suctioned away so the body does not have to absorb it. This contrasts with LipoDissolve injections, which cause the fat cells to die, and probably other cell types too, and rely on the body's inflammatory response to mop up and absorb the dead tissue products into the body.

Dr. Alan Matarasso, a New York plastic surgeon and expert in body contouring surgery, cautions: "To ensure some level of safety before using phosphatidylcholine in mesotherapy, it would be prudent to know the products of dissolution, whether or not free fatty acids are released into the patient's bloodstream, whether the injected chemical is absorbed into the bloodstream, the effects on the liver and other organs, the appropriate dose, and so on."

LipoDissolve is not inexpensive. A series of treatments, usually 5-10, costs about the same as liposuction. Are the results comparable? Before-and-after photographs tend to be poor quality and are not standardized. The results appear inferior to what can be accomplished with liposuction and even its proponents admit that mesotherapy is no substitute for liposuction. Clearly, the volume of fat removed by a single liposuction procedure exceeds what can be achieved with repeated, multiple LipoDissolve spot treatments. Liposuction remains the only treatment that can provide comprehensive and continuous contouring for all areas of the body.

Clearly, the volume of fat removal by a single liposuction procedure exceeds what can be achieved with repeated, multiple LipoDissolve spot treatments.

After a burst of advertising and expansion into several states, the Advanced LipoDissolve (later called "Fig.") company filed for bankruptcy in 2008, a vivid demonstration that no service can flourish on hype alone. Results matter.

Procedure-driven marketing is familiar in plastic surgery. Other examples are SmartLipo™, QuickLift™, and Lifestyle Lift®. This is a marketing-oriented business strategy that starts with the procedure and works backward to the patient, rather than starting with the patient and deciding what treatment best suits his or her needs (more about this in *Ideal Facelift*). Unfortunately, this approach predictably leads to patient dissatisfaction.

External Ultrasound

An effective noninvasive treatment for body contouring would have huge marketing potential, not to mention the potential to put plastic surgeons out of business! The external ultrasound technique makes use of ultrasound waves administered externally, like the familiar obstetrical ultrasound, but using higher energy settings in an effort to dissolve fat. There are no skin incisions. Such devices have been tried since ultrasound was first used internally to assist liposuction. However, the results have been underwhelming. There is also the issue of the fate of any fat that is degraded. Similar to mesotherapy, there is no suction component to remove the dissolved fat from the body. Whether fatty acids and other degradation products that enter circulation might have any deleterious effects is unknown. While external ultrasound is a topic that comes up perennially at plastic surgery meetings, it has failed to gain popularity.

Abdominal "Etching"

Liposuction can make the underlying abdominal definition much more visible (See P.K., Patient Photographs) by reducing the thickness of the fat layer between the muscle and the skin. Some operators have claimed that they can use liposuction to etch the abdominal six-pack, by concentrating the liposuction on the borders of the muscle compartments (called tendinous intersections). Such claims are overstated. Any attempt to artificially simulate muscle definition by suctioning fat may cause contour irregularities that can be hard to fix. Most operators perform liposuction evenly over the abdomen. A uniform reduction of the fat layer gives the most natural result and avoids complications.

It is important for prospective patients to know that not everyone is lucky enough to have a six- or an eight-pack. You need to be genetically fortunate to have well-demarcated abdominal muscles in the first place. On top of that, you need to be lean, and there is no easy way to do it, despite what the fitness magazines might say. Strict dieting and weight loss are mandatory. Muscular development increases with exercise. Liposuction complements the result by reducing the fat layer and making the muscle definition more visible. It provides the icing on the cake, so to speak.

Anesthesia

Patients, especially those in the medical and nursing professions, are generally aware of the importance of the anesthetic. In appropriate patients, liposuction itself is unlikely to be life-threatening. However, anesthetic factors such as airway management, fluid administration, and medication effects can be potentially life-threatening. When I discuss complications with my patients, I often describe many of the details of the anesthetic, modifications that make it safer, and how patients are monitored during surgery.

Liposuction may be performed under local anesthesia (the area is numbed with anesthetic); conscious or unconscious intravenous sedation (the patient is sedated partially or fully); or a traditional general anesthetic, in which the patient is unconscious with a tube down the trachea ("intubated"), paralyzed, and on a breathing machine ("ventilated"). This represents the spectrum of anesthesia from lighter to heavier.

Local anesthesia	**Local anesthesia + I.V. sedation ("Total Intravenous Anesthesia")**	**Traditional general anesthesia**
Awake	Asleep	Asleep
Injection of lidocaine	Propofol infusion Oxygen Laryngeal Mask Airway (LMA) Spontaneous breathing	Paralysis Oxygen and anesthetic gas Endotracheal intubation Ventilator
"Lighter"		"Heavier"

Local Anesthesia

"Local" anesthetic is a medication that is injected directly into the tissues to numb them. Many practitioners, particularly dermatologists, use local anesthesia exclusively. The patient is awake during liposuction under local anesthesia.

After allowing some time for the anesthetic to take effect, liposuction is performed. Advantages to the patient include the avoidance of a deeper level of anesthesia, less expense, and virtually no recovery time. Patients can usually drive home afterward. A practical advantage for nonsurgeons is that it allows them the capability of doing liposuction in an office setting rather than an ambulatory surgery center or hospital, where they would not have surgical privileges. Office procedures also avoid additional costs and scheduling issues.

A disadvantage of local anesthesia is the patient discomfort and anxiety associated with long procedures in which multiple areas are treated. One memorable television report showed a patient casually talking on the telephone (it was so old there was a cord on the phone) while having liposuction, but this is not the typical experience! Patients who have had previous liposuction elsewhere under local anesthesia tell me it was not a day at the beach. They welcome the idea of a short I.V. anesthetic and often sigh with relief when they are informed that we prefer our patients to be asleep for surgery.

Patients who have had previous liposuction elsewhere under local anesthesia tell me it was not a day at the beach.

I use local anesthesia only for small liposuction cases, such as a touchup liposuction of one or two areas. Patients tolerate this well and have minimal discomfort, like a trip to the dentist. The cost is minimal.

It is inadvisable for any nonsurgeon to perform a substantial amount of liposuction as an office procedure under local anesthesia alone. Liposuction is a serious surgical procedure that should be done by a qualified surgeon in an operating room in an outpatient surgery center or hospital. Ideally, liposuction is done by a plastic surgeon experienced in body contouring surgery who has the capability to perform other cosmetic procedures if they are indicated, such as an abdominoplasty, and treat complications. Anyone performing liposuction should also be an expert in performing fat injection, the remedy for overtreatment. As a rule in surgery, the operator should be capable of treating his or her surgical complications.

Furthermore, local anesthesia is not necessarily the safest type of anesthesia. The patient may not have intravenous access for administration of fluids or medications. She may not have an oxygen monitor, continuous measurement of vital signs, EKG, and the uninterrupted attention of an attending anesthetist. A conscious patient who is uncomfortable or in pain can develop variations in respiratory rate, pulse, and blood pressure, including hypertension, all of which are undesirable during surgery. The patient may lose consciousness (faint) or become restless, requiring the operator to interrupt surgery to attend to the patient. Consequently, the operator cannot devote all of his or her attention to performing the surgery and may need to limit the treatment out of concern for patient comfort and safety.

Intravenous Sedation (Total I.V. Anesthesia)

Understandably, some patients may be fearful of being asleep during surgery. They may have never had an anesthetic before, and the thought of the anesthesia makes them more nervous than the surgery itself. However, once the anesthesia is explained to them, and its safety, they readily understand its advantages, and are less anxious about it. The best remedy for apprehension is education, so the patient knows what to expect.

The best remedy for apprehension is education, so the patient knows what to expect.

Many physicians consider any anesthetic that renders a patient unconscious a "general" anesthetic. However, there are some important technical points that distinguish a "deep" or unconscious sedation (commonly called total I.V. anesthesia, or TIVA), from a traditional general anesthetic. The anesthetist administers the medication through the I.V. tubing and uses an infusion pump to provide a continuous delivery of a short-acting anesthetic called propofol ("Diprivan"). This "wonder drug" has made traditional general anesthesia unnecessary for many types of surgery that were previously done exclusively in hospitals. Many patients are already familiar with its use for a variety of out-patient procedures such as colonoscopy, knee arthroscopy, and dental procedures.

If propofol is a wonder drug, then the LMA™, short for "laryngeal mask airway," is a "wonder airway." Designed by a British anesthesiologist in 1983, it provides a reliable airway without the need for an endotracheal tube. Supplemental oxygen is provided without a need for the anesthetist to hold a mask over the patient's face. This ingenious but weird-looking device lodges in the back of the throat and protects the airway, without extending down between the vocal cords. The LMA eliminates the need for intubation, which can be difficult in some patients and occasionally traumatic to the vocal cords. A rare patient may still need to be intubated, such as one with symptomatic esophageal regurgitation, but the majority may be safely treated with an LMA.

Once the patient is asleep, I inject a dilute solution of local anesthetic and epinephrine ("infusion solution") into all the areas that I plan to treat with liposuction. The reader might ask, "Why inject local anesthetic if the patient is asleep already? " These are the reasons:

- The anesthetist can use smaller amounts of propofol. The less medication needed to keep the patient asleep during the surgery, the faster he or she will wake up after surgery.

- There is minimal pain for the first several hours after surgery, making the recovery phase more comfortable, and reducing the need for pain killers after surgery. This pain relief after surgery is called postoperative analgesia.

- With fewer pain killers, there is less risk of side effects, such as nausea, sedation, constipation, and respiratory depression (particularly for patients with sleep apnea). These side effects are not trivial. Nausea is frequently cited by patients as the most distressing recollection of their recovery after traditional general anesthesia. For patient comfort, it should be prevented as much as possible.

A total intravenous anesthetic, with the addition of local anesthetic injected into the tissues once the patient is asleep, is the preferred type of anesthesia used at our facility for all plastic surgical procedures.

General Anesthesia

The traditional general anesthetic calls for a muscle relaxant (for paralysis), intubation, a breathing machine ("ventilator"), and an inhalational anesthetic agent ("gas"). Patients are paralyzed to allow mechanical ventilation—positive-pressure ventilation using an endotracheal tube.

This type of anesthesia certainly provides an unconscious, motionless (except for mechanical respirations) patient. This level of anesthesia is necessary for major surgical procedures that require mechanical ventilation such as intra-abdominal surgery. But it is a deeper level of anesthesia than is needed for plastic surgical procedures, even for an abdominoplasty.

Why not use a traditional general anesthetic anyway? Because of these additional risks:

- Anesthetic gas can cause nausea, irritate the bronchial linings, may have a depressant effect on the cardiovascular and respiratory systems, and can rarely be toxic to the liver and kidneys.

- Muscle relaxants, such as succinylcholine, reduce the sympathetic tone to the leg veins, possibly setting the stage for blood clots; can rarely prolong the recovery time in patients with an enzyme deficiency (pseudocholinesterase deficiency); can rarely trigger malignant hyperthermia, which is a potentially fatal complication; and may allow unrecognized awakening in surgery.

- Endotracheal intubation can occasionally damage teeth or the vocal cords.

- Positive pressure mechanical ventilation can sometimes cause a pneumothorax.

This is just a partial list of possible problems with traditional general anesthesia. Even if such problems are few and far between, a risk of zero is always preferable to a risk of 1 in 50,000. As a general principle, any opportunity to eliminate a risk factor is worthwhile to keep the odds in favor of patient safety and comfort. This is part of the well-known KISS principle (Keep It Simple, Stupid). The perpetuation of a technique that has a risk without a benefit should be questioned. Rituals need to be examined. This is not easy for any surgeon who has developed habits, including myself, but a fresh look at old habits is part of the culture of patient safety.

One anesthetist who clearly understood the economics of a good anesthetic remarked, "Have 'em wake up happy and they'll come back for more."

Recovery

After working for a long time with the same surgeon, anesthesia providers learn just how stimulating certain procedures are to the patient and can anticipate anesthetic requirements accordingly. For example, lifting the muscle during a breast augmentation is more stimulating than liposuction, which is more stimulating than sewing the eyelid skin. The anesthetist learns how much anesthetic to give and when to turn up or down the propofol infusion rate and administer I.V. medications such as Versed and fentanyl. I work with anesthetists who can make these judgments so accurately that the patient often awakens within seconds of my last stitch, sometimes asking when the operation will begin. This capability is a sign of anesthesia virtuosity—a pilot might say "greasing the landing." The goal is to have the patient awaken quickly and easily in the recovery room. Ideally, within minutes after surgery the patient is awake and lucid. Within half an hour, she can get up and walk to the bathroom with assistance. A short time later, perhaps an hour after surgery, she is getting dressed to go home. A quick recovery is not just good patient care—it's good for business. One anesthetist who clearly understood the economics of a good anesthetic remarked, "Have 'em wake up happy and they'll come back for more."

Avoidance of Nausea

Sometimes a patient's biggest concern in having elective procedures is not so much the surgery as the anesthesia. This is particularly true for smaller patients, or those who are simply more susceptible to the effects of anesthesia, who may have required a few hours to wake up after operations they had in the past, and they still remember the nausea. Indeed, such unpleasant experiences can leave indelible memories. In fact, anesthesia-related nausea may be more memorable than postoperative pain. By contrast, some of our patients have a euphoric reaction to the anesthesia and ask facetiously if they could come back for just the anesthesia (at least I think they are being facetious). The avoidance of gas, the use of propofol, the routine administration of antinausea medications, and local anesthesia to reduce the need for narcotics—all reduce the risk of the dreaded nausea.

Antinausea medications are selected that work on different receptor sites. At our surgery center, we routinely use three different medications in an effort to eliminate nausea. This might seem to be redundant, but not to anyone who has experienced postoperative nausea. With this proactive approach, what was once the scourge of postoperative recovery is now a rare occurrence.

Can I Wake Up in Surgery?

When I explain intravenous sedation to patients, their eyes sometimes widen and I know what question comes next: "With this type of anesthesia, doc, is it possible for me to wake up during surgery?" They may have heard about the problem of an anesthetic wearing off during surgery from sensational tabloid stories. Intraoperative awakening was even the theme of the 2007 movie *Awake*, although it is hard to imagine that this subject would be of sufficient interest for a successful feature film, which may explain why it wasn't.

In such a situation, the patient is paralyzed and cannot move, so she cannot alert anyone that the anesthetic has worn off. The patient feels every cut and every stitch. This is certainly a nightmarish scenario, one that might interest Stephen King or Robin Cook (on second thought, maybe not that bad!). Also called "recall," it is a rare occurrence after elective surgery, occurring more often in emergency situations in which the desired level of anesthesia needs to be balanced against a life-threatening condition (for example, an emergency cesarean section when the baby's life is at risk).

Fortunately, intraoperative awakening is very unlikely to happen when an I.V. sedation anesthetic is administered because the patient is never paralyzed. If the level of anesthesia were to "lighten" during surgery, the patient would start moving and alert the staff. In fact, we *expect* the patient to move a little during surgery, and this happens commonly. I stop operating for a minute or so while the anesthetist administers more I.V. medication or adjusts the rate of the propofol infusion. Even if a patient lightens a little, like moving in her sleep, she is still anesthetized. She remains unconscious and has no recollection of surgery.

I prefer this level of anesthesia, with the patient moving slightly from time to time, because this slight movement assures me that she is receiving just enough anesthesia to keep her asleep and no more. Some surgeons are used to operating on a motionless patient and are upset if the patient moves at all. But with a little patience they learn to tolerate little movements from time to time, recognizing that this is a signal their patient is not over-sedated. She is likely to wake up quickly after surgery and recover faster.

Positioning in Surgery

Avoidance of Prone Positioning

A common practice among surgeons is to place the patient face down ("prone") on the operating table for liposuction. This is also the anesthetist's least favorite position for some very good reasons. The airway is more difficult to manage. Endotracheal intubation, paralysis, and mechanical ventilation are mandatory if the patient is prone. If the endotracheal tube comes out, it's a serious problem because the patient is face-down and difficult to reintubate. Furthermore, pressure on the face can potentially cause problems. Pressure at the hips caused by rolls used to bolster the hips may interfere with venous return from the legs (with possible relevance to blood clotting). There is a period of inactivity, as much as 20 minutes, in the operating room while the patient is turned from a face-up to a face-down position on the operating table. Often the patient needs to be reprepped and draped because of loss of sterility.

The patient is treated for about 30 minutes in a supine position, followed by 30 minutes on one side, and then 30 minutes on the other side.

Position Changes during Surgery

Prolonged motionlessness can cause problems. Nerves can be damaged by unrelieved pressure. Skin breakdown can occur at pressure points. Therefore, it is advantageous to move patients during surgery. Our patients start supine on the operating table, but are then moved to one side and then the other side while the anesthetic solution is injected. This turning routine is repeated when liposuction is performed. The patient is treated for about 30 minutes in a supine position, followed by 30 minutes on one side, and then 30 minutes on the other side (See Illustration, Incisions). This rotation of positions ensures that there is no prolonged pressure on any body parts. Intraoperative movement of the lower extremities may also be helpful to avoid blood pooling in the calves ("venous stasis") which can cause deep vein blood clots.

Supine and lateral positioning have several other advantages. The patient never needs to be positioned face-down. Intubation, paralysis, and mechanical ventilation are eliminated. There is no delay in surgery to reposition a prone patient. Operating time and efficiency are improved. This turning routine also enables full, circumferential access to the body, facilitating treatment of all areas by liposuction.

Blood Clots

The development of blood clots in the legs is a major concern and a frequent topic of discussion at plastic surgery meetings. These clots can develop even without surgery. This is the reason flight attendants have passengers get up and move around the cabin on long flights. Prolonged inactivity raises the risk of blood pooling in the legs, called venous stasis. If a piece of this blood clot breaks off, it travels to the heart and then to the lungs, and where it becomes a pulmonary embolus—a potentially fatal complication. Accordingly, it is important to take the steps to prevent this complication.

Preventive measures start with reducing periods of immobilization. Long surgery times (over six hours) and bed rest after surgery are avoided. It makes sense to avoid muscle relaxation, including the use of paralytic agents that are part of a traditional general anesthetic. Avoidance of a general anesthetic likely reduces the risk of a pulmonary embolus. Surgeons who avoid general anesthesia report low incidences of this dangerous complication.

Movement of the patient's legs, frequent position changes during surgery, and the use of sequential compression devices also make sense. Patients are not placed in a prone position, so there is no external pelvic pressure. Early ambulation after surgery is important. Getting up to go to the bathroom after surgery gets the legs moving. Out-patient surgery forces the patient to ambulate during the first 24 hours. I usually see patients the day after surgery, so that I know they are getting up and moving around. The trip to the doctor's office helps. *The objective is to reduce the risk of blood clots to a level as close as possible to the baseline risk that exists without surgery.*

Some surgeons have recommended the use of blood-thinners such as heparin or Lovenox®, but these agents may increase the risk of bleeding. Whether their presumed advantage compensates for increased risk is open to question. For most plastic surgeons, including me, the balance has to be decidedly favorable before we will consider an intervention that has serious risks. *Primum non nocere.*

Intraoperative Photographs – Ultrasonic Liposuction

1. Liposuction is getting started in the operating room. The patient has been prepped and draped. The intravenous anesthetic has started, and she has just gone off to sleep. As the anesthetist looks on, I infuse the abdomen with the anesthetic solution, which has just been taken out of the warming compartment. It is seen in the foreground hanging from an I.V. pole.

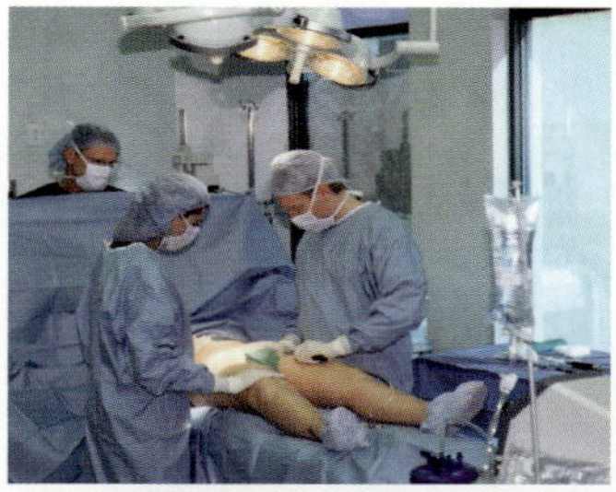

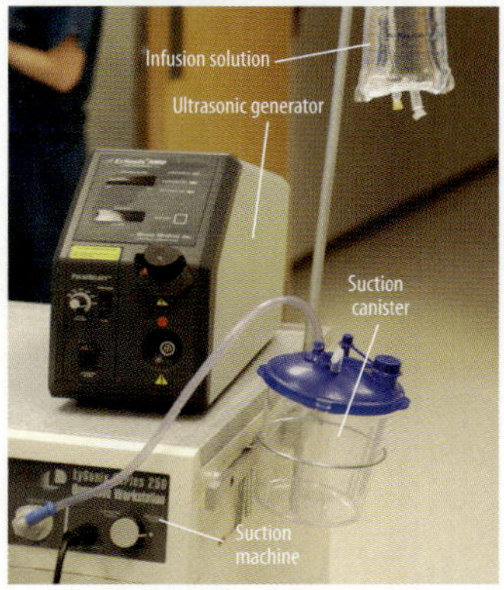

2. The ultrasonic generator converts electrical energy into a high-frequency sound wave.

3. (*Right*) For demonstration purposes, a globule of fat has been taken out and placed on a sterile sheet. (*Far right*) The fat dissolves into liquid as it is exposed to the ultrasonic energy. The connective tissue component is left behind.

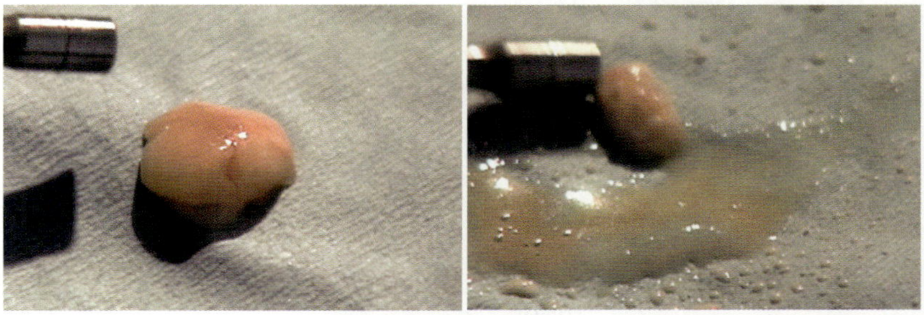

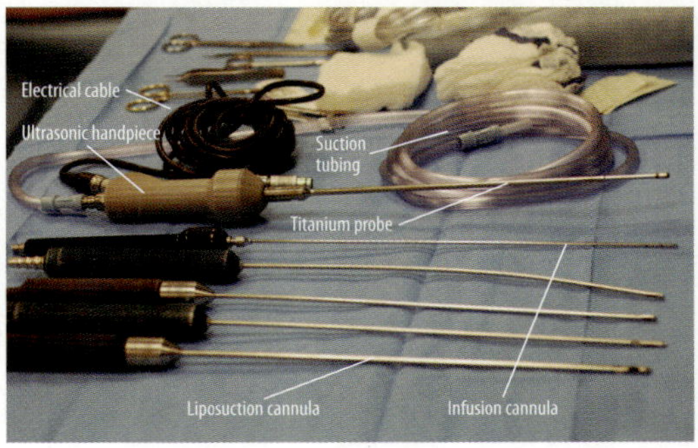

4. The ultrasonic handpiece and attached hollow titanium probe are shown on the operating table, along with the thin infusion cannula, used to inject the infusion solution, and the various liposuction cannulae, used to suction the dissolved fat.

5. The fat is seen filling a 3-liter canister. There is very little blood mixed in with the fluid, called the infranatant, at the bottom of the container.

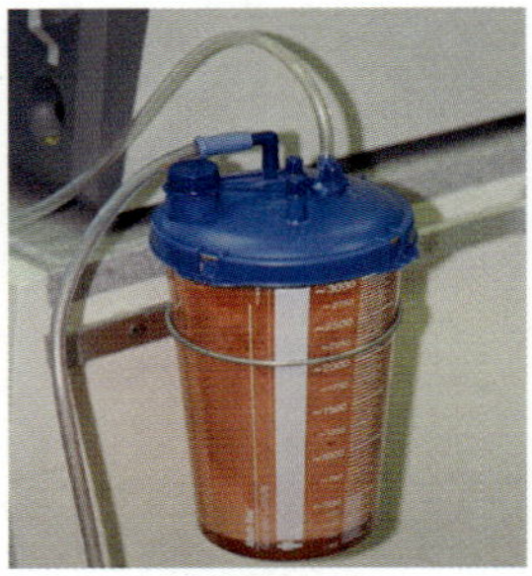

Ultrasonic Liposuction Is a 3-Step Process

	1. Infusion	2. Ultrasound	3. Liposuction
Abdomen	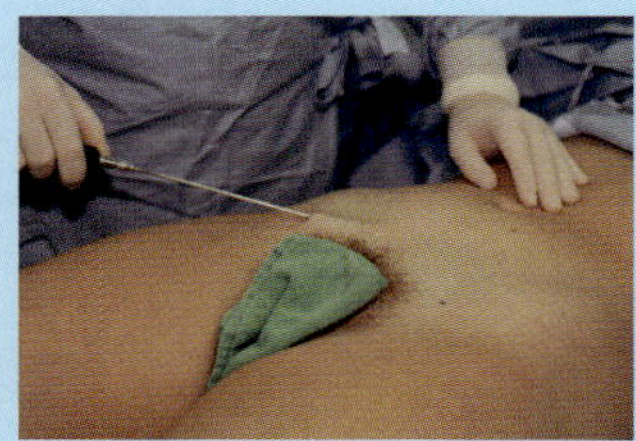	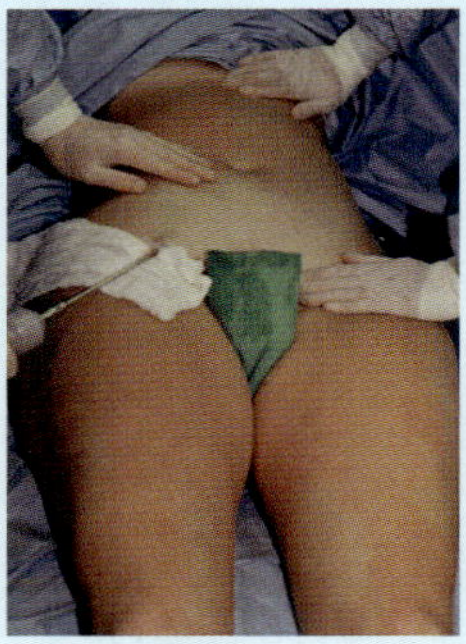	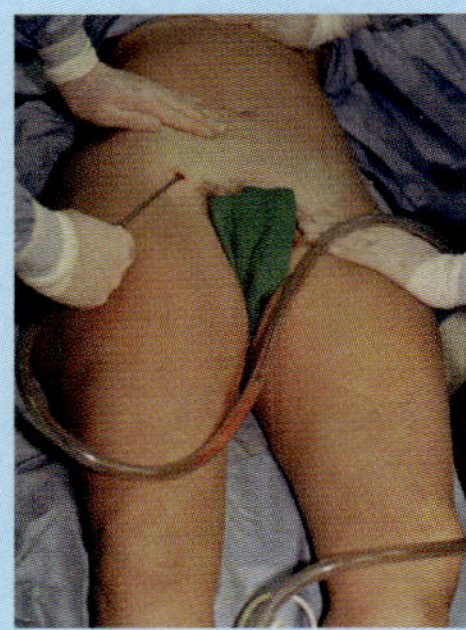

Treatment Areas

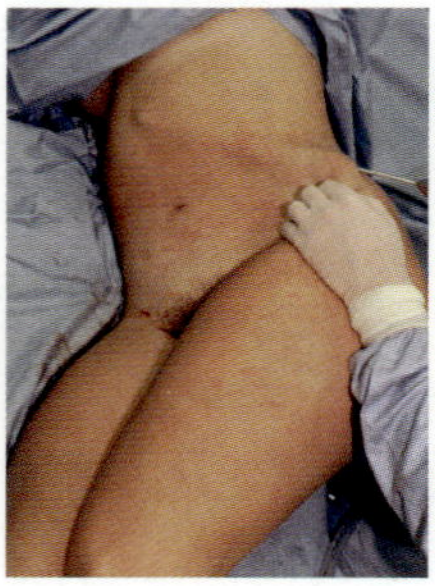

Abdomen

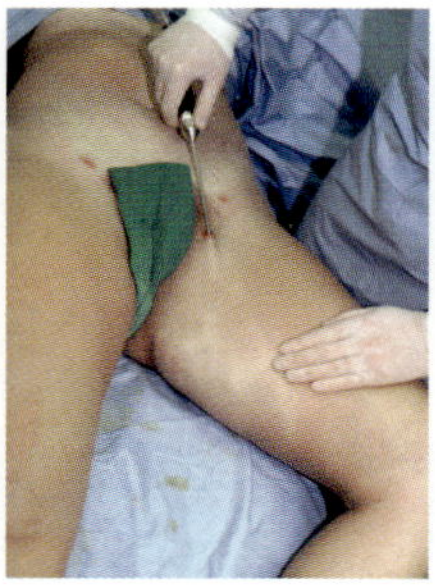

Inner thigh

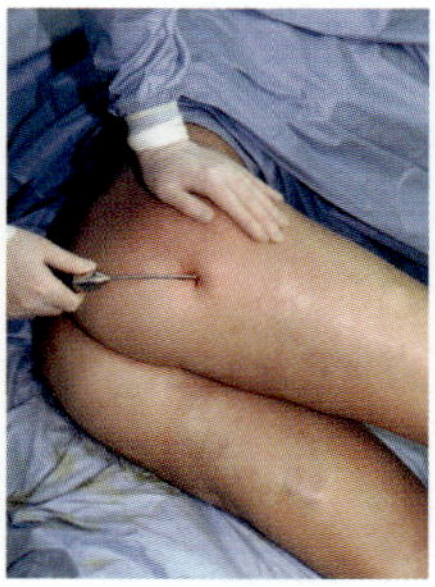

Outer thigh

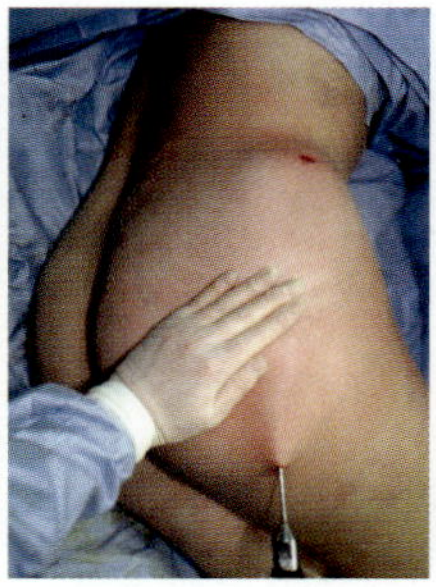

Buttock

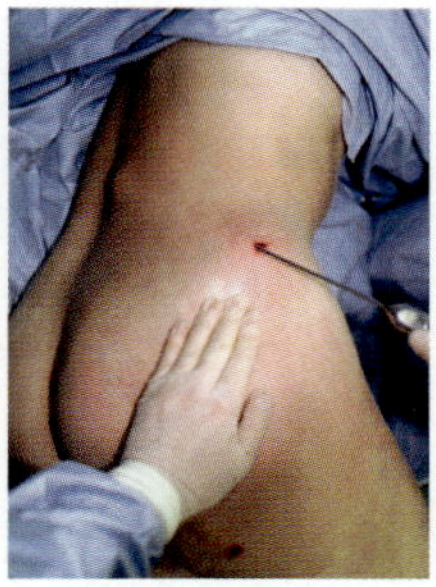

Flank

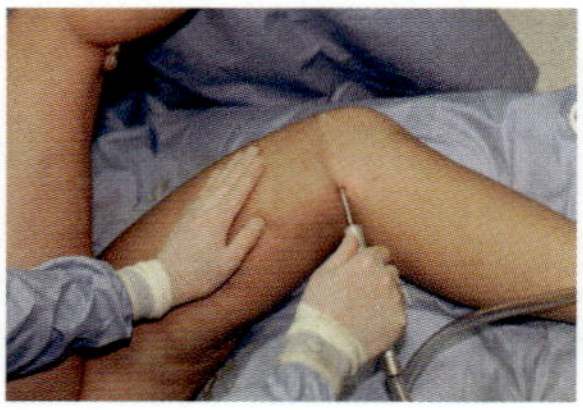

Knee

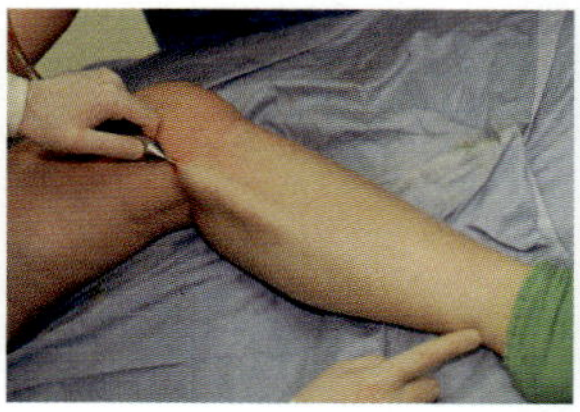

Calf

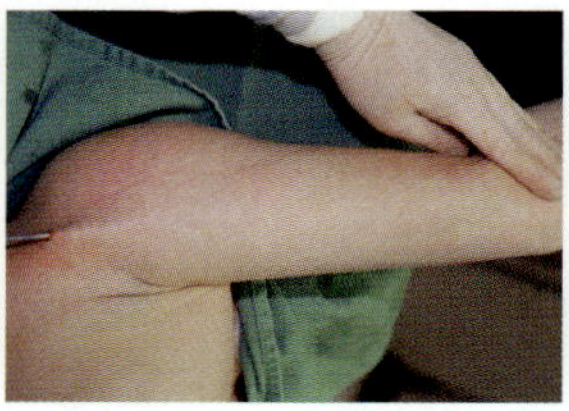

Arm

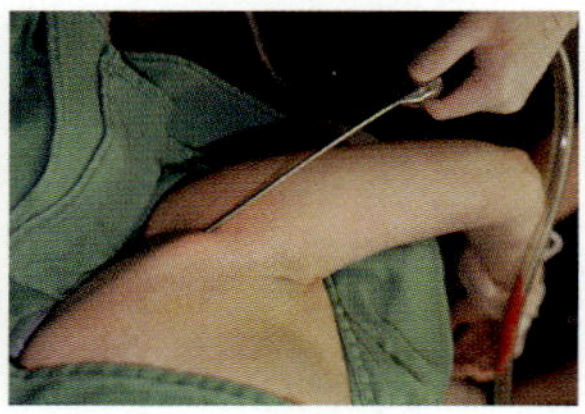

Axilla (Underarm)

Incisions

I use as few incisions as possible to access the areas I need to treat. When treating the abdomen and flanks, I use an incision on either side of the pubic area and on each flank (See Illustration). These are placed so that they would typically be hidden by a bikini. The access incisions for the thighs are in the groin crease on each side and on the lower buttock. The knee incision is tucked in the crease just below and on the medial side of the knee. These incisions can be seen in the intraoperative photographs. The small scars fade with time and are usually inconspicuous. Any that are objectionable may be revised. I do not use incisions placed midway along the arms, thighs, or calves, where they might be visible, or outside the bikini area on the abdomen and hips. The cannulae are long enough to permit such limited incisions and still access all the areas.

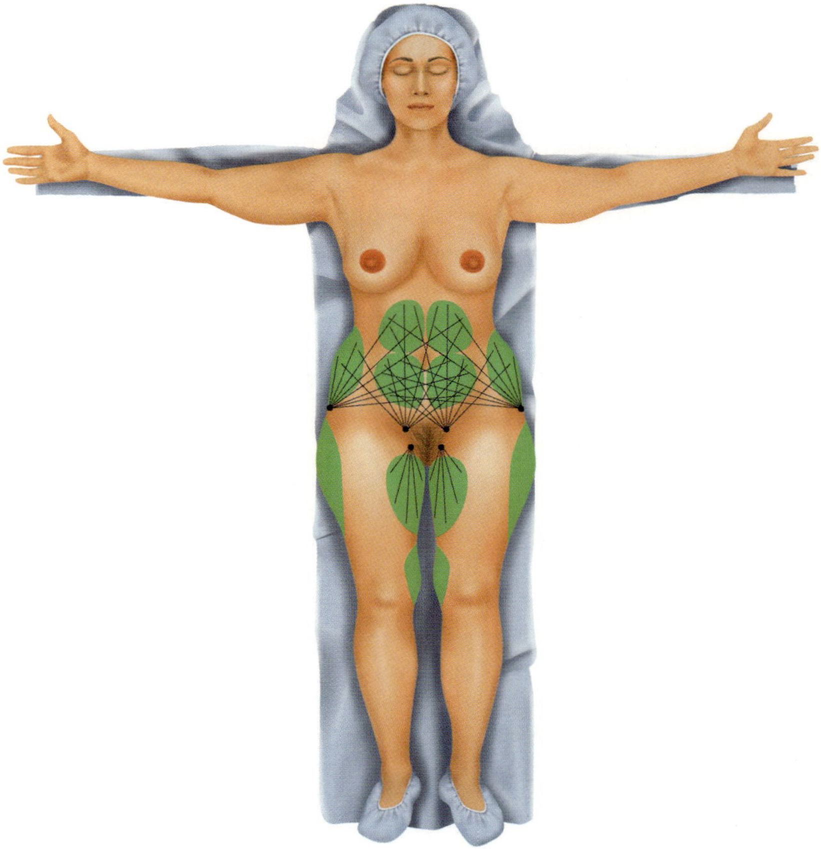

Incisions and Positioning in Surgery
The patient starts out supine on the operating table and is moved from side to side during surgery to inject the areas with local anesthetic solution and then to perform liposuction.

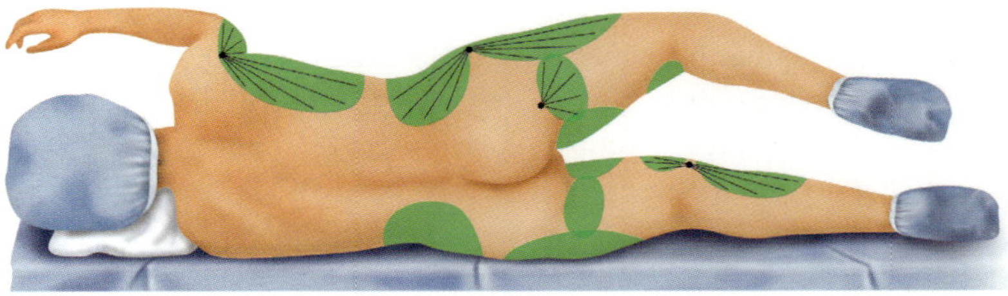

How Much Fat Do You Take Off?

This is a very common question asked by patients. I do not know beforehand exactly how much fat will come off in surgery, but I can usually provide an approximate volume. Depending on body characteristics, I may estimate one to 1-1.5 liters or 2-2.5 liters, for example. Touchup volumes are significantly less, as you might expect, often about one-third of the original aspirate volume.

The volume removed from each area is measured in cubic centimeters (cc). Often there is more fatty tissue on one side than the other so that it is common for these volumes to be different. During surgery, I assess how much fat to remove visually by looking at the treated area and by feel, using my free left hand to judge the contour and assess thickness. My right hand holds the instrument, allowing me to judge the resistance of the tissues as I move the cannula. (In certain areas, I change hands to hold the instrument with my left hand and assess thickness with my right hand.) As more fat is removed, there is less resistance. Another factor is the volume removed from each area, which the nurse records in real time and reports to me.

Of course, the volume removed is related to the patient's body characteristics and how much extra fat is present to start with. At first, the fat comes out readily, a stream of fat globules traveling down the suction tubing that is gratifying to watch and listen to, as the fat globules reverberate down the suction tubing and spill into the canister (this gives plastic surgeons great satisfaction, seeing the fat depart and watching the areas become trimmer). Gradually, the fat stream slows to a trickle.

An experienced surgeon knows how far to "push the envelope." This is the art of performing liposuction. It is important to take off as much excess fat as possible to produce the best result for the patient, but it is even more important not to overdo the treatment. If the surgeon persists in trying to take off another 10% or so after the fat stream has been reduced to a trickle, this may cause unnecessary tissue trauma, more bruising, and increase the risk of skin irregularities or poor skin contraction. It is far better to avoid such skin problems and return for a touchup later if necessary.

Many patients, immediately before surgery, tell me to take as much fat off as possible, saying, "Don't hold back, doc!" Nothing personal, they tell me, but they'd rather not come back for more surgery. Yes, they want the surgery to be safe, but they also want as dramatic a result as possible.

I tell my patients that I will take off as much fat as I can without overdoing it and increasing the risk of complications. I also reassure my patients that I will not undertreat them either. The possibility of doing a touchup later does not mean I'm going to leave to another time something I can do today. I treat them as if they may not have an opportunity to come back.

Maximizing Efficiency

Treatment of the abdomen and flanks takes about an hour. Lower body liposuction takes about an hour and a half. When the arms and underarms are included, the operation may take two hours. It is not unusual for me to treat the fat pad under the chin ("submental fat pad") at the same time, adding another 20 minutes or so. By prepping the patient circumferentially at the beginning and then infusing all areas before starting liposuction, efficiency is maximized. This operative sequence allows me to safely treat multiple areas in a comprehensive fashion without unduly long operating times. The efficient use of operating time allows more time for other cosmetic procedures, such as an abdominoplasty or breast augmentation, which may be done safely under the same anesthetic.

The Terms

Although patients sometimes refer to their "stomach," this is obviously not precise, the stomach being an internal organ. The terms "abdomen" or "tummy" are preferred.

The "love handles," located just above the waist on each side, are called the flanks and the "saddlebag" areas are called the outer thighs. When talking with patients, plastic surgeons tend to use these quaint popular expressions because everyone knows what they mean (although it doesn't occur to us, plastic surgeons must appear a little silly at meetings talking seriously about the treatment of "love handles"). The use of the term "hips" can cause confusion because sometimes people use "hips" to refer to their outer thighs. For this reason, plastic surgeons often speak of "flanks" instead of "hips" when referring to the fat deposits above the waistline on either side, and when they do use the term "hips" it is synonymous with flanks.

In plastic surgery usage, the "axilla" is the area below the armpit extending down the shoulder blade (also called the scapular area). The small area in front of the armpit that can cause a bulge above the breast is also included in this anatomic area (more precisely the "anterior axilla"). Women sometimes refer to axillary fat as "bra fat" when describing the fat bulges above and below their bra on either side. The term "axillae" is the plural, referring to both sides.

The "arms" are the upper extremities between the shoulder and elbow, synonymous with "upper arms." The fat that accumulates along the lower border (with the arms held horizontally) is commonly treated with liposuction. The upper extremities below the elbows are the "forearms"—areas that are rarely treated with liposuction and are therefore not especially relevant to body contouring surgery.

The calves are, of course, the regions between the knees and the ankles. The popularly-labeled "cankles," or fat above the ankles, are included. Technically, the "legs" are just the portion of the lower extremities below the knees. We speak of "thighs" when referring to the lower extremities above the knees. By "knees," plastic surgeons mean the medial aspect of the knees, where there is commonly a fat pad that can cause a knock-kneed appearance, interrupting the preferred streamlined look of the feminine leg (or rather "lower extremity").

These treatment areas are all depicted in the illustrations in the preceding section.

All body weights presented here were recorded by our nurses using the same hospital scales in the office. Some patients treated outside the study period do not have postoperative weights. Dress and pant sizes, where available, were provided by patients themselves at the time of their postoperative interviews. All available data are included. Patients are presented in order of liposuction aspirate volume. To convert to pounds, simply multiply the volume in liters by two (e.g., 2,000 cc = 2 liters = 4 lbs.).

Ethnicity does influence body shape, but not so much the performance of liposuction. However, patients do ask to view others of the same ethnic group, so ethnicity is indicated where it is not Caucasian.

Female Liposuction – Abdomen and Flanks

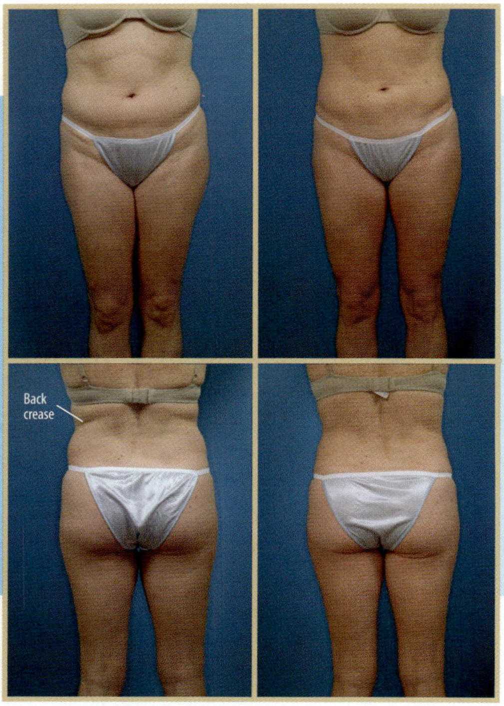

before *4 months after*

Ultrasonic liposuction of abdomen and flanks.

Comments: This patient ran six miles three times a week, but was unable to improve the contour of her tummy and flanks. She was concerned about postoperative nausea because she experienced vomiting after an appendectomy. She was gratified that she had no nausea after the liposuction. At her one-week postoperative appointment, she asked about lumpiness she could feel in the lower abdomen. I reassured her that this was swelling and would soften with time. She was pleased with the improvement in her shape. The creases of the upper flanks, seen on the back view, are almost eliminated.

Height: 5′6″
Weight before: 142 lbs.
BMI: 22.6
Children: 0
Weight after: 135.5 lbs.
Liposuction volume: 1,000 cc
Dress size before: 8
Dress size after: 8
L.M., age 39, dog groomer

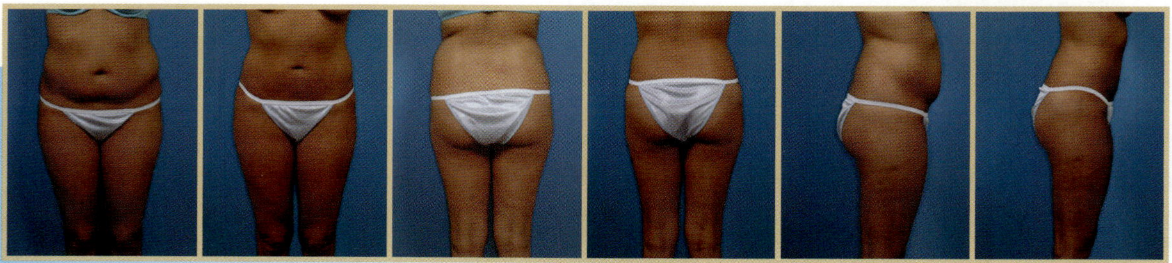

before *3 months after* *before* *3 months after* *before* *3 months after*

Ultrasonic liposuction of abdomen, flanks, and axillae.

Comments: This patient felt uncomfortable wearing a bikini before surgery. She was in a bikini before her one-month follow-up visit and said she already "loved" the result. She reported a major improvement in self-esteem.

Height: 5′4″
Weight before: 127 lbs.
BMI: 21.5
Children: 0
Liposuction volume: 1,300 cc
Dress size before: 4/6
Dress size after: 2/4
J.J., age 24, student

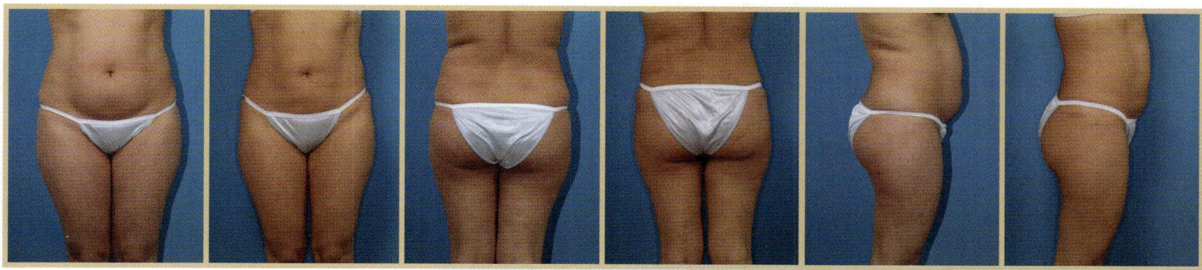

before *6½ months after* *before* *6½ months after* *before* *6½ months after*

Ultrasonic liposuction of abdomen and flanks.

Comments: This Hispanic patient had always been bothered by excess fullness of her tummy and hips. She was apprehensive because she had never had surgery before. She waited two years before scheduling her liposuction.

Height: 5'2"
Weight before: 139 lbs.
BMI: 25.0
Children: 0
Weight after: 124 lbs.
Liposuction volume: 1,500 cc
Dress size before: 8/9
Dress size after: 8/9
C.M., age 31, real estate agent

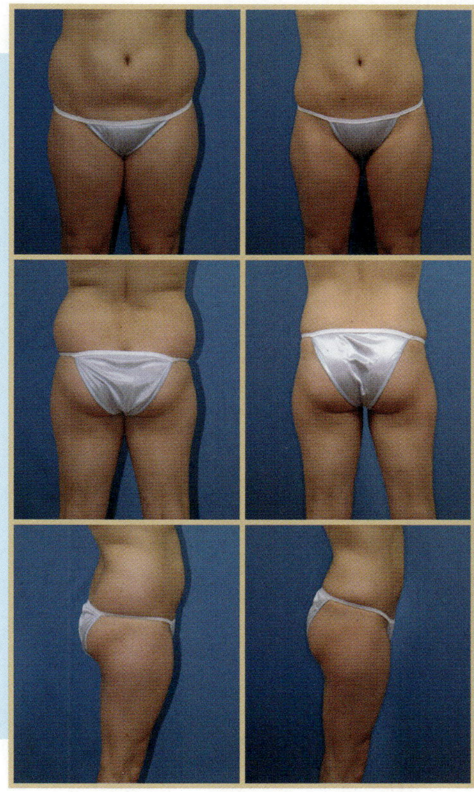

before *1 year after*

Ultrasonic liposuction of abdomen, flanks, inner thighs, arms, and axillae, and submental lipectomy.

Comments: This patient had excess fat deposits of the trunk and inner thighs, sparing the outer thighs that are so commonly affected in women. This is an example of the "apple" fat distribution, as opposed to the more common "pear" distribution. She had a hypertrophic scar at the site of a scar revision of the right lower abdomen (the scar was left over from removal of an old skin lesion), which I revised later under local anesthesia. Not surprisingly, the change in body shape bolstered this student's self-image. She noticed an improvement right away, even with the swelling.

Height: 5'4"
Weight before: 150 lbs.
BMI: 25.3
Children: 0
Weight after: 128 lbs.
Liposuction volume: 2,400 cc
M.C., age 22, student

Female Liposuction – Lower Body

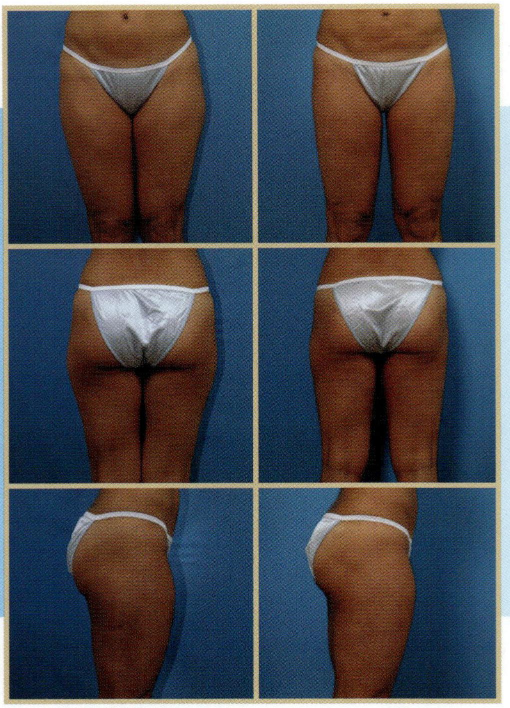

before *1 year after*

Ultrasonic liposuction of thighs. Second procedure, 6 months later: ultrasonic liposuction of abdomen, flanks, and knees, and touchup liposuction of thighs.

Comments: This patient had liposuction in stages. First she had her thighs treated. Then she returned for liposuction of the other areas of the lower body. Liposuction of the peripheral areas has provided a more flattering appearance of her buttocks. Her recovery was easier than she anticipated. She told me she went out for dinner with her husband and another couple the day after her second procedure.

Height: 5′2″
Weight before: 118.5 lbs.
BMI: 21.3
Children: 2
Weight after: 122.5 lbs.
Liposuction volume: 550 cc,
Second procedure: 1,100 cc
Dress size before: 2/4
Dress size after: 2/4
J.P., age 44/45

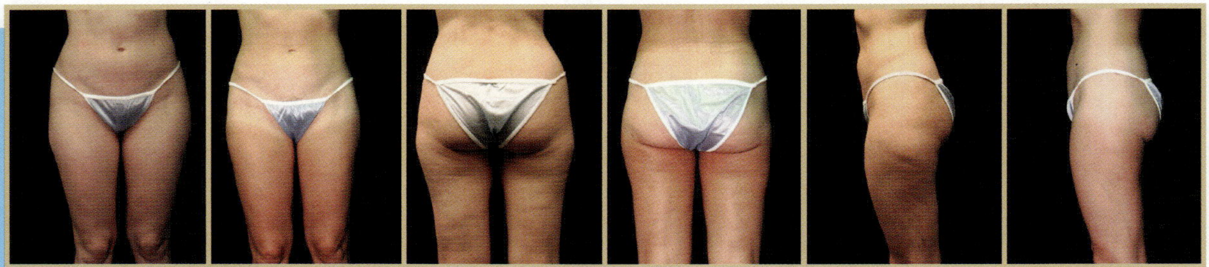

before *3½ months after* *before* *3½ months after* *before* *3½ months after*

Ultrasonic liposuction of lower body.

Comments: This patient had an excellent skin response after ultrasonic liposuction, in addition to correction of her areas of fatty excess. Her waist measurement dropped from 71 cm to 66 cm (two inches). Her thigh circumference also dropped five centimeters on either side. Cellulite of the outer and posterior thighs is noticeably improved.

Height: 5′ 8″
Weight before: 128 lbs.
BMI: 19.2
Children: 0
Weight after: 126.5 lbs.
Liposuction volume: 1,875 cc
Dress size before: 6
Dress size after: 6
K.K., age 28, physical therapist

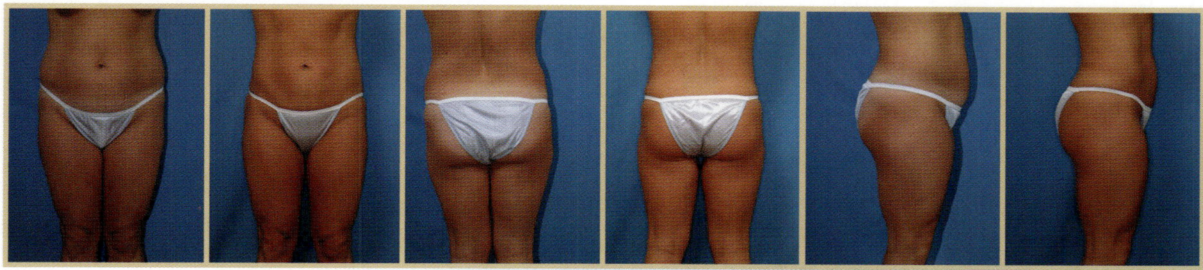

before *8 months after* *before* *8 months after* *before* *8 months after*

Ultrasonic liposuction of abdomen, flanks, inner thighs, arms, excision of multiple skin lesions of neck and body, breast lift, and breast implants. Touchup, 5 months later: abdomen, flanks, and inner thighs.

Comments: This 32-year-old mother-of-three was 5'2" tall. After liposuction and a breast lift, she looks leaner. Her torso appears longer and she looks taller. She has improved muscle definition.

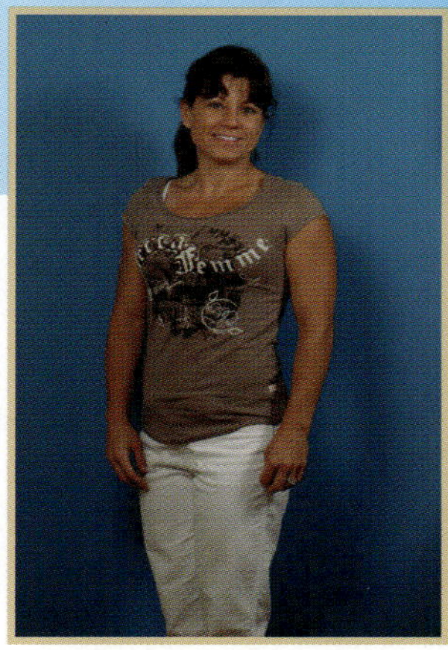

A.L.

Height: 5'2"
Weight before: 149 lbs.
BMI: 26.8
Children: 3
Weight after: 137 lbs.
Liposuction volume: 1,475 cc, touchup: 600 cc
Dress size before: "tight 12"
Dress size after: "loose 10"
A.L., age 32/33, bartender

Ultrasonic liposuction of lower body.

Comments: This patient said her upper body had never been the same size as her lower body. Her proportions are now balanced. There is a modest improvement in her cellulite.

Height: 5'7"
Weight before: 166 lbs.
BMI: 25.6
Children: 0
Weight after: 167.5 lbs.
Liposuction volume: 2,450 cc
Dress size before: 12
Dress size after: 12
N.W., age 33, consultant, part-time aerobics instructor

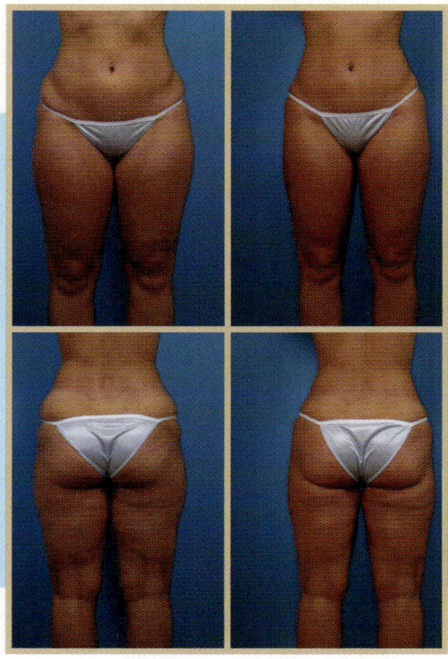

before *3 months after*

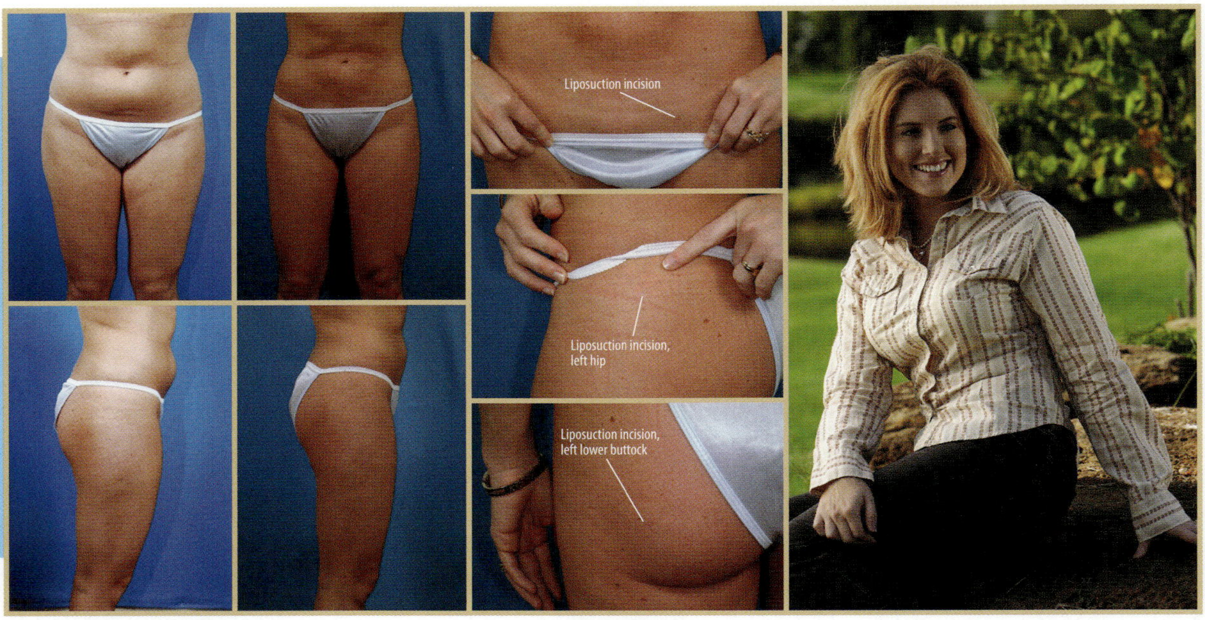

before ***9 months after*** ***close-up of incisions*** ***K.M.***

Ultrasonic liposuction of lower body, and breast augmentation. Touchup, 4 months later: abdomen, flanks, inner thighs, and left outer thigh.

Comments: This 27-year-old nurse dropped from a size 8 to a size 4. She had a simultaneous breast augmentation. She was pleased that the incisions were almost invisible.

Height: 5'3"
Weight before: 130 lbs.
BMI: 22.6
Children: 0
Weight after: 129 lbs.
Liposuction volume: 1,800 cc, touchup: 700 cc
Dress size before: 6/8
Dress size after: 4
K.M., age 27, registered nurse

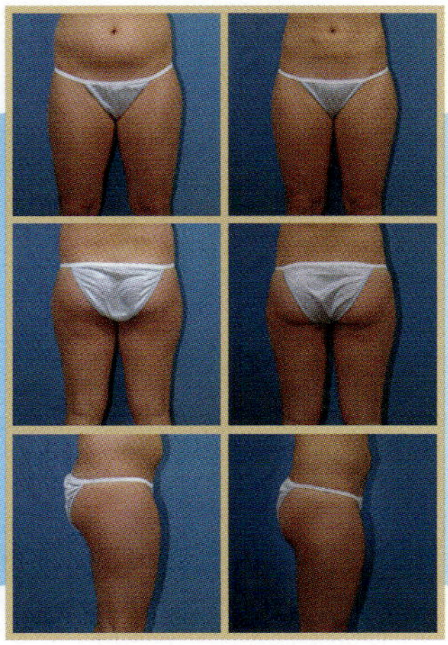

before ***2 months after***

Ultrasonic liposuction of lower body and submental lipectomy.

Comments: This college student was very athletic, played varsity basketball, but could do nothing about her unflattering bulges. After surgery she thought she looked more attractive and could wear clothing that complemented her feminine form. Her parents were glad to see her stop wearing baggy, loose-fitting clothes.

Height: 5'5"
Weight before: 157 lbs.
BMI: 25.7
Children: 0
Weight after: 150 lbs.
Liposuction volume: 2,700 cc
Dress size before: 6
Dress size after: 6
E.G., age 21, student

Liposuction of lower body. Touchups, 1 year later: liposuction of thighs and hips, and touchup liposuction of posterior thighs (local anesthesia).

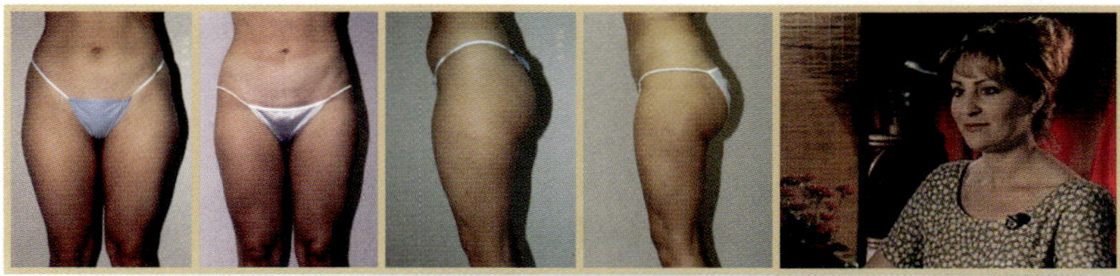

before *13 months after* *before* *13 months after* *C.G.*

Testimonial: "I have always worked out and tried to maintain the same type of body weight that is good for me and just through heredity, I got a couple of areas that I did want to change. What I couldn't do physically I changed surgically. I would tell anyone interested to go ahead and take the plunge."

Height: 5' 8"
Weight before: 144.5 lbs.
BMI: 21.7
Weight after: 140 lbs.
Liposuction volume: 2,475 cc, touchups: 450 cc, 225 cc
C.G., age 30, yellow pages sales rep.

Liposuction – 10 Years Later

Liposuction of lower body (no knees). Touchup, 1 year later: lower buttocks.

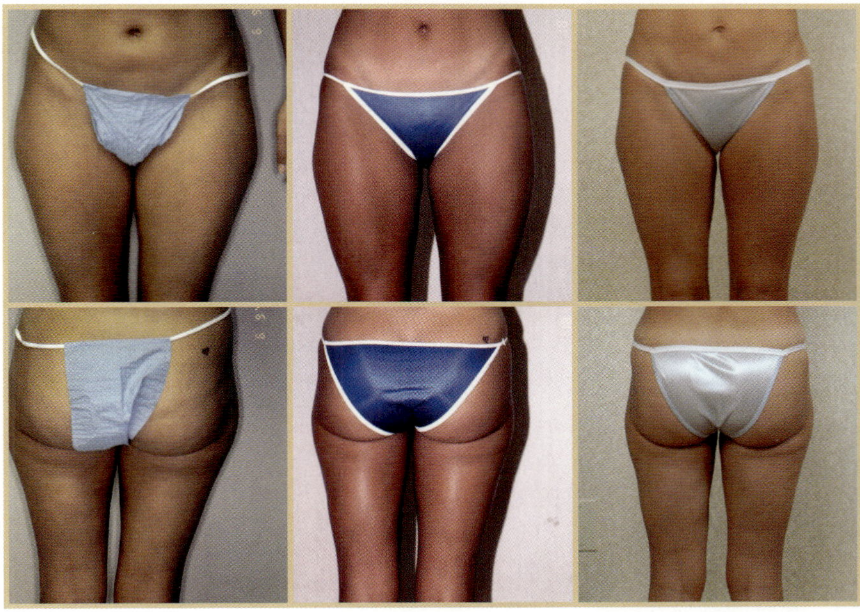

before *2 years after* *11½ years after*

Testimonial (6 years after): "I was uncomfortable wearing a bathing suit. I could lose weight everywhere except in my thighs and bottom. To try to get rid of the extra fat, I would lose weight and my face would get thin and drawn. My friends thought I was looking too thin and I didn't feel good either.

In high school and college I did some modeling part time. But I had trouble with the clothing. From my appearance, people thought I was smaller than I really was and it was embarrassing not being able to fit the clothes, but what could I do?

Liposuction seemed to be the only answer. The surgery wasn't as painful as I thought it would be. After liposuction, I went from a size six to a size four, which I think is my natural size. Now I find when I lose weight, I lose it all over. I had my liposuction six years ago and have since gotten married and had a baby girl. After my pregnancy, I am still a size four. The extra fat has not come back. I'm 13 weeks pregnant now with my second child. I'm very happy that I had this done."

Comments: This part-time model was embarrassed asking for a size eight. She dropped to a size four/six after liposuction. She is seen two years and 11 years after liposuction. Between the times of these follow-up photos she had two babies. These photographs demonstrate that future pregnancies do not detract from the results of liposuction, although obviously the abdominal skin and muscles are stretched. Pregnancy does not create more fat cells, so the benefit of liposuction is not compromised.

Height: 5'5½"
Weight before: 128 lbs.
BMI: 20.6
Children: 2 (after liposuction)
Weight after: 120 lbs.
Liposuction volume: 2,600 cc, touchup: 425 cc
Dress size before: 8
Dress size after: 5
H.E., age 22,25,34, real estate agent and mother

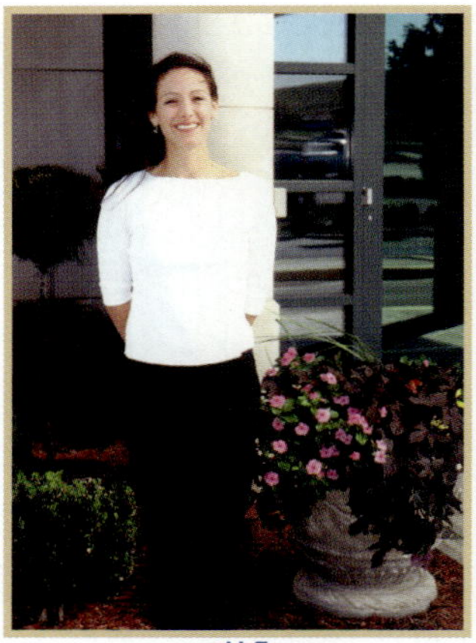

H.E.

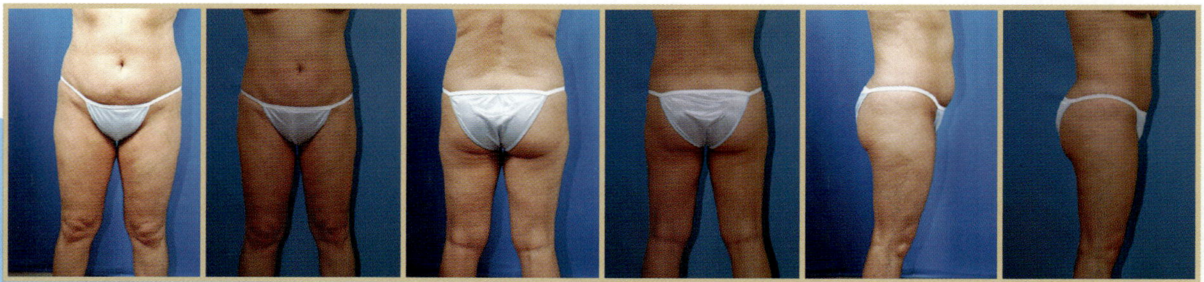

before | 16 months after | before | 16 months after | before | 16 months after

Ultrasonic liposuction of lower body, arms, and axillae, breast augmentation, scar revision of upper chest, and excision of facial skin lesion.

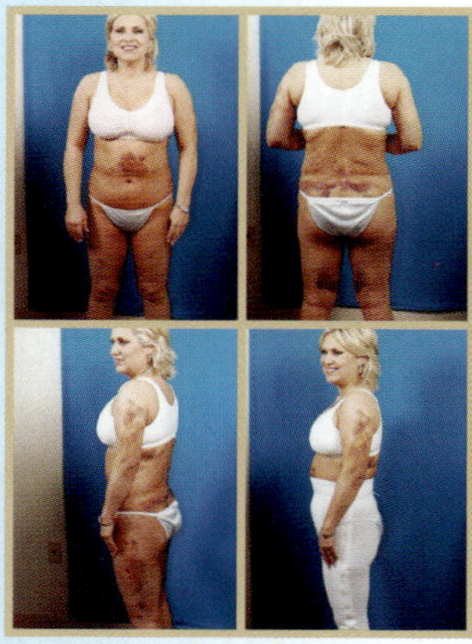

6 days after

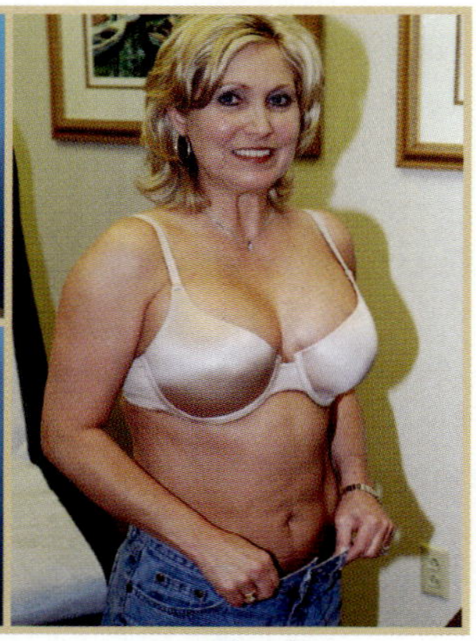

6 weeks after

Comments: This patient had a simultaneous breast augmentation. She requested a large breast size to restore volume lost after her pregnancies. She did not take any prescription pain killers after the first day after surgery. She is wearing the garment and bra and has the expected degree of bruising six days after surgery. Six weeks after surgery, her jeans fit much more loosely. Three months after surgery, she had dropped from a size eight to a size four. Her skin tone before surgery was not ideal—she had moderate laxity consistent with her age and four children. After ultrasonic liposuction, her skin tone has noticeably improved.

Height: 5'3"
Weight before: 138 lbs.
BMI: 23.9
Children: 4
Weight after (16 months): 142 lbs.
Liposuction volume: 3,250 cc
Dress size before: 8
Dress size after: 4
B.D., age 42/43, realtor

"Muffin top"

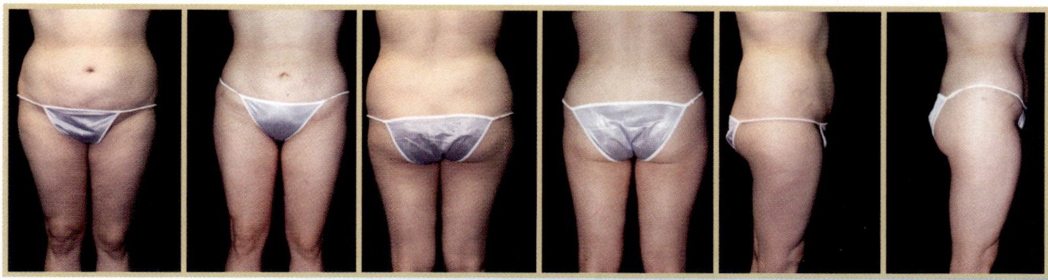

before | 9 months after | before | 9 months after | before | 9 months after

Ultrasonic liposuction of abdomen, flanks, inner thighs, and arms, and submental lipectomy.
Touchup, 6 months later: abdomen and flanks.

Comments: This 23-year-old pharmacist was embarrassed by her body shape. She had excess fullness of the flanks, which created a bulge just above her waistline. This overhang is popularly, but not affectionately, called a muffin top. Liposuction eliminated this bulge, making her buttocks appear more curvaceous. She can now wear tight-fitting pants without embarrassment. An abdominoplasty would have eliminated the skin laxity and stretch marks, but she planned to have children in the future, so this procedure was deferred. Despite poor skin elasticity, she demonstrates reasonable contraction of the abdominal skin, although she still has stretch marks. At the time of her postoperative appointment, her weight was 143 pounds, representing an 8.5 pound weight loss, which corresponds to the weight of the fat tissue removed. This means her caloric consumption versus expenditure after surgery remained just about even, and the difference in body shape is a true representation of the results of liposuction without any superimposed weight gain or loss.

Height: 5′ 5½″
Weight before: 151.5 lbs.
BMI: 24.4

Weight after: 143 lbs.
Volume: 3,150 cc, touchup: 625 cc.
Dress size before: 10

T.N., age 23, pharmacist

Ultrasonic liposuction of lower body, arms, and axillae, and excision of skin lesion of right flank.

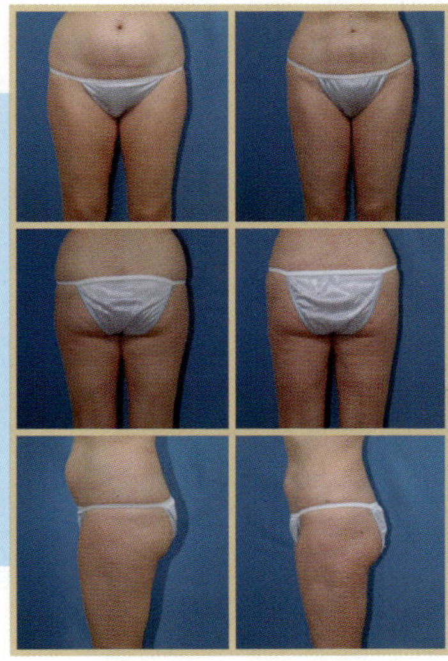

before | 3 months after

Comments: This 54-year-old woman decided to have liposuction after seeing what it did for her husband (this was a little different—wives usually go first). She has excellent skin tone afterward. (It is remarkable to consider that at one time plastic surgeons were hesitant to perform liposuction on patients over 50 out of concern for skin resilience.) She was pleased to be able to fit pants that she had not worn in years. Her contours are improved from top to bottom and from every angle. This is the advantage of comprehensive liposuction of the lower body, which is performed circumferentially from the level of the ribcage down to the knees.

Height: 5′7″
Weight before: 145 lbs.
BMI: 22.3
Children: 0
Weight after: 144 lbs.

Liposuction volume: 3,800 cc
Dress size before: 10
Dress size after: 6/8
M.H., age 54, homemaker

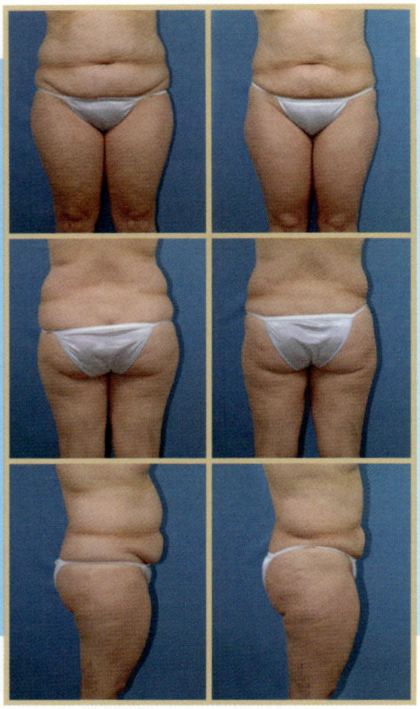

before *3½ months after*

Ultrasonic liposuction of lower body, arms, and axillae.

Comments: This patient had five children, aged 15 to 28. She decided to have liposuction after her daughter had it done. She was aware that liposuction would reduce her areas of extra fat, but would not treat her skin laxity, and that she was a candidate for an abdominoplasty. She dropped two dress sizes after surgery. She still has skin laxity, but it has not been made worse by liposuction, and there appears to be a modest degree of skin contraction. She is considering having a breast augmentation and tummy tuck in the future.

Height: 5'5"
Weight before: 187 lbs.
BMI: 30.6
Children: 5
Weight after: 184 lbs.
Liposuction volume: 4,300 cc
Dress size before: 20
Dress size after: 14/16
D.S., age 49, assisted living administrator

Ultrasonic liposuction of lower body, arms, and axillae, and submental lipectomy.

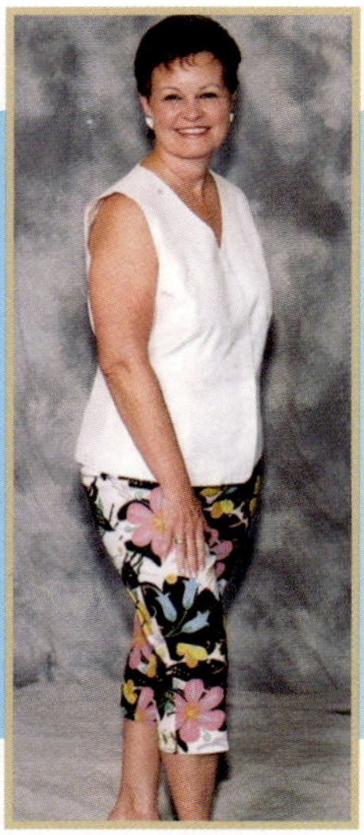

1 month after

Testimonial: "I go to Hawaii regularly and spend a lot of time in a swimming suit. It seemed I was always on a diet. I was frustrated and thought it was time to stop the endless dieting. My sisters encouraged me to go ahead with liposuction. I decided to have my arms and chin treated at the same time as my tummy and thighs. The new carpeting at home would just have to wait.

I'd had trouble before with nausea after anesthetics. So when I woke up after surgery, my first thought was, 'Oh, good. I'm not feeling sick.' The first three days were the only tough part. After that, I didn't need the pain killers anymore. I felt like I needed to wear the girdle. Sometimes I would feel pulling at the small incisions under my arms but now this has gone away.

It's been a month now since my surgery. I started as a size 14 and I'm down to a size 10 already. I'm wearing things I haven't been able to fit in years. The results are actually better than I expected. Everywhere seems to be smaller. I love it. I feel like I'm 40. My husband says he married Miss America. I don't know about that, but I think my whole body looks good now."

Height: 5' 5"
Weight before: 157 lbs.
BMI: 25.7
Children: 2
Liposuction volume: 4,350 cc
Dress size before: 14
Dress size after: 10
C.H., age 52, massage therapist

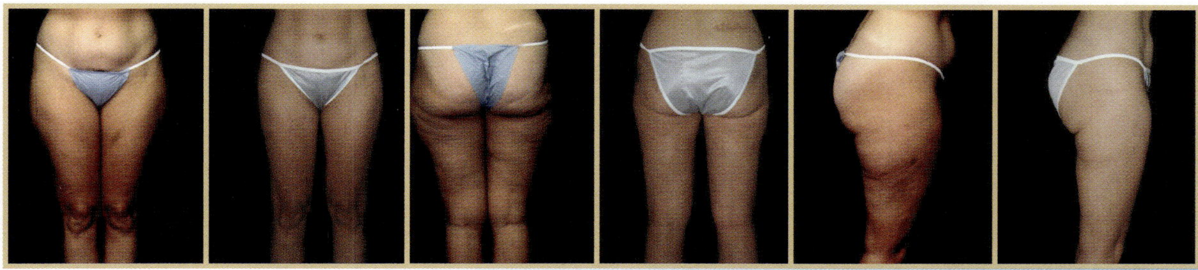

before *19 months after* *before* *19 months after* *before* *19 months after*

Liposuction of lower body. Touchup, 5 months later: outer thighs and scar revision of right hip.

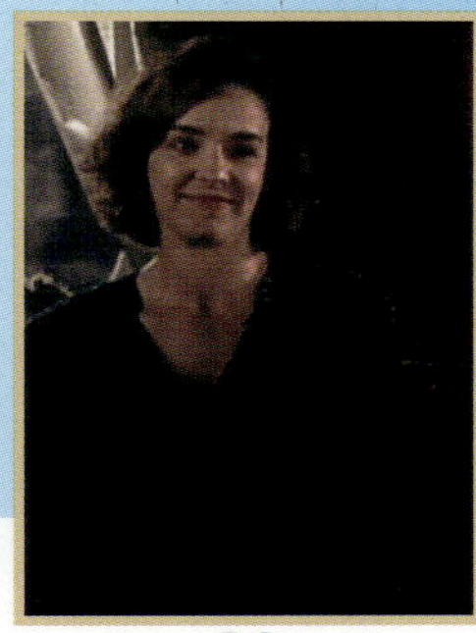

E.G.

Testimonial: "I wanted to get rid of the saddlebags on my thighs. My husband and I scuba dive and the wet suit was always tight on the bottom and loose on top. After surgery, before the swelling set in, I got a glimpse of what I was going to look like and I thought, Wow! This is going to be great. I was really pleased with what I was seeing in the mirror. Now I'm the same size top and bottom.

The surgery was 18 months ago and I love my new body. It does wonders for my self-confidence. I got my first new swimsuit a month ago. Shopping for it was actually fun. My saddlebags are gone and I just feel better about myself!"

Height: 5'3"
Weight before: 125 lbs.
BMI: 21.7
Children: 2
Weight after: 117 lbs.
Liposuction volume: 4,100 cc, touchup: 450 cc
E.G., age 33, dental hygienist

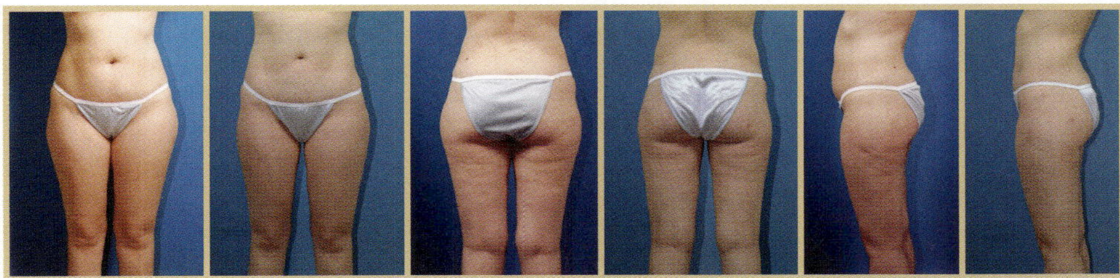

before *1 year after* *before* *1 year after* *before* *1 year after*

Ultrasonic liposuction of lower body, excision of skin lesions of left flank and perineum, and revision of umbilical scar. Touchup, 11 months later: lower body.

Comments: This patient demonstrates the common pear-shaped fat distribution. Women often point to the roll just below the buttock. This bulge has the tropically inspired name "banana roll." She reported receiving numerous compliments when I saw her in follow-up three months after surgery. She wondered if plastic surgery was "addicting" (we like to think in a good way). She returned for a breast augmentation and had a touchup liposuction simultaneously.

Height: 5'4"
Weight: 137.5 lbs.
BMI: 23.2
Children: 2
Liposuction volume: 3,650 cc, touchup: 1,150 cc
A.S., age 28/29, claims adjuster

Liposuction – African-American

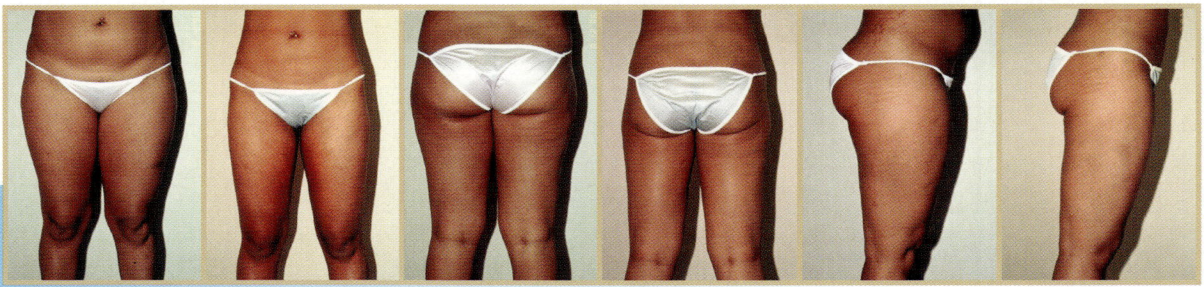

before *11 months after* *before* *11 months after* *before* *11 months after*

Liposuction of lower body and submental lipectomy. Touchup, 6 months later: abdomen, hips, inner thighs, and right posterior thigh.

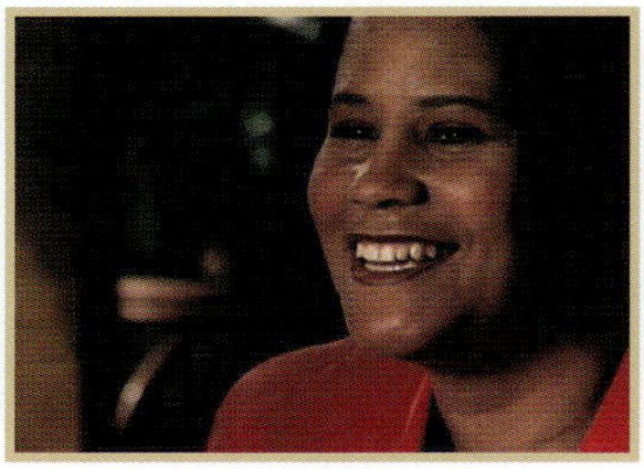

T.F.

Testimonial: "I was interested in lipo after I had a disease where I had to be on prednisone. I gained weight and couldn't fit in any of my clothes. I wanted to see what could be done for me. The procedure helped a lot. My clothes fit again. It's an ego boost. It makes you feel a lot better. I feel like I have more control over my life and can make it better. This is an incentive to exercise and get even more in shape. I was feeling I couldn't make a difference. Now things are falling into place. I feel a lot better when I go shopping. It's an elective surgery but it's still surgery. You can't expect that you'll get the inches off and not have to do anything. You still have to work at it. I can exercise without wearing a big old sweatsuit."

Height: 5' 7"
Weight before: 166 lbs.
BMI: 25.6

Children: 0
Liposuction volume: 4,225 cc, touchup: 950 cc
T.F., age 26, registered nurse

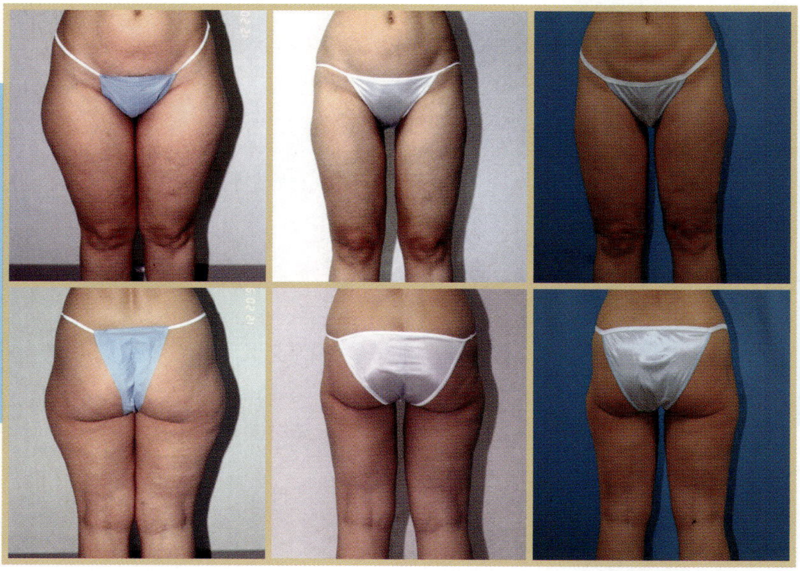

before *1½ years after* *8 years after*

Liposuction of lower body including calves and breast augmentation.

Testimonial: "I vividly remember in third grade noticing that my sisters were tall and lanky. Not me. I wanted bigger breasts and lankier legs. I was always very self-conscious about my body and embarrassed by it.

I was doing this strictly for myself. As an adult, I could make this decision. I interviewed several surgeons. I had a little bit of pain, but the outcome was well worth it.

After my surgery, my self-esteem really increased a lot. I had surgery two years ago. I still feel a lot better about myself. I don't have to have my clothes altered anymore. I have a lot more self-confidence. I feel better about my body. I feel like I'm at least worth looking at now.

I had an old scar on my abdomen from a car wreck when I was 17. It was wide and long. Dr. Swanson did a scar revision. Now it lays down. I can even wear a two-piece swimsuit. I'm really pleased with the results.

After lipo, my clothes fit much better. I'm a perfect size four now. I wish I could have done this when I was 19. It would have changed my life."

Comments: This patient was 5'2" tall and weighed 125 pounds, but her inherited pear-shaped fat distribution made her look much heavier. At surgery, about 10 pounds of fat were removed, but it looks like much more. A breast augmentation was done simultaneously, further improving her proportions and defeating the pear shape that had plagued her. She had an old abdominal scar from previous surgery. Her shape and skin tone are unchanged eight years later. She has had no touchups.

Height: 5' 2"
Weight before: 125 lbs.
BMI: 22.5
Children: 1
Weight after: 126 lbs. (8 years)
Liposuction volume: 5,325 cc
T.M., age 34/35/42, office manager

Male Liposuction

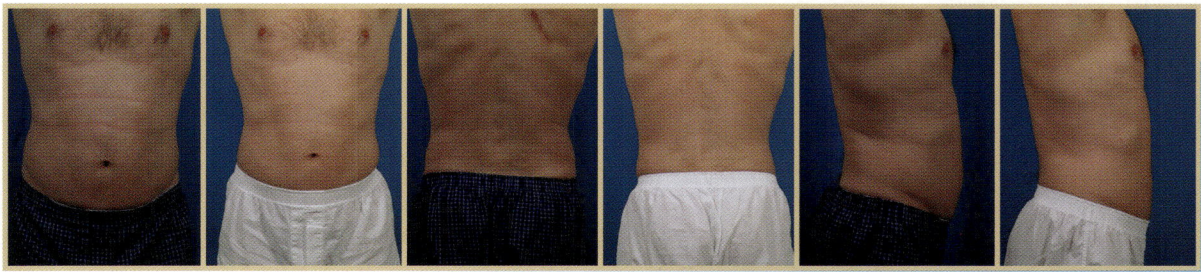

before | *6 months after* | *before* | *6 months after* | *before* | *6 months after*

Ultrasonic liposuction of abdomen and flanks, and submental lipectomy.

Comments: This patient worked out regularly but could not seem to get rid of extra fat of the abdomen and flanks. He dropped from a 35 inch waist to a 33 inch waist after liposuction. He started walking on a treadmill one week after surgery.

Height: 5'11"
Weight before: 198 lbs.
BMI: 27.2
Weight after: 190 lbs.
Waist before: 35"
Waist after: 33"
Liposuction volume: abdomen 400 cc, flanks 500 cc, total 900 cc
J.T., age 45, sales

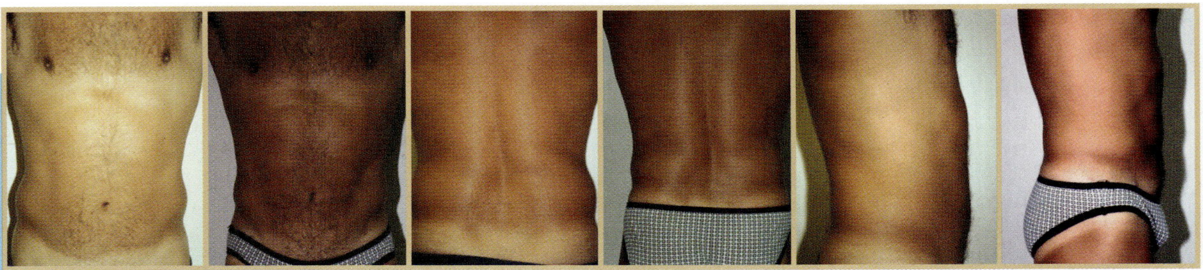

before *6 weeks after* *before* *6 weeks after* *before* *6 weeks after*

Liposuction of abdomen and flanks.

Comments: This 39-year-old former "Mr. Atlanta" had continued to work out regularly. He kept lean, and his body fat was only 8%. Many men (not to mention women) would accept his "before" appearance, but he was a perfectionist. He wanted a ripped abdomen and no more love handles. The improved definition is visible six weeks after surgery. His incisions are still visible, but are starting to fade already.

Height: 5′ 9″
Weight: 193 lbs.
BMI: 28.0
Liposuction volume: 925 cc
J.C., age 39, medical sales

Male Liposuction – Bodybuilder

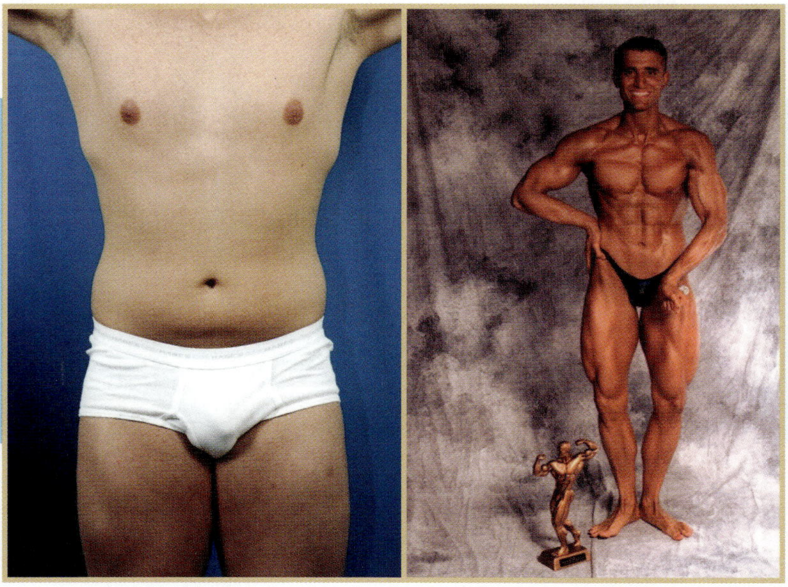

before *1 year after*

Ultrasonic liposuction of abdomen and flanks. Touchup, 7 months later: abdomen and flanks.

Comments: Despite a 12% body fat, this fitness director and personal trainer could not get the abdominal definition he wanted. After liposuction and additional training, he won his category in a bodybuilding competition.

Height: 6′0″
Weight: 200 lbs.
BMI: 26.6
Liposuction volume: 850 cc, touchup: 750 cc
P.K., age 24/25, personal trainer, bodybuilder

Ultrasonic liposuction of abdomen, flanks, and breasts.

Testimonial: "I work out all the time and I still couldn't get rid of the love handles around my waist. I'd heard about liposuction, but waited a year before I finally made an appointment with the surgeon. Now I wish I'd had it done sooner because it's great. I can now wear spandex to ride my bike. And I didn't mind when I had to buy new jeans because I'd lost two inches around my waist."

Height: 5'7"
Weight before: 165 lbs.
BMI: 25.4
Weight after: 171.5 lbs.
Liposuction volume: abdomen 700 cc, flanks 800 cc, breasts 300 cc, total 1,800 cc
Waist before: 34"
Waist after: 31/32"
J.N., age 31, store manager

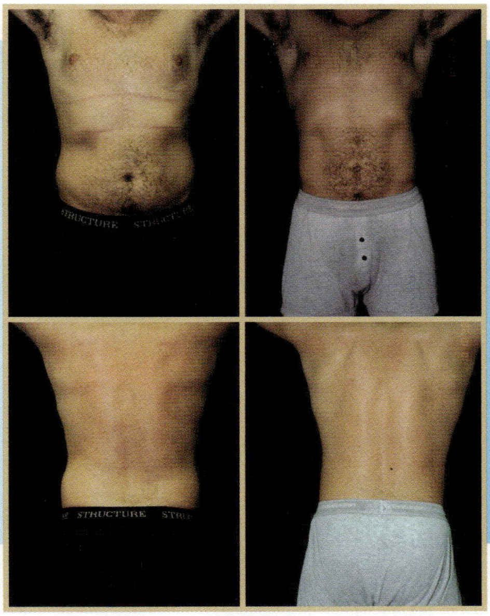

before *9 months after*

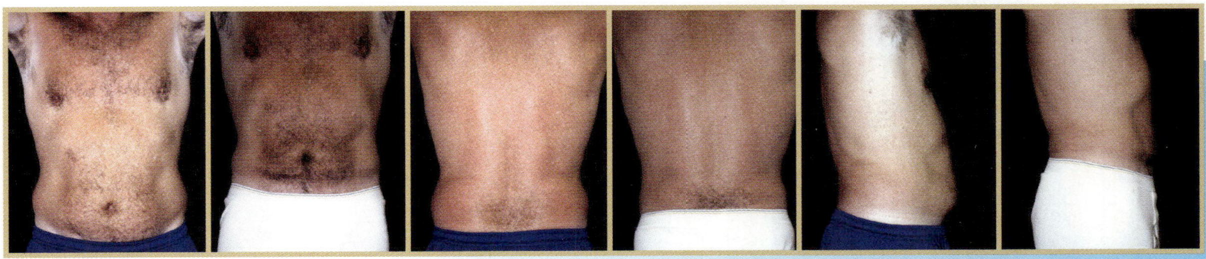

before *2 months after* *before* *2 months after* *before* *2 months after*

Ultrasonic liposuction of abdomen and flanks.

Testimonial: "At 53, I thought I was doing alright. I worked out with a punching bag three times a week. Nevertheless, I couldn't get rid of extra fat around my abdomen and sides. I was sore and swollen for awhile, but I got back to work after only a few days. One month after surgery, I had dropped from a 36 waist size to a 33. The love handles were gone. Now I look like I'm in good shape. I'm looking forward to wearing a bathing suit again."

Height: 5'11"
Weight before: 198 lbs.
BMI: 27.2
Liposuction volume: abdomen 850 cc, flanks 975 cc, total 1,825 cc
Waist before: 36"
Waist after: 33"
K.H., age 54, art gallery owner

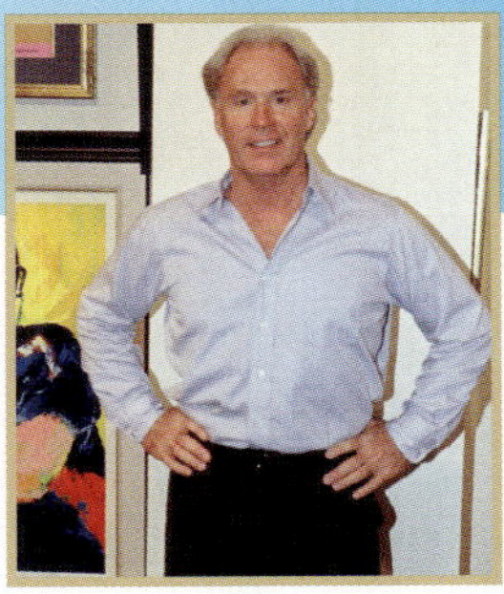

K.H.

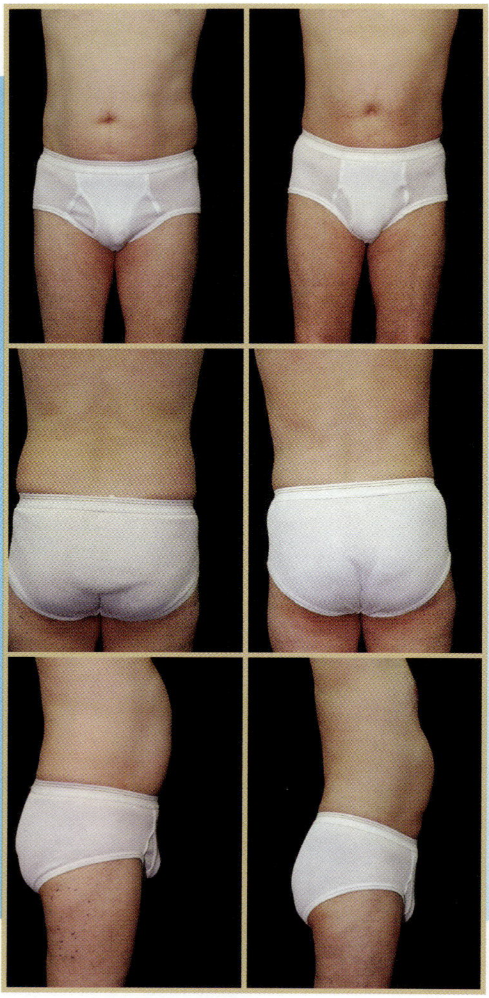

before *4 months after*

Liposuction of abdomen, flanks, inner and outer thighs, and knees.

Testimonial: "I had liposuction on my flanks, my abdomen, and my inner thighs. About 10 years ago, I began to accumulate a lot around my waist and other areas where I wasn't getting much exercise, so I got to the point where I was really miserable. I had grown out of all of my pants. I couldn't get any of them on any more except for new ones. I couldn't bend over without just feeling really miserable and hardly being able to get my breath. I really hadn't had very much success as far as dieting or exercise, although I had done both, and never had any immediate or lasting results from it, so I thought this might be a tough way to go, but I got it done and have it behind me, and hopefully it would be what I was looking for.

Now that it is over I am really glad that I had it done. Anytime I am able to get into another pair of trousers that I had grown out of, I more or less decided, that just discounts my bill. I am able to get back into most of the clothes that I wasn't able to wear any more and I have gotten away from that full feeling and not being able to bend over comfortably and I feel a lot better about myself too. We were in Cancun about a year ago and when I put on my swim suit I felt like I was just draping out all over my suit and that is definitely changed, so I am looking forward to going back again this fall.

To anyone who is hearing or seeing me, I would say that if you have a problem like that, growing out of your wardrobe or just feeling miserable because you cannot get rid of extra fat through dieting or exercise alone, although I think those are two components that need to accompany even liposuction after it is all done, I think a person needs to stay in shape and not allow the ravages of time to take effect and lose the benefit that you have achieved. I think it is a viable solution for anyone that has those things in mind. The first two days you feel like you have been beat up and run over by a truck, but it is definitely worth it and I think, you know with the medications that you can take. Of course you can imagine I was pretty anxious to see what the results were going to be and I was really gratified when I first put on my trousers after I had healed up and I pulled my belt up five notches beyond where I had worn it before and, after measuring, I discovered that I had gone from about a 38 to about a 33 on the waist."

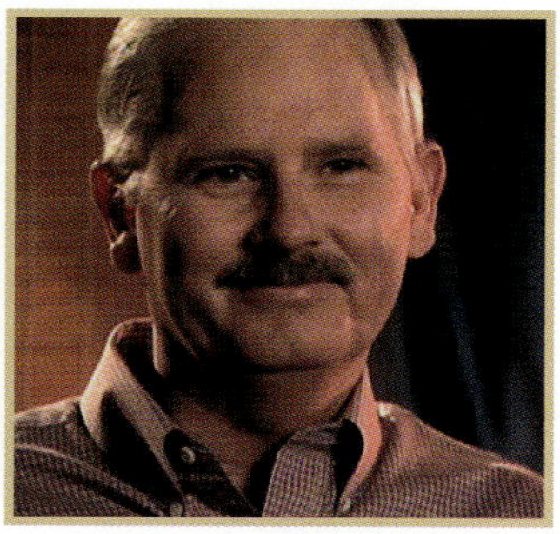

J.S.

Height: 5'10"
Weight before: 164 lbs.
BMI: 23.2
Liposuction volume: abdomen 800 cc, flanks 625 cc, inner thighs 200 cc, outer thighs 125 cc, knees 100 cc, total 1,850 cc
Waist before: 38"
Waist after: 33"
J.S., age 59, small-business owner

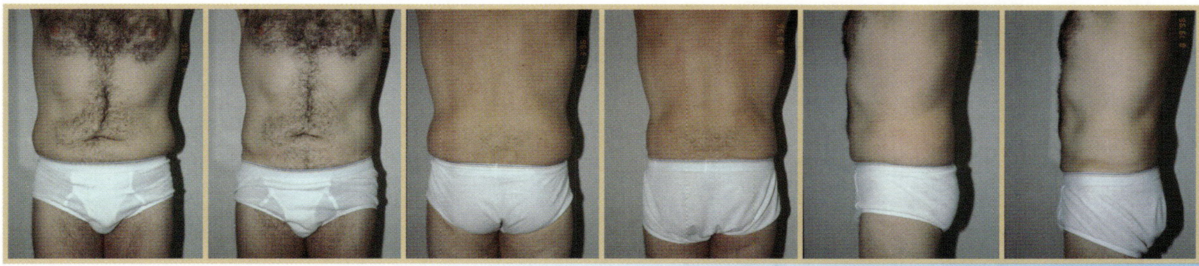

before *4 months after* *before* *4 months after* *before* *4 months after*

Liposuction of abdomen and flanks.

Comments: This 45-year-old male had lost weight recently. He demonstrated the expected loss of skin tone of his abdomen. In the past, I may have recommended an abdominoplasty. However, his abdominal skin contracted nicely after liposuction alone. He commented that his result was "nothing short of miraculous."

Height: 6'2"
Weight before: 195 lbs.
BMI: 24.6
Liposuction volume: abdomen 625 cc, flanks 1,300 cc, total 1,925 cc
D.D., age 45, auto assembly worker

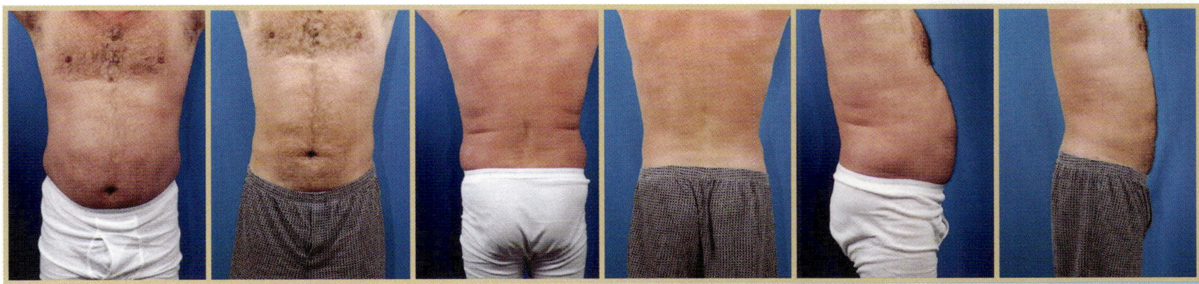

before *6 months after* *before* *6 months after* *before* *6 months after*

Ultrasonic liposuction of abdomen and flanks, submental lipectomy, and jawline implant.

Comments: This patient also had a submental lipectomy and a jawline implant. He felt good enough to drive himself to his appointment the day after surgery (not generally recommended, and certainly not when taking prescription pain killers). He said that now that he was seeing some results, he was very motivated to stay in shape. The love handles were eliminated along with the skin creases. It now appears that he "has a butt." In both men and women, liposuction of the flanks reduces these bulges, giving the welcome illusion of a fuller butt.

Height: 6'0"
Weight before: 238 lbs.
BMI: 31.6
Weight after: 204 lbs.

Liposuction volume: abdomen 525 cc, flanks 1,475 cc, total 2,000 cc
Waist before: 40"
Waist after: 37"
L.M., age 37, restaurant owner

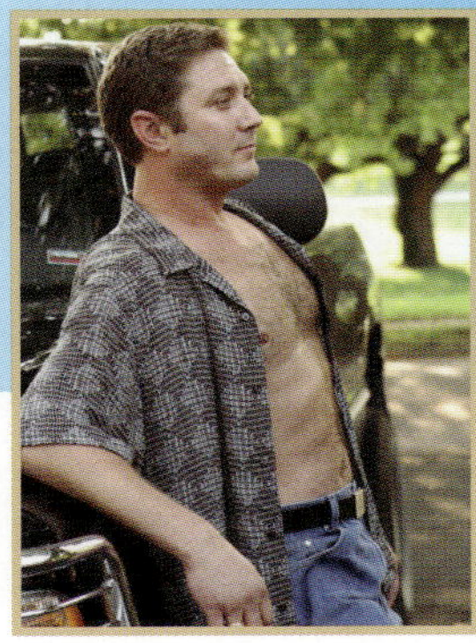

L.M.

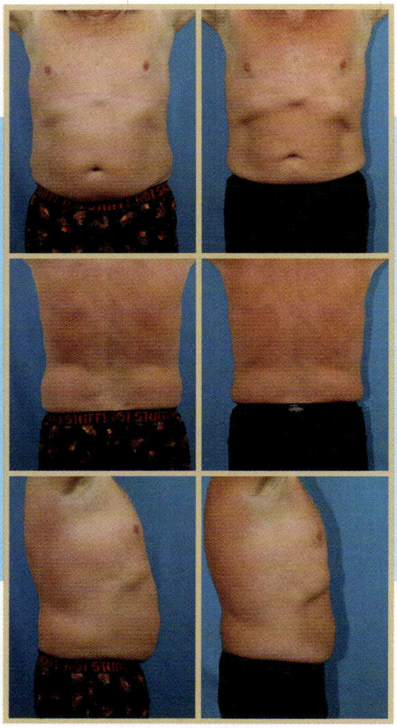

before 5 months after

Ultrasonic liposuction of abdomen, flanks, and breasts.

Comments: This 55-year-old teacher and part-time farmer had recently lost his wife to cancer. He said he had been undergoing some lifestyle changes. He quit smoking and started watching his diet and exercising. He had liposuction before the spring break so he could take a week off. At his appointment four days after surgery, he admitted he had been driving his tractor and doing some work around the farm. He wore snug-fitting "Under Armour®" garments. At his last follow-up appointment, he told me he was dating a much younger woman. No doubt that provided some extra motivation.

Height: 6′1½″
Weight before: 232 lbs.
BMI: 29.4
Weight after: 210 lbs.
Liposuction volume: 2,050 cc
Waist before: 40″
Waist after: 36″ "loose"
S.P., age 55, teacher and farmer

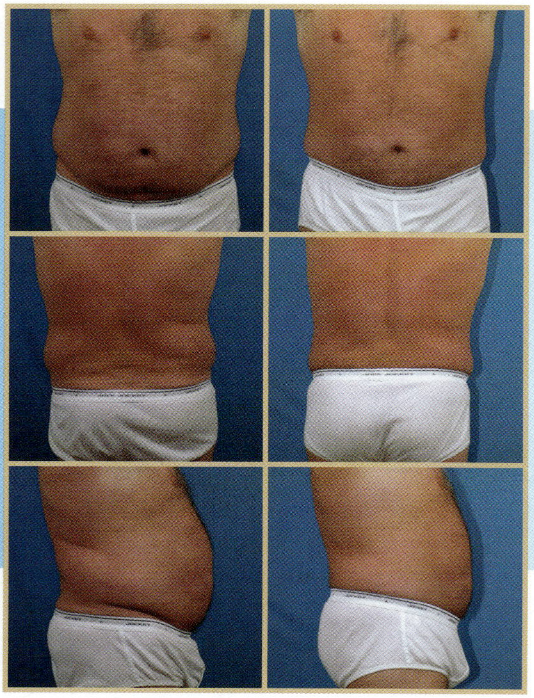

before 3 months after

Ultrasonic liposuction of abdomen and flanks, and submental lipectomy.

Comments: This patient was aware that he was overweight. He said that even when he was lighter, he had these areas of excess fullness. He understood that a combination of weight loss and liposuction was needed. He returned to work five days after surgery.

Height: 5′10″
Weight before: 217 lbs.
BMI: 30.7
Weight after: 210 lbs.
Liposuction volume: abdomen 850 cc, flanks 1,300 cc, total 2,150 cc
Waist before: 38
Waist after: 36
W.C., age 50, sales

Ultrasonic liposuction of abdomen, flanks, breasts, and axillae, subcutaneous mastectomies, submental lipectomy, and jawline implant.

Comments: This 40-year-old male also had excess breast tissue, called gynecomastia, which was treated simultaneously with an excisional procedure, "subcutaneous mastectomies," in addition to ultrasonic liposuction. The two techniques are commonly used together to provide a smooth chest contour.

Height: 5'8"
Weight before: 170 lbs.
BMI: 25.5
Weight after: 156 lbs.
Liposuction volume: abdomen 850 cc, flanks 900 cc, breasts 450 cc, total 2,200 cc
Waist before: 34"
Waist after: 32"
J.G., age 40, VP educational resources

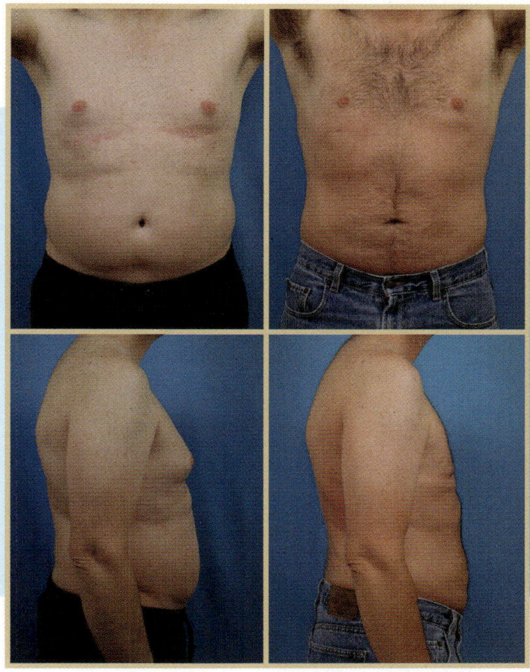

before *3 months after*

Repair of Umbilical Hernia

Sometimes, patients have a bulge in the belly button, where the abdominal fat is protruding through a weakness in the abdominal wall. This hernia may be repaired using an inconspicuous incision along the inside border of the umbilicus. It is common for me to repair such a umbilical hernia at the same time as liposuction or (particularly in women) an abdominoplasty.

Ultrasonic liposuction of abdomen, flanks and breasts, repair of umbilical hernia, and submental lipectomy.

Comments: This patient's umbilical hernia had been present for about 10 years. He said it caused him discomfort from time to time and he thought it was getting worse. It was corrected at the time of his liposuction.

Height: 6'0"
Weight before: 222 lbs.
BMI: 29.5
Liposuction volume: 1,650 cc
A.W., age 38, bricklayer

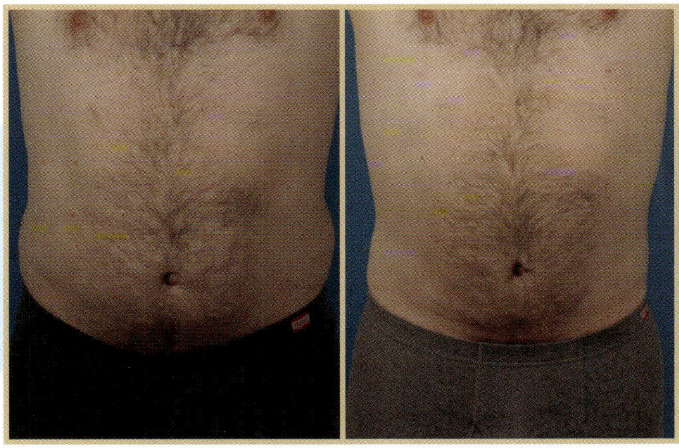

before *3 months after*

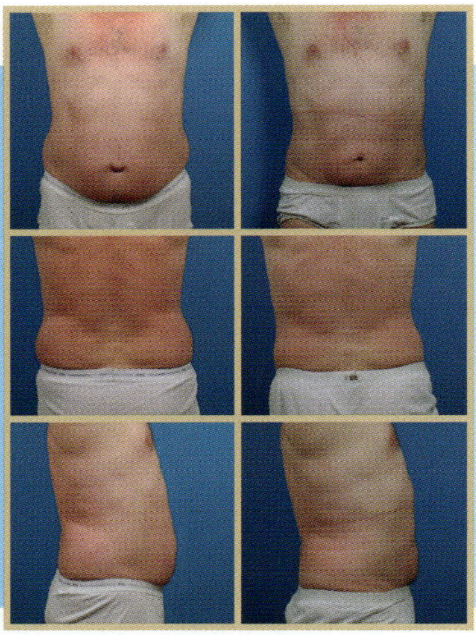

before *1 month after*

Ultrasonic liposuction of abdomen and flanks, repair of umbilical hernia, and upper and lower blepharoplasties.

Comments: This patient is seen only one month after surgery, before he moved out of town. The umbilical hernia was corrected. Even with the swelling, there is already a gratifying improvement in his contours after liposuction.

Height: 5'6"
Weight before: 190.5 lbs.
BMI: 30.3
Liposuction volume: 1,725 cc
K.W., age 47, letter carrier

Liposuction of Arms

Introduction

The arms are a favorable area for liposuction. Commonly, I treat the arms and underarms (axillae) at the same time as liposuction of the lower body. Women often complain about extra "flub" in their arms and shake this area to demonstrate it to me (both this maneuver and the shaking up and down of a tummy fat roll are not done outside a plastic surgeon's private examining room). They are embarrassed by it and avoid wearing sleeveless tops during the summer.

Most women are understandably concerned about what will happen to the skin after the fat is suctioned away. They don't want to end up with a lot of loose skin hanging down. Fortunately, the skin often responds surprisingly well, even in older patients (See Patient Photographs, Liposuction of Arms – Over 50). In patients with existing skin laxity, the skin tone may be no better after liposuction, but it is unlikely to be worse, and the removal of the extra fat improves the contour. It is always possible for the patient to return to have the extra skin removed with arm lifts ("brachioplasties") if necessary. However, I have treated plenty of women over 50 with compromised skin tone using liposuction alone and very few have returned for brachioplasties. It is a plus to avoid a brachioplasty scar because this scar, which goes down the back (posterior) border of the arm, cannot be completely hidden.

It is a plus to avoid a brachioplasty scar because this scar, which goes down the back border of the arm, cannot be completely hidden.

In patients who have lost a great deal of weight and have loose skin hanging to start with, brachioplasty is the better option, a skin excisional procedure that is often done in combination with liposuction. There is a limit after all to skin contraction after liposuction. The brachioplasty scar is preferable to loose skin that is sometimes called a "bat wing." (This label, like "witch's chin," does tend to inspire a patient to schedule surgery at the earliest opportunity.)

Axillary Fat ("Bra Fat")

Women often reach around and grab a roll of fat just lateral to their breasts when I see them in consultation. This is commonly called the bra fat. This fat can bulge around the bra, which is not very attractive. Even though this area is actually below the axilla, plastic surgeons refer to it as the axilla, or sometimes the scapular area.

The same armpit incision that is used to treat the arms may be used to access the axillary area to treat the bra fat. There is often a crease between this fat roll and the love handle below it. By treating the extra fat in the roll above and below this crease, the crease may be softened or sometimes eliminated (See L.M. and J.J., Patient Photographs, Female Liposuction – Abdomen and Flanks).

How It's Done

An incision is made in the armpit. The area is first injected with anesthetic solution, the same way that liposuction is performed in other areas, using the superwet technique. The second step is the introduction of the ultrasonic probe to dissolve fat cells. The third step is removal of the fat using liposuction. This is the familiar three-step process.

Some surgeons have been reluctant to treat the arms or calves because of concerns about complications. However, if the superwet technique is used, ultrasonic times are kept to a few minutes at the most, incisions are limited, and overtreatment avoided, these become very favorable areas to treat, with minimal risk.

It is unusual for me to treat just the arms and axillae. Most women also have concerns about the lower body, so these areas are treated at the same time as liposuction of the lower body. The exception is the patient who has liposuction of the lower body and then returns to have the arms treated. (Ideally these areas are treated in one operation.) Because men have a different fat distribution, very few men require liposuction of the arms, although I frequently treat the axillary areas when I perform liposuction on male breasts.

Patient Photographs

Ultrasonic liposuction of abdomen, flanks, inner thighs, arms, and axillae, and submental lipectomy.

Comments: This student had an apple body type (See M.C., Patient Photographs, Female Liposuction–Abdomen and Flanks). Her arms and axillae were treated simultaneously.

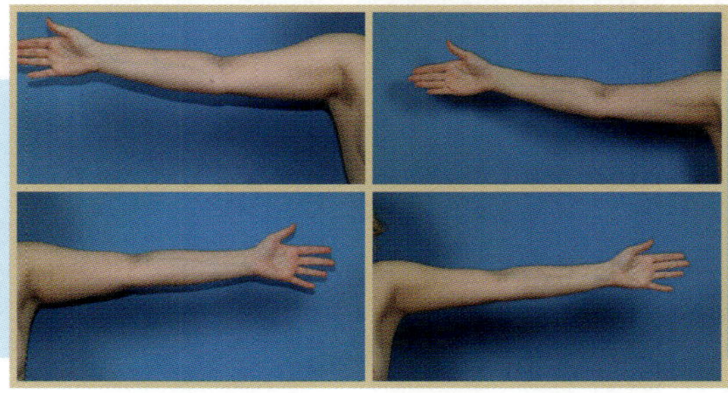

before *1 year after*

Height: 5'4"
Weight before: 150 lbs.
BMI: 25.3
Children: 0

Weight after: 128 lbs.
Liposuction volume: right arm 100 cc, right axilla 100 cc, left arm 125 cc, left axilla 75 cc
M.C., age 22, student

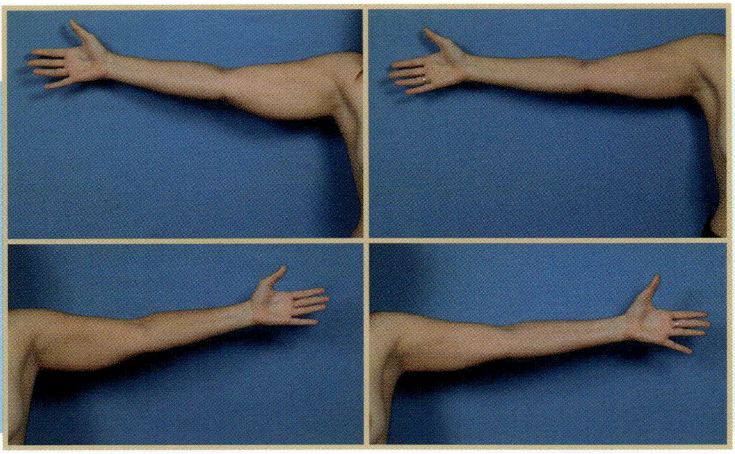

before 3 months after

Ultrasonic liposuction of arms and axillae.

Comments: This actress had a sleeveless role coming up. She wondered how saggy the skin would be if she just had liposuction. She informed me that she had checked out about *300 Web sites*! She was aware that her right arm was slightly larger than her left. One week after surgery she told me she thought she would be very happy and I needed to promote this procedure more.

Height: 5'6"
Weight before: 153 lbs.
BMI: 23.6
Children: 0
Weight after: 140.5 lbs.
Liposuction volume: right arm 275 cc, right axilla 125 cc, left arm 250 cc, left axilla 100 cc
S.C., age 32, actress

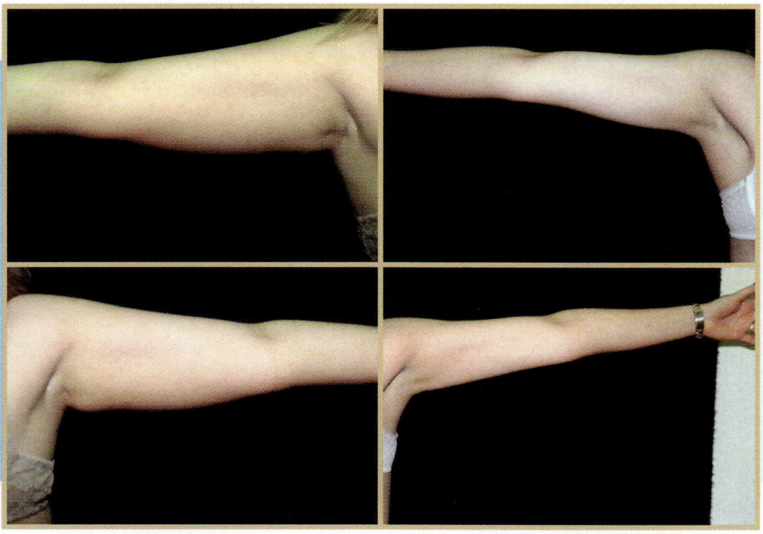

before 3 months after

Ultrasonic liposuction of lower body and arms.

Comments: This patient was self-conscious about her arms and would not wear sleeveless tops, so she had liposuction of the arms at the same time her lower body was treated. She demonstrates an excellent skin response after ultrasonic liposuction.

Height: 5'8"
Weight before: 155 lbs.
BMI: 23.3
Weight after: 160 lbs.
Liposuction volume: right arm 150 cc, left arm 175 cc
S.H., age 34

Ultrasonic liposuction of lower body, calves, arms, and axillae. Touchup, 4 months later: lower body, arms and axillae.

Comments: This patient has an excellent result after liposuction of her arms, which were treated with a touchup at the same time as a touchup liposuction of her lower body.

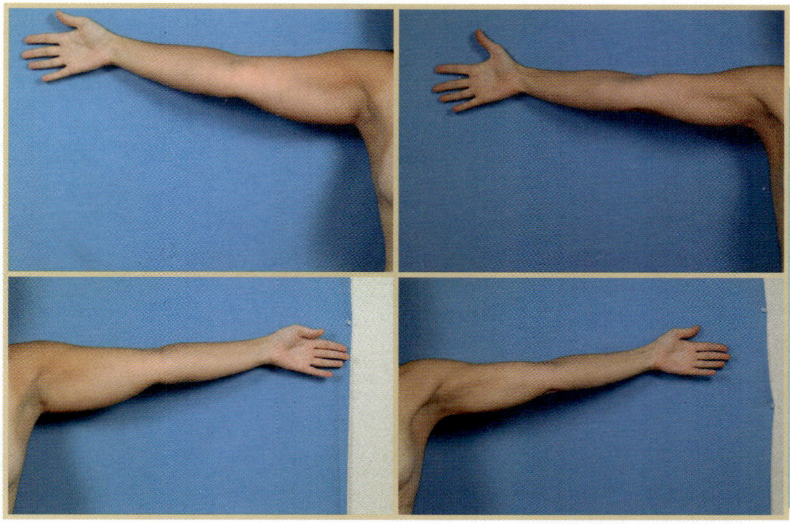

before *1 year after*

Height: 5′7″
Weight before: 157 lbs.
BMI: 24.2
Children: 0
Weight after: 134.5 lbs.
Liposuction volume: right arm 100 cc, right axilla 150 cc, left arm 125 cc, left axilla 150 cc,
touchups: right arm 25 cc, right axilla 25 cc, left arm 25 cc, left axilla 25 cc
E.B., age 39/40, computer consultant

Liposuction of Arms – Over 50

Ultrasonic liposuction of lower body, arms, and axillae.

Comments: This 58-year-old patient's skin contracted nicely after liposuction.

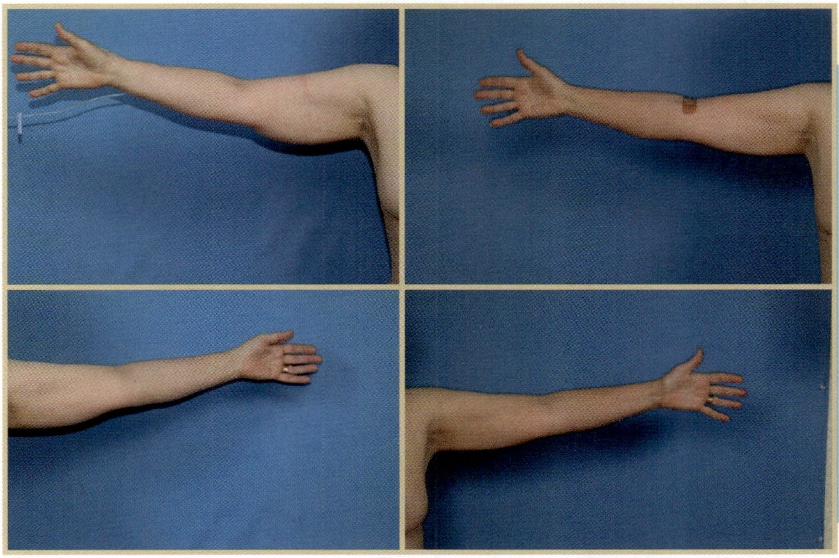

before *1 year after*

Height: 5′2″
Weight before: 148.5 lbs.
BMI: 26.7
Weight after: 135.5 lbs.
Children: 0
Liposuction volume:
right arm 100 cc,
right axilla 100 cc,
left arm 125 cc,
left axilla 100 cc
C.H., age 58/59,
freelance illustrator

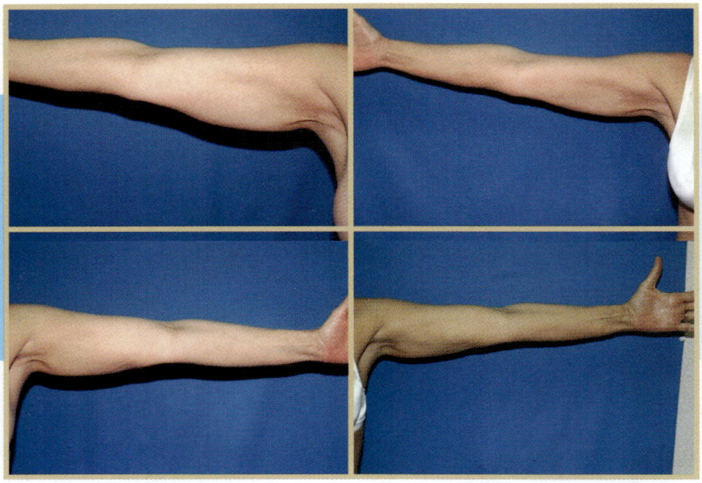

before *3 months after*

Ultrasonic liposuction of lower body and arms.

Comments: This patient did not like the "flabby" appearance of her arms. Her skin tone was reasonable, so brachioplasties were not recommended. Despite her age, her skin responded well to ultrasonic liposuction.

Height: 5' 4½"
Weight before: 142 lbs.
BMI: 23.6
Children: 1
Liposuction volume: right arm 200 cc, left arm 150 cc
L.B., age 61, director of government agency

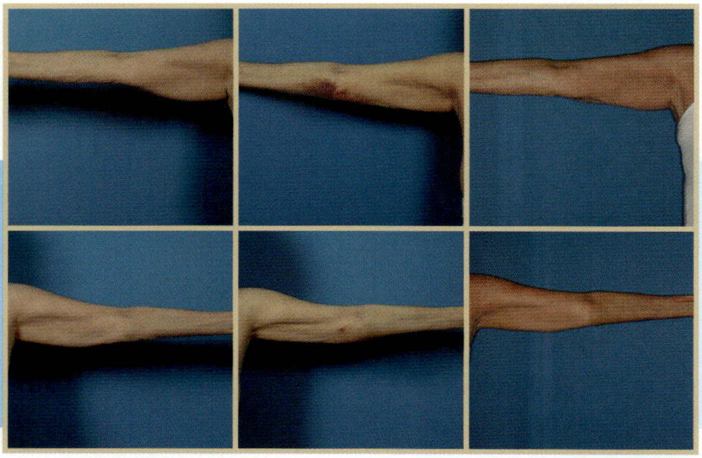

before *8 days after* *5½ months after*

Ultrasonic liposuction of arms and axillae.

Comments: This 66-year-old was at ideal body weight and had never been overweight. She had excess fatty tissue of her arms and skin laxity due to aging. In the past, I might have considered brachioplasties to remove loose skin, at the expense of a long scar on the back of the arms. Partly because I don't like scars in visible areas, and partly because of improved results with ultrasound, I find myself doing fewer brachioplasties. This woman's skin responded well to ultrasonic liposuction alone and there are no burnt bridges—she can always return for brachioplasties if necessary. But this is rare.

Height: 5'7"
Weight before: 131 lbs.
BMI: 20.2
Children: 3
Liposuction volume: right arm 165 cc, left arm 140 cc
S.D., age 66/67, retired former model

Our Survey Says

	Female (168 patients)	Male (51 patients)
Pain (1-10)	6.6	4.6
Pain killers (days)	4.5	3.7
Need assistance (days)	2.8	1.1
Driving (days)	5.1	2.4
Time off work (days)	6.7	2.9
"Back to normal" (days)	31	20
Exercise again (days)	35	29
Sleep comfortably (days)	16	4.7
Result (1-10)	7.7	8.0
Dress size (women), Pant size (men)	1.7 sizes	1.4"
Improved self-esteem	83.3%	80.4%
Do it again	93.3%	94.1%

Survey results confirm that liposuction in males is less painful and the recovery is much faster than in females. Doctors (including male plastic surgeons, but only under direct questioning) know this gender difference is *not* because men are more stoic than women! In fact, we suspect the reverse. Women have more discomfort, on average, simply because they typically have more areas treated and greater volumes are removed. Women who have the abdomen and flanks treated alone (the areas most commonly treated in men), without treating the thighs, knees, axillary areas or arms, have recovery experiences similar to males. There is also considerable variability between individuals. The range of pain ratings was 1-10 for both sexes. Some patients experienced virtually no pain; others rated it 10—*the worst possible pain they could imagine*. Reassuringly, patient satisfaction was similar for men and women, and the vast majority would have the surgery again.

Women dropped an average of 1.7 dress sizes (a drop from a 14 to a 10/12 would be 1.5 sizes). Men reported an average reduction of 1.4 inches around the waist.

MRI Studies

How much does the fat layer go down and how long does it take?

Patients often ask how much reduction in the fat layer they may expect to see after liposuction. This is a very reasonable question. They would also like to know how long it will take the swelling to go away. The answer may have practical implications, such as whether patients can still go on a cruise one month after surgery (anyone asking that question is doing alright, basically). Surprisingly, until recently, we have not had good, data-based answers to these basic questions. In the absence of good data, patients are given all kinds of answers, based mainly on vague perceptions, hunches, and marketing. Sometimes the recommendations are simply ridiculous (for example, You can go dancing the night after your liposuction!).

To better answer these questions, our center undertook a study using MRIs. This test is harmless because there is no radiation. Three of our patients completed MRIs before and at various times after liposuction. (I am grateful to these patients because, although harmless, MRIs can make people feel claustrophobic). The purpose of this study was to assess the reduction in the fat layer at three sites—the abdomen, flank, and outer thigh. Patients were studied at different follow-up times to determine how long it takes for the swelling to go down. The sample size was admittedly small, and there were no untreated controls, but the use of multiple sites, and both sides of the body, added to the statistical reliability of the results.

What were the results? At one month, the fat layer had been reduced 30%; at 3 months, 40%; and at 9 months, 45% (See Illustrations, next page). These reductions were all statistically significant. *This data showed that liposuction significantly reduced the fat layer, by almost half.* Furthermore, two-thirds of the full reduction occurred in the first month, and about 90% by three months after surgery. Looking at it the other way, patients still had about one-third swelling at one month and 10% swelling three months after surgery.

As it turns out, these findings are very much in line with our clinical perceptions, and support our historical practice of waiting three months or more before doing final "after" photographs, to allow enough time for almost all the swelling to go down. Many patients have told me that they noticed an improvement after more than three months had elapsed, and this study confirms that, indeed, there may be another 10% reduction to be expected after their three-month follow-up appointments.

Patients readily understand, and the patient photographs demonstrate, that a 50% reduction is a dramatic change (See Illustration). After all, we do not want to remove *all* the fat. Even in lean individuals, there is still a layer of fat between the skin and muscle. Without it, the skin would stick down to the muscle and this would look and feel very unnatural. The fat does have a purpose in providing cushioning for the skin.

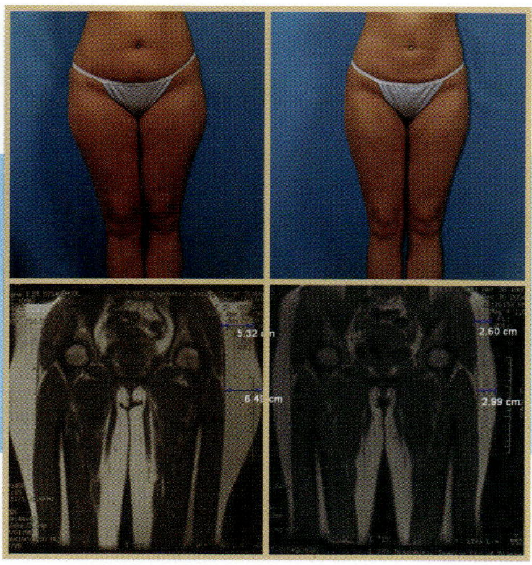

before ***6 months after***

Patient Photographs and MRIs

Ultrasonic liposuction of lower body, arms, and axillae, submental lipectomy, and breast augmentation.

Comments: This patient's photographs and MRI studies were taken at the same times, before and six months after surgery. Both demonstrate a reduction in the thickness of the fat layer in the treated areas.

Height: 5′6″
Weight before: 156 lbs.
BMI: 24.8
Children: 1
Weight after: 136 lbs.

Liposuction volume: 3,250 cc
Dress size before: 14
Dress size after: 8/10
T.S., age 24

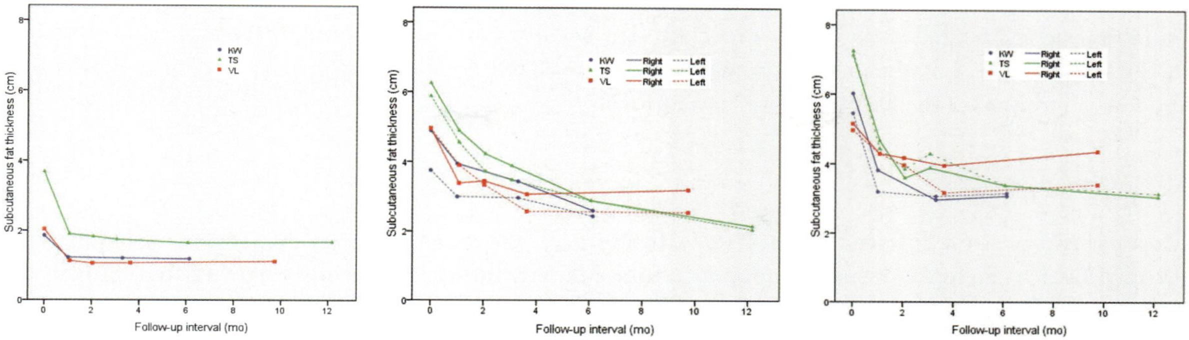

Abdomen **Flank** **Outer thigh**

Reduction in fat layers of the abdomen, flank, and outer thigh, at various follow-up times after surgery. The thickest point was measured.

Discomfort

Postoperative discomfort relates to the extent of liposuction and the number of areas treated. There is usually a generalized soreness and some stiffness due to swelling. Pain is usually well-controlled with medication, which is taken during the first several days after surgery.

I have heard stories from patients who have been treated elsewhere under local anesthesia, telling me how painful the procedure was. Some patients have friends who reported a lot of pain after liposuction. No doubt, liposuction can be a painful procedure. However, there are ways of reducing the pain. One way is by doing the surgery with the patient asleep, which is preferred for all but small touchup liposuction procedures.

Local anesthetic is injected into the tissues as part of the tumescent (superwet) technique. The local anesthetic works for several hours, so patients are not in pain waking up after surgery. Also, tissue trauma is minimized using the ultrasonic technique, less traumatic blunt cannulae, and by avoiding overaggressive treatment. These precautions allow for superior results with manageable pain levels. Most patients report that the pain level was what they thought it would be. It does not surprise them. It is tolerable and controlled by prescription pain killers.

There is a range of patient experiences. Some patients take liposuction in stride, even returning to work the next day. Others give me a somewhat accusatory look (maybe I'm reading too much into it) and tell me, "I feel like I've been run over by a truck!" The number of areas treated is relevant. Most men have the abdomen and flanks treated, which makes for a relatively easy recovery. Some say the soreness compares to a tough workout in the gym. Most women also have their thighs treated. Treatment of the thighs does cause more discomfort, particularly when sitting down.

Numbness

Numbness in the treated areas is to be expected. The small sensory nerve endings have been traumatized by the surgery. There may also be unusually sensitive areas; this is called "hypersensitivity." It typically takes about two months for the feeling to return to normal.

Swelling

Most patients notice a difference immediately after surgery. However, swelling develops during the first few days, which can make the areas temporarily look fuller than they were before surgery, particularly in lean patients. For this reason, we recommend that patients wear loose-fitting clothing right after surgery. Although swelling is variable from patient to patient, our MRI studies suggest that two-thirds of the swelling is gone in a month. Ninety percent of the swelling is gone in three months. This is important for patients to know, because they may otherwise be disappointed at their one-month follow-up appointment, thinking that they are seeing their final result, when in fact they still have a significant amount of swelling at this point.

Many patients call the office several days or a week after surgery to report that their feet and ankles are swelling more. They have difficulty putting on shoes. They wonder if this is normal. They figure the swelling should be getting better by now, not worse. But this finding is normal. The calves and ankles often swell more a week after surgery because of the effects of gravity, even when the calves are not treated with liposuction. Bruising may extend all the way down to the toes. This swelling may be alleviated by elevating the legs on an ottoman. If one leg swells conspicuously more than the other, this could signal a blood clot in a leg vein (deep venous thrombosis), which is a serious complication requiring prompt investigation and treatment.

The Garment

At the end of the operation, while patients are still asleep, a compression garment is applied. This is either a simple Velcro® binder that goes around the abdomen and flanks (commonly used in men), or a girdle that goes from the level of the upper abdomen down to the thighs, either above or, more commonly, just below the knees.

The patient can remove the garment for short periods to bathe and shower, and it may be worn under regular clothing. Bruising usually disappears within one month. Patients may then wear shorts or a bathing suit. The stitches dissolve on their own.

The purpose of the garment is not to smooth body contours. The remaining fat cells do not move around, which is why surgical expertise in removing the fat cells evenly is important. Rather, the garment is used to limit swelling and help the swelling to go down more quickly. Most patients also find it more comfortable to wear the garment; they feel that they need the support. It may be washed, although it should be dried in a no-heat cycle to avoid shrinking. It is difficult for women to put on the girdle at first. But after changing it a few times, it becomes easier. One trick is to leave the bottom end of the garment at the knees zipped for several inches so that it does not become tangled when it goes in the wash.

I recommend wearing the garment for one month. It is concealed under clothing, except during the summer when capri pants may be needed to conceal the knee-length girdle (when the knees are treated). However, two weeks after surgery patients may wear spandex instead, such as cycling shorts or an aerobics outfit. They can alternate wearing the garment and wearing spandex. The principle is gentle compression. Some patients are never comfortable with the garment and make the switch to spandex earlier. Fitting too loose is better than too tight. Without the garment, the result would be the same, but it would take longer for the swelling to go down. I recommend wearing slightly compressive athletic garments when exercising (Under Armour® is an example). These garments are useful even after the one-month visit for comfort and to reduce swelling, which can be aggravated by physical activity.

Time off Work

Time off work depends on the areas treated, how physical the job is, and the patient's own pain tolerance. For women, who usually have the lower body treated (thighs included), one week off is recommended for office jobs. However, plenty of my patients return to work sooner. For jobs that involve standing for long periods (working in a pharmacy, for example), a week off is recommended. Otherwise, patients are likely to swell more at the end of the day. Prolonged sitting is uncomfortable after having the thighs treated. It helps to get up frequently and move around. Women who have very physical jobs (examples: server, flight attendant, massage therapist) are best accommodated with two weeks off, although many cannot afford to miss this much work and make do with less time off.

Men usually recover quickly because fewer areas are treated. They are often back to an office job in three or four days. Some men return to work the day after surgery. For more physical jobs, such as plumbing or construction work, one week off is recommended. If the job is very physical, involving such activities as going up and down ladders, two weeks off is better.

Exercise

Most people want to know when they can get back to exercising. Many work out on a regular basis, some every day. The most difficult aspect of the surgery may be interruption of their exercise routine. I tell them not to exercise for two weeks, and they give me a look that I recognize well—maybe for other patients, doc, but not me. I explain that they will be sore after surgery and that if they do work out, they will have more swelling and will hurt more afterward (not while they are working out, but afterward). Patients can return to nonvigorous exercise, walking for example, but any vigorous exercising that raises the blood pressure will make the swelling worse. The use of an elliptical trainer or exercise bike should wait until about three weeks after surgery. All exercises may be resumed four weeks after surgery. Their bodies will help them know when they are ready. I tell patients to start with a light workout, maybe 50% of normal, and then see how they feel the evening after exercising. If there is no problem, the exercise routine may be increased the next day. If patients jump back in and do their usual workout, they are likely to swell and hurt more afterward. This does not jeopardize the final result, but the swelling may take longer to subside.

Another common question is, "When can I go on a vacation?" Some of my patients have gone on Caribbean vacations as early as several days after surgery, but most people want to look and feel their best. One month after surgery, the bruising and most of the swelling are gone. There are no restrictions at this point, so a minimum of one month of recovery time is recommended before going on such a vacation.

The Arms

There is no garment that is applied to the arms. However, some patients wear a snug athletic shirt that has sleeves to provide some gentle compression (Under Armour® makes a good one). Swelling and bruising are to be expected. The bruising may extend down the forearms because of gravity. There are areas of numbness that can take a few months to return to normal. The arms are sore, but the pain is tolerable. A caretaker may grab the arm to help, not realizing that it is sore. Because the arm is at a higher level than the heart, arm swelling tends to go down more quickly after liposuction than leg swelling. Liposuction of the arms does not seem to add much to the amount of postoperative discomfort, and treats an area that is visible and responds favorably, so it is common for women to have the arms treated simultaneously with the lower body.

Body Weight and Lipid Level Changes after Liposuction

Our study found a modest, but statistically significant ($p < 0.05$), average weight loss of 2.2 pounds three months after surgery for all liposuction patients. Patients with liposuction volumes of 3,000 cc or more experienced a greater average weight loss, dropping 5.2 pounds three months after surgery.

Most notably, there was a highly significant drop in the fasting triglyceride level ($p<0.001$) after liposuction. Triglyceride levels dropped from an average of 152 mg/dL to 113 mg/dL for all liposuction patients. The decrease was even more impressive for patients with liposuction volumes over 3,000 cc, whose average fasting triglyceride level dropped from 186 before surgery to 118 after! There was no significant change in total cholesterol, LDL (the "bad" cholesterol), or HDL (the "good" cholesterol). Also, there were no significant changes in control patients tested at the same time intervals, confirming that these changes are caused by liposuction.

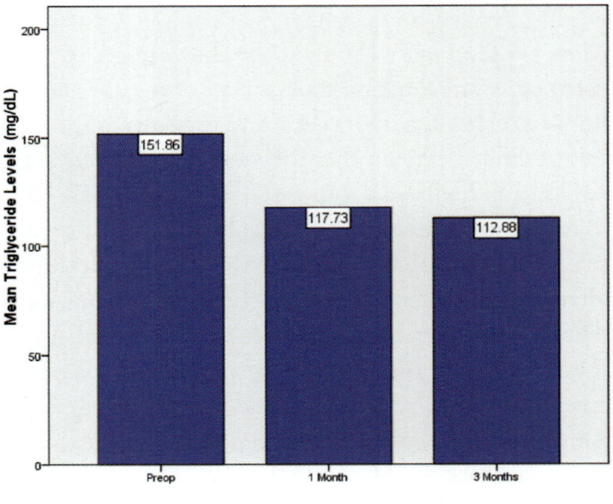

Triglyceride Levels in Patients after Ultrasonic Liposuction

Triglycerides are molecules that contain glycerol and three chains of fatty acids. They are stored by fat cells. They are a major component of VLDL (very low density lipoproteins).

How meaningful are these findings? The American Heart Association classifies triglyceride levels below 150 mg/dL as normal and above 150 as borderline-high risk. Patients with triglyceride levels over 150 are more likely to develop metabolic syndrome, increasing the risk of atherosclerosis. Plaque buildup in arterial walls can lead to coronary artery disease, stroke, and peripheral vascular disease. Metabolic syndrome also raises the risk of Type II insulin-resistant diabetes. Although liposuction is not a substitute for a healthy lifestyle, this remarkable drop in circulating triglycerides appears to be a favorable metabolic effect of liposuction.

Hemoglobin Levels after Liposuction

Patients are sometimes told there is very little blood loss with liposuction when the tumescent technique is used. As it turns out, this statement is only partly true, and (as is usually the case in matters that are partially true) the part that is not true is of more interest. Our study showed a drop in hemoglobin—the oxygen-carrying molecule contained in red blood cells—level immediately after surgery, as expected. Three months after surgery, hemoglobin levels were back to normal. This drop in hemoglobin is not primarily due to *external* blood loss at surgery (the fluid in the canister is highly dilute), but rather due to *internal* blood loss into the tissues, which accounts for the bruising. Surgeons call this "third space blood loss," and it can be significant.

The body gradually absorbs these breakdown products of hemoglobin and the red cell level gradually returns to normal. Iron supplementation can help, particularly in patients who feel especially fatigued after surgery.

Patients feel better and recover faster if blood loss is kept to a minimum. The natural hormone, epinephrine, is administered in the infusion solution to reduce blood loss by constricting blood vessels. At our center, we use a more effective concentration of epinephrine (1:500,000 rather than the traditional 1: 1,000,000), and limit the infusion volume to less than five liters to avoid toxicity. Also, we infuse all treatment areas before starting liposuction, so the epinephrine has time to be maximally effective. We rarely remove more than five liters at one setting (very few nonobese patients have five liters or more of excess fat anyway). These measures help prevent an excessive drop in hemoglobin, keeping the procedure safe and the recovery not too onerous for patients.

Blood Tests after Liposuction

Our study showed that levels of circulating anesthetic agents given in the anesthetic solution—lidocaine and bupivicaine (used for abdominoplasty patients)—remain below toxic levels. There are no significant changes in liver enzymes or blood sugar. These tests confirm there is no harmful effect of ultrasonic liposuction on liver function. Of course, this finding is not unexpected. The liquefied fat is suctioned out of the body and does not depend on circulatory absorption to be cleared. Fasting blood sugars are unchanged after liposuction, also an expected finding.

Skin Excess

Liposuction is primarily a procedure to remove excess fat. It does not remove extra skin. Patients who have extra skin causing rolls in the abdomen are usually better served with a tummy tuck (abdominoplasty) performed simultaneously with liposuction. However, there are areas where the scars from skin excisional procedures are more obvious than the lower abdomen, such as the arms and inner thighs. Here we often perform liposuction even in the presence of loose skin, hoping that a modest degree of skin contraction will suffice. It is possible to come back later and remove extra skin if necessary. However, it may be best to accept some skin looseness and avoid the scars of excisional procedures such as brachioplasties or inner thigh lifts. This is often a judgment call made by both the patient and surgeon.

Cellulite

Although liposuction is a reliable technique to remove extra fat cells and improve proportions, it is not consistently helpful for treating cellulite. In fact, there is no treatment available today that is good for treating cellulite, despite claims to the contrary (See Illustration) and machines that are marketed and "FDA approved" for this purpose. Patients are disappointed to hear this news. Cellulite is a big, unsolved problem. In some patients, it may be possible to achieve a modest improvement (See A.S., K.M., B.D., in Patient Photographs, Female Liposuction – Lower Body) in certain areas treated with ultrasonic liposuction, but patients should not count on this. Fortunately, liposuction does not usually make cellulite *worse*, except for situations of poor skin laxity, where an excisional procedure such as a tummy tuck or thigh lift may be more appropriate.

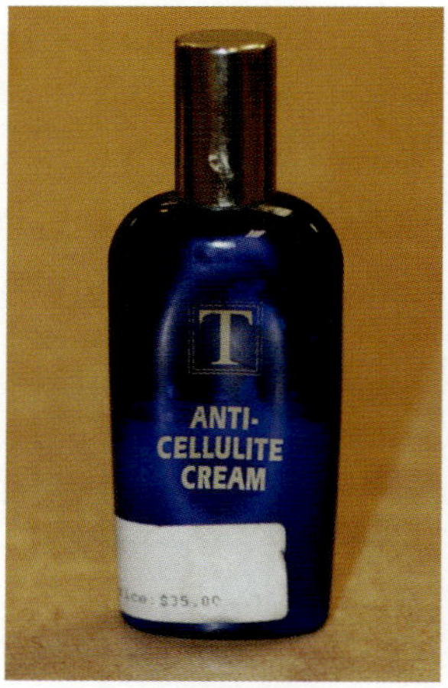

Example of skin cream marketed to treat cellulite.

The type of cellulite that is improved by pulling up on the skin (called "secondary" cellulite, as opposed to "primary" cellulite, which does not seem to respond as much to skin tightening), can be improved with a lifting technique such as a thigh/buttock lift, but this is a major procedure that leaves a long scar along the hip line. A thigh/buttock lift (when combined with a tummy tuck, this is called a lower body lift) is typically recommended for patients after major weight loss, or in patients whose cellulite is so severe that it prevents them from wearing shorts in the summer.

Skin Loss

Skin loss can happen if the blood supply to the skin is jeopardized. For example, if a patient has old scars, these scars can reduce the blood supply to an adjacent area of skin by acting as barriers to blood vessels. Liposuction may cause just enough trauma to jeopardize blood supply to the adjacent skin (See Illustration, next page). Skin loss from burns is rare, particularly if the operator protects the entrance site and moves the cannula so as to avoid causing too much heat buildup in one area (like ironing clothes). Also, limiting the duration of ultrasonic treatment to a few minutes per area helps prevent complications, such as burns or seromas.

Touchup ultrasonic liposuction of abdomen, hips and thighs, and scar revision of left posterior thigh.

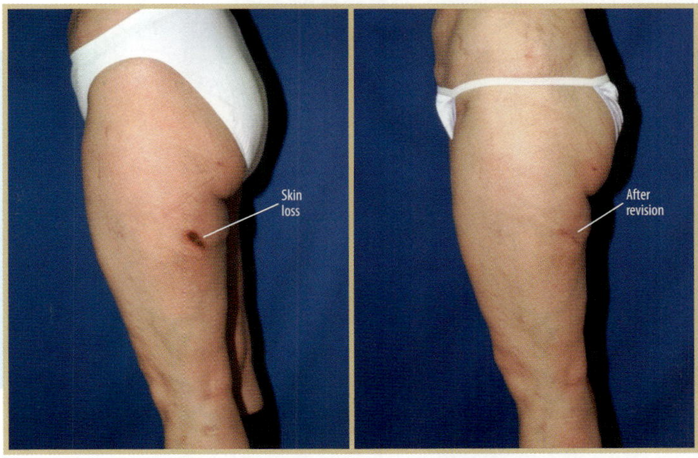

scar 5 weeks after touchup

5 weeks after scar revision

Comments: This patient developed an area of skin loss after a touchup ultrasonic liposuction treatment of the thighs. She had previous surgery to remove varicose veins, leaving scars on the posterior thighs. This area of skin necrosis was located lateral to one of the old scars. It was revised under local anesthesia in the office. She is seen five weeks after revision (10 weeks after the touchup liposuction). This is an unusual problem after ultrasonic liposuction and in fact this is one of only two small areas of skin loss I have encountered after ultrasonic liposuction. In both cases, the wounds healed nicely after revision.

C.B., age 46, registered nurse

Asymmetry

During surgery, measurements of the amount of fluid injected, ultrasound time, and the volume removed ("aspirate volume") are recorded. This information helps to ensure symmetrical treatment. Of course, asymmetrical fat distribution is common, so it is not unusual for me to remove more volume from one side than the other. It is also important to recognize any existing skeletal asymmetry, such as scoliosis, which of course is unchanged after surgery.

Seroma

If ultrasound times are kept short and excessive tissue trauma is avoided, seromas are rare. They tend to occur more frequently in areas that are simultaneously undermined, creating a pocket in which fluid may accumulate, such as under the chin after a submental lipectomy, or the abdomen after an abdominoplasty.

Overtreatment

Overtreatment with liposuction is much more difficult to manage than undertreatment. It is not difficult to return to do more liposuction. However, if too much fat is removed, restoring normal contours is a challenge. Fortunately, fat injection is available and can be used to fill in small defects.

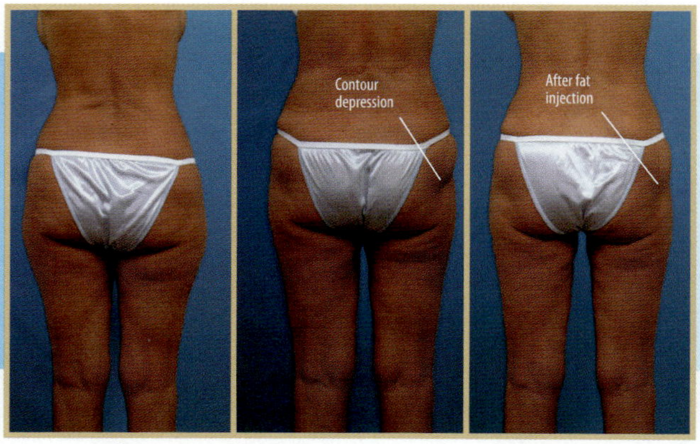

before *3 months after* *1 year after*

Abdominoplasty and ultrasonic liposuction of lower body. Second procedure, 8½ months later: fat injection of lateral gluteal depressions.

Comments: This 54-year-old woman was happy with her tummy tuck and the overall improvement from liposuction, but was concerned about depressions on the sides of her buttocks ("lateral gluteal depressions"). This appearance is called the violin deformity. Although she was very lean, additional fat was available in the outer thighs and was used to fill in these depressions.

Bowel Perforation

Patients occasionally ask about the risk of puncturing an organ during liposuction. The most important safety consideration is the surgeon's experience. The cannula is passed horizontally in the subcutaneous plane, where there is minimal resistance. It is usually not difficult for the surgeon to stay in this plane. Operator experience, the superwet technique, ultrasonic assistance, and blunt cannulae all help reduce risk. Previous surgery with scarring of the subcutaneous plane or undiagnosed hernias may increase the risk.

Fat Embolism

Normally some fat is released into the bloodstream during liposuction and travels to the lungs, which effectively filter it from the circulation. In the rare but potentially dangerous "fat embolism syndrome," fat is released into the arterial circulation (possibly through shunts in the lung tissue) and can cause organ damage and even death.

One concern about techniques that do not remove the dissolved fat from the body (LipoDissolve, for example) is the fate of free fatty acids that are liberated by the destruction of fat cells. What happens to this fat? Evaluation of circulating triglyceride levels after ultrasonic liposuction shows that these levels actually decrease after ultrasonic liposuction, an important safety consideration. Furthermore, there has not yet been a reported case of fat embolism syndrome after *ultrasonic* liposuction. We can only speculate as to whether this finding is due to reduced tissue trauma, improved liquification of the fat, or simply a fortunate statistical coincidence.

Care after Surgery

- Drainage from the incisions is normal during the first 24-48 hours. This may cause blood-staining of the garment.
- You can shower and bathe after your appointment the day after surgery.

- When getting ready to shower, remove the garment and then sit down for several minutes before getting up. This gives your body a few minutes to adjust because your blood pressure drops a little with the garment off. When you are up, if you feel faint, immediately lie down and this problem will correct itself. After a few days, light-headedness is unlikely to be a problem.
- You will probably need some help taking off the garment and putting it back on during the first few days. Then you will get the knack of doing it yourself.
- Swelling and bruising are to be expected. Remember, bruising is affected by gravity. Areas such as the flanks and the back of the thighs tend to bruise more because you sleep on your back. If your thighs are treated, the swelling and bruising can go down your legs, even to your ankles and feet. Usually, when the abdomen is treated, there is swelling and bruising of the pubic area, often going down to involve the genitalia. Don't worry about bruising and swelling of this area. It is normal.
- Wear the garment day and night. Take it off to bathe, and wash the garment at the same time. Wash the garment in a gentle cycle in cold water and line dry or use the air-fluff dryer setting. Leave the knees zippered for a few inches so it doesn't get tangled.
- After two weeks, you can alternate and wear spandex for periods of the day, which is likely to be more comfortable. Aerobics outfits or cycling shorts usually contain this material, which provides compression. The principle is uniform compression of the treated areas for comfort and to reduce swelling. You should wear the garment for a month.
- The small bandages can come off after two days, or sooner if they are saturated. Leave the Steri-Strips™ on another couple of days (but don't worry if they come off with the bandages). Usually, you don't need to apply another bandage unless there is still some drainage or the incision is in an area that might be subject to friction from the garment. The sutures dissolve on their own.
- Contact the office if you experience excessive fainting, nausea, swelling, pain, or a fever over 101.0°F or 38.5°C. Swelling of the feet and ankles is normal if you had your thighs and knees treated. But if the swelling seems to be much greater on one side than the other, this may signal a blood clot and you need to come in to the office to have this assessed.
- Bruising can take up to a month to go away. Swelling takes longer. About two-thirds of the swelling is gone in a month, and 90% of it is gone in three months. We usually wait three months or more before taking "after" photos to allow the swelling to go down fully.

Frequently Asked Questions

Q: Does it hurt?

A: The pain level is moderate and usually well-tolerated. Patients tell me it is about what they expected.

Q: Does the fat come back?

A: The fat cells removed by liposuction are gone forever. Fat cells that are left behind can swell with weight gain and shrink with weight loss, but the numbers are reduced forever. Liposuction provides a permanent improvement in body proportions.

Q: Where do you put the incisions?

A: I use as few incisions as possible to cover the areas I need to treat. When treating the abdomen and flanks, there is one on either side of the pubic area and one for each flank. These are placed so that they would typically be hidden by a bikini. The access incisions for the inner thighs are hidden in the groin crease on each side. The outer thighs are accessed using the same incisions used to treat the flanks plus an incision on each lower buttock. The knee incisions are tucked in the crease just below and on the medial side of each knee. (See Intraoperative Photographs) The scars fade with time and are usually inconspicuous. Objectionable scars may be revised later.

Q: Do you leave the incisions open?

A: Some patients have heard that the incisions are left open to allow fluid to drain out. However, most plastic surgeons prefer to close them and allow any remaining fluid on the inside to be absorbed. This makes it easier for the patient because it is not as messy after surgery. Also, the incisions heal better and with less scarring if they are sutured, as opposed to leaving them to heal in on their own.

Q: Do I have to wear a girdle?

A: Wearing a girdle sounds onerous, but most patients feel more comfortable in the garment after surgery. The garment helps limit swelling. You wear it for a month after surgery.

Q: Will liposuction help my cellulite?

A: You should not expect much improvement in cellulite. Liposuction removes fat and improves proportions but is not primarily for smoothing skin irregularities. We still do not have a good treatment for cellulite. There are patients whose cellulite is better after liposuction, but I am careful not to promote liposuction as a cellulite treatment. It is a body shaping treatment. If my patient has an improvement in cellulite, that's great, but she should not expect it.

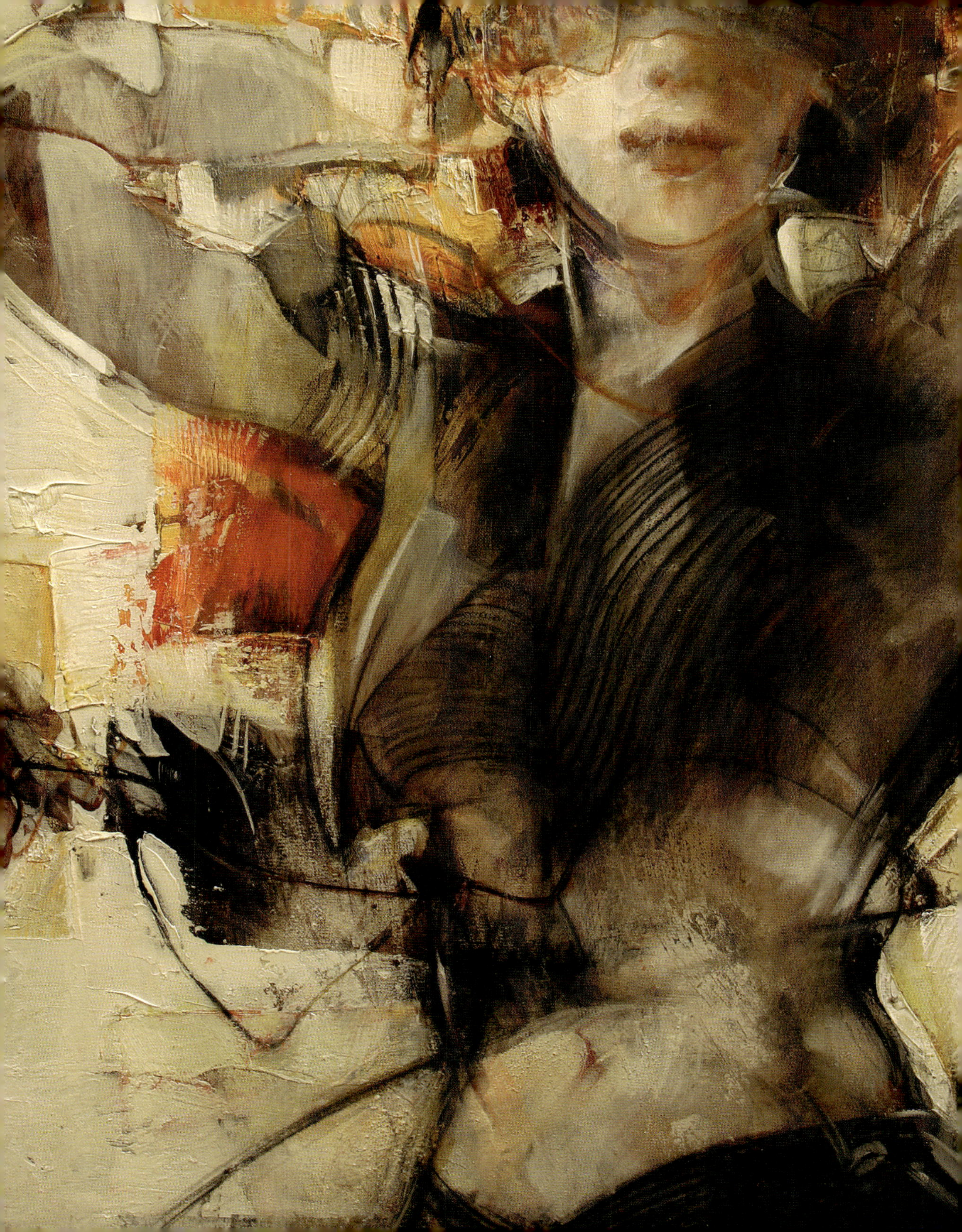

CHAPTER TWO

Ideal Buttocks

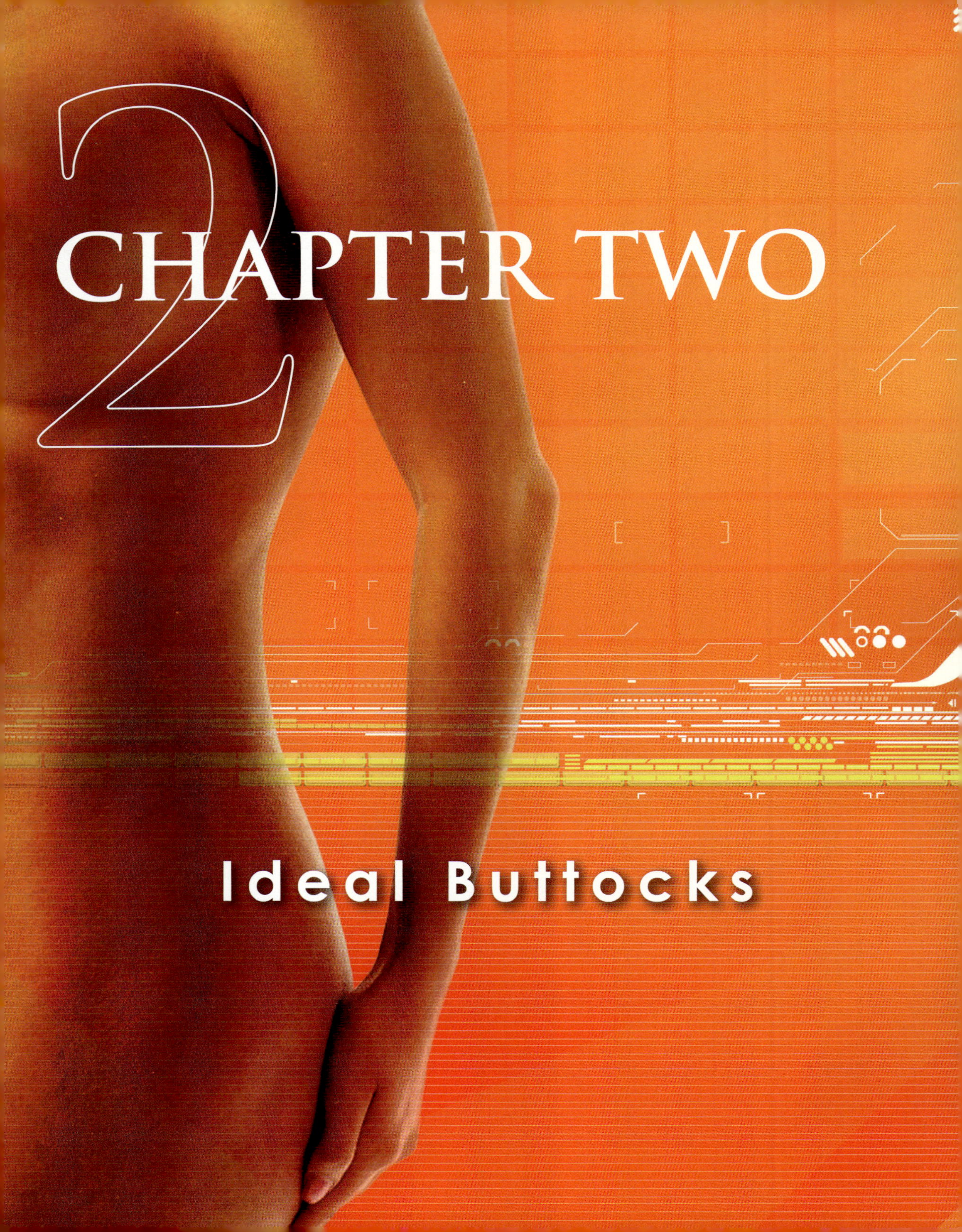

Ideal Buttocks

Not overlooked in the appreciation of human form is the appearance of the butt. This area of anatomy had been largely neglected by plastic surgeons until the last decade. No longer. Now entire books are devoted to the human butt. Several years ago, "butt cleavage" made its debut among female singers, although (thankfully) this trend does not appear to be catching on. Jennifer Lopez has a world-famous butt, and her name invariably comes up in discussions of butt aesthetics, like Pamela Anderson for breasts and Angelina Jolie for lips. Tabloid magazines include a "best butt" category the same way they include "best abdomen" or "best breasts," and this particular recognition is no doubt highly prized. In fact, surveys suggest that men rate the importance of the aesthetics of female buttocks on par with their breasts. Sir Mix-A-Lot immortalized fine (and large) buttocks in the memorable 1992 hip-hop song "Baby Got Back." George Carlin for years lamented his lack of buttocks, saying his black friends chided him, "Man, where's your ass at?" Ideal buttocks have many of the same qualities that make them look good in both men and women—full, rounded cheeks and no sagging, or "high and hard," as Joan Rivers puts it. In fact, Rodney Dangerfield once asked men in the audience, "Ever stare at a butt and then realize it was a guy?"

It is becoming more common to incorporate fat injection at the time of liposuction or lifting procedures of the buttocks and thighs.

Obviously, there is a racial influence on buttock size. Black women tend to have, and desire, full buttocks. Latino women clearly have a preference for fuller buttocks, as evidenced by the popularity of the "Brazilian butt lift," which is not really a lift procedure, but rather fat injection of the buttocks. Many white women notice some flattening of the buttocks with aging, and particularly after weight loss. Rather than discarding the fat, it is becoming more common to incorporate fat injection at the time of liposuction or lifting procedures of the buttocks and thighs. Men can also benefit.

Buttock Implants

Like breasts, implants would seem to be a natural choice for buttocks to provide volume, firmness, and roundness. However, implants have a much higher complication rate when used in the buttocks than when used in the breasts. These complications include wound opening ("dehiscence"), infection, seroma, capsular contracture, and malposition. Buttock implants can produce an unnatural "bubble butt" appearance. Most surgeons in the United States avoid using buttock implants, and opt for fat injection instead, accepting a lesser degree of augmentation for fewer complications.

Liposuction

Properly-performed liposuction can improve the appearance of the buttocks by reducing excess fat in adjacent areas. Liposuction must be done with the eye of a sculptor to achieve attractive buttocks. The center of the buttock is usually not treated; no one wants a flat butt. Most of the liposuction is done around the periphery of the buttocks—the flanks, back of the thighs, and the lower pole of the buttocks. This sculpting makes the buttocks appear tighter and more rounded (See A.L., Patient Photographs). Both women and men benefit from reduction of the love handles, which accentuates their buttocks and improves their figures (See T.N., Female Liposuction and L.M., Male Liposuction).

Fat Injection

The buttocks lend themselves nicely to fat injection. In the past, fat obtained by liposuction was usually discarded. We now recognize that there is a limited amount of fat cells available, and it is a shame to discard this limited resource if it can be put to good use. It is much more common now to save this fat and inject it where we want it, typically the face and the buttocks.

How It's Done

The areas to be injected are marked before surgery. Also, the donor sites where fat will be harvested are marked. The donor sites are the areas of fat excess, which usually include the flanks because subtraction of fat from these areas helps to accentuate the curve of the buttocks, a pleasing synergy. The other typical donor areas are the tummy and the thighs.

The LipiVage™ system, which separates the fat while it is being suctioned, makes this procedure much easier and more efficient than it was in the past because it eliminates the need to centrifuge small syringes of fat. The use of the centrifuge (a spinning device) to separate fat is very time consuming and may increase the risk of infection by subjecting the fat to more handling, so this is a worthwhile advantage.

The fat is injected into the central part of the buttock, measuring to ensure equal amounts are injected on each side (See Illustration). The fat is injected through the same incisions used to perform liposuction of the flanks, so there are no additional scars.

Ultrasonic assistance is still used, but only after the fat has been removed for transfer, so that the ultrasound does not break up the fat cells, which must be preserved intact to survive in their new location. Fragmented fat cells would be quickly absorbed.

Intraoperative Photographs

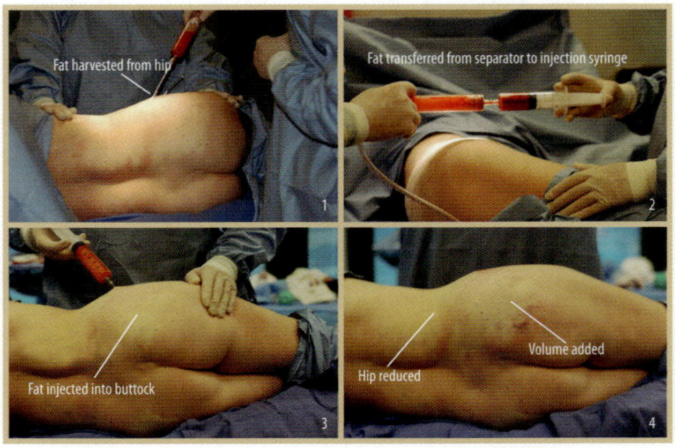

(*Above, left*) Fat is harvested from the right hip. (*Above, right*) Fat is transferred from the LipiVage collection system to the injection syringe. (*Below, left*) Injection of fat into the buttock. (*Below, right*) Improved proportions, with increased volume of the buttock and reduction of the flank.

Ultrasonic liposuction of abdomen, flanks, and axillae. Second procedure, 2 years later: touchup ultrasonic liposuction of abdomen, flanks, and axillae, and fat injection of buttocks and lips.

Comments: This 26-year-old inherited extra fullness around her midsection. She underwent liposuction of the abdomen, flanks, and axillae (See J.J., Patient Photographs – Female Liposuction). Two years later, she returned for fat injection of the buttocks and a simultaneous touchup liposuction. After surgery, she said she now feels comfortable in a bikini.

Height: 5'4"
Weight before: 127 lbs.
BMI: 21.5
Children: 0
Weight after: 135 lbs.
Liposuction volume: 1,300 cc, touchup: 850 cc
Fat injection: 200 cc per buttock
J.J., age 24/26, sports management

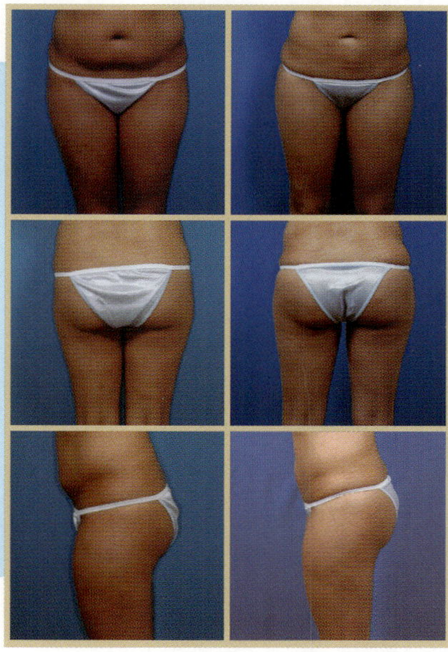

before *2½ years after*

Buttock Fat Injection – Asian

Ultrasonic liposuction of abdomen, flanks, and inner thighs, and fat injection of buttocks. Touchup, 3 months later: abdomen and flanks.

Comments: This 33-year-old Asian female wished to have a more pleasing shape. Despite her best efforts and an ideal body weight, she had been unable to lose extra fullness in the flanks. She requested fuller buttocks. After surgery she has a more desirable hourglass shape, and her flank creases have disappeared.

Height: 5'5"
Weight before: 128 lbs.
BMI: 20.9
Children: 2
Weight after: 132 lbs.
Liposuction volume: 1,600 cc, touchup: 580 cc
Fat injection: 100 cc per buttock
Touchup: 40 cc per buttock
M.M., age 33/34

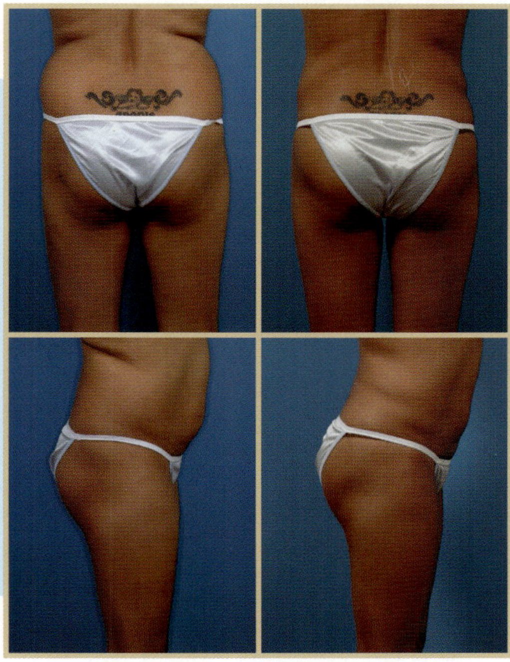

before *1 year after*

What to Expect after Surgery

Like fat injection anywhere, there is a variable degree of fat take. However, any degree of improvement is a welcome addition. It is possible to have additional fat injected at a subsequent procedure if desired, and some patients return for more. The procedure is not painful. The same garment used for liposuction is worn for fat injection, providing gentle circumferential pressure.

The buttocks feel firm at first because of both the transplanted fat and the swelling. As the swelling goes down, the firmness starts to soften. The consistency returns to normal in about a month.

It is probably best to avoid prolonged pressure directly on the transplanted fat so as to optimize fat take. There are no special instructions for sleeping. The normal changes in position during sleep are likely sufficient to prevent uninterrupted pressure on the injected areas.

There is little in the way of scientific data on fat take after surgery, so postoperative instructions are based on first principles only. It makes sense to avoid exercise to minimize movement of the fat globules, which might jeopardize fat survival. It is reasonable to limit periods of sitting, although most of the transplanted fat is situated slightly above the area of the buttocks exposed to pressure during sitting. Although sometimes recommended by plastic surgeons, it is impractical to avoid sitting entirely. It is likely that by one month after surgery, any fat that is going to be absorbed by the body has already been absorbed. There are no restrictions on activities after one month.

Complications

Irregularity

The fat is injected evenly in tunnels using a radial (like spokes of a wheel) technique and measuring both sides to ensure symmetry. Contour irregularities are unusual, and may be treated with a touchup fat injection.

Touchup

The buttocks may be treated later with another fat injection. I have not yet encountered a patient who thought she had too much fat injected in her buttocks (which might be remedied by liposuction), but some patients desire more volume, and these patients may consider a second procedure.

Care after Surgery

- Instructions for the areas treated by fat injection are identical to those postoperative instructions for liposuction. In fact, all patients who have buttock fat injection also have liposuction because it is necessary to harvest fat from another location and simultaneous liposuction of adjacent areas accentuates the buttocks.
- Avoid prolonged pressure on the buttocks. The pressure should be evenly spread out. Get up frequently. Avoid sitting for long periods.

Frequently Asked Questions

Q: How much of the fat that you inject will take?

A: We estimate about 50%, but the answer is not really known. It varies from patient to patient. Most of the swelling is gone in one month and any fat that is going to be absorbed has likely been absorbed by then, so you can assess the result at that time.

Q: What happens if I gain weight?

A: Because there are now more fat cells in the buttocks, your buttocks will be fuller at any given weight than they would have been without fat injection. If you gain weight you will notice these areas become fuller, in proportion with other areas of the body.

Q: Can you freeze fat and inject it later?

A: No. Freezing causes the fat cells to die. It is surprising to sometimes hear someone advocate freezing fat. There are also risks involved in storage and patient identification, similar to a blood bank.

CHAPTER THREE

Abdominoplasty

Patient Motivation

The tummy tuck ("abdominoplasty") is one of the most gratifying procedures for patients and plastic surgeons, with patient satisfaction ranking right at the top with breast augmentation, because of the immediacy of the result and the profound effect on self-esteem. An unattractive tummy is a very common problem, especially for women. Surveys indicate that 57-71 percent of women are dissatisfied with their midtorso!

A protuberant abdomen is a source of embarrassment. Women typically hide their tummies by leaving their tops hanging out or wearing jackets for camouflage. It does seem unfair that motherhood's reward should be a stretched-out, unattractive midsection. Similarly, women and men who have lost weight recognize that there is a limit to the contractility of abdominal skin. No amount of exercise or dieting can cause this skin to contract. Despite what patients are sometimes told by their personal trainers and others, such efforts are futile.

An unattractive tummy can have a great deal of psychological significance for women, often more than their husbands realize.

Women are motivated by feelings of inadequacy. They are not typically being pressured by their husbands to have surgery. Our survey indicated that 89% of patients are doing it for their own reasons and 11% are doing it for both themselves and someone else. An unattractive tummy can have a great deal of psychological significance for women, often more than their husbands realize. Many women have told me they need to have the lights off when they are undressed around their husbands.

The deformity affects clothing options. Loose skin may cause a rash to form under the skin fold. Some women can literally grab the extra apron of tissue and shake it up and down to demonstrate. The extra weight can place additional unbalanced torque on the lower spine, contributing to back pain.

Women are candidates for an abdominoplasty far more often than men, of course, because of the stretching effect of pregnancy. In fact, most women who have had multiple pregnancies can likely benefit from a tummy tuck. However, occasionally I treat women who have not had children but have developed laxity of the abdomen anyway, often coincident with menopause. Men who have lost a great deal of weight (usually greater than 75 pounds) may find they have an extra roll of tissue to deal with too.

This procedure is very reliable in meeting patient expectations. Despite the name "tummy tuck," which sounds simple and almost trivial, it is a major procedure that produces major results. Women are freed to wear form-fitting dresses. No more bubble dresses and swing jackets. There is no need to hide the midsection. Some of my patients are able to show off their tummies for the first time in decades (See J.G., Patient Photographs), since before they had children. They can tuck in their tops and wear belts (See C.B., Patient Photographs) with no unsightly bulge. This is a huge advantage for dressing and enjoying fashion.

Stretch Marks

Stretch marks are an unsolved cosmetic problem, like cellulite. Although lasers have been used to treat stretch marks, the results have been disappointing. No doubt this failure is due to the fact that stretch marks resemble scar tissue on a microscopic level. The normal dermal anatomy is missing. No amount of laser resurfacing can change a scar into skin, which is a very different and more complex tissue. If such a treatment were successful, it would represent modern alchemy—you might as well expect to turn lead into gold, although if my patients are any indication, getting rid of stretch marks may be more profitable!

The only effective treatment is to remove stretch marks surgically and bring skin edge to skin edge, which is what happens in a tummy tuck. This is unwelcome news to patients who call the office asking about how to remove stretch marks. They are looking for a cream or laser treatment; they are disappointed that a major (and costly) procedure is their only option.

Fortunately, abdominal stretch marks are often contained on the excess skin flap that is removed by an abdominoplasty. A welcome side effect of the skin tightening is stretch mark removal.

Like wrinkle and cellulite treatment, the lack of a good nonsurgical remedy for stretch marks provides the therapeutic vacuum for hucksterism to fill. Literally hundreds of products are marketed to relieve stretch marks. Women can easily invest a great deal of time and money in skin creams; spa treatments, such as body wraps; personal trainers; and exercise programs that are supposed to relieve stretch marks. They all have the same thing in common—they do not work.

Fortunately, abdominal stretch marks are often contained on the excess skin flap that is removed by an abdominoplasty. A welcome side effect of the skin tightening is stretch mark removal. Stretch marks below the belly button are eliminated. Any stretch marks on the skin of the upper abdomen, above the level of the belly button, are moved down to the lower abdomen. Stretch marks on the flanks and thighs, where there is no skin removal, remain unchanged.

"Mommy Makeover"

The expression "mommy makeover" has gained popularity, referring to surgery to treat stretched-out tummies and deflated breasts after pregnancy. This makeover usually includes a tummy tuck, breast augmentation, breast lift, and some degree of liposuction. Fortunately, with modern techniques and anesthesia, it is usually possible to perform these procedures in combination, so that women can benefit from having one operation and one recovery period. Combination treatment also reduces the cost.

How It's Done

Tissue Removal

A horizontal elliptical excision is performed, removing the skin and fat from the lower abdomen. All the skin from the level of the belly button (umbilicus) to the pubic area is removed. The skin flap is released from the underlying muscle all the way up to the lower border of the rib cage ("costal margin") to allow the remaining skin of the upper abdomen to be pulled like a bed sheet down to the lower incision, which is tucked just inside the bikini line (See Illustration). This technique avoids a vertical scar. It is necessary to flex the patient's hips to do this (the operating table is adjusted to flex the hips). The lower the incision line, the more the hips must be flexed to allow this flap to reach.

Operative Sequence – Abdominoplasty

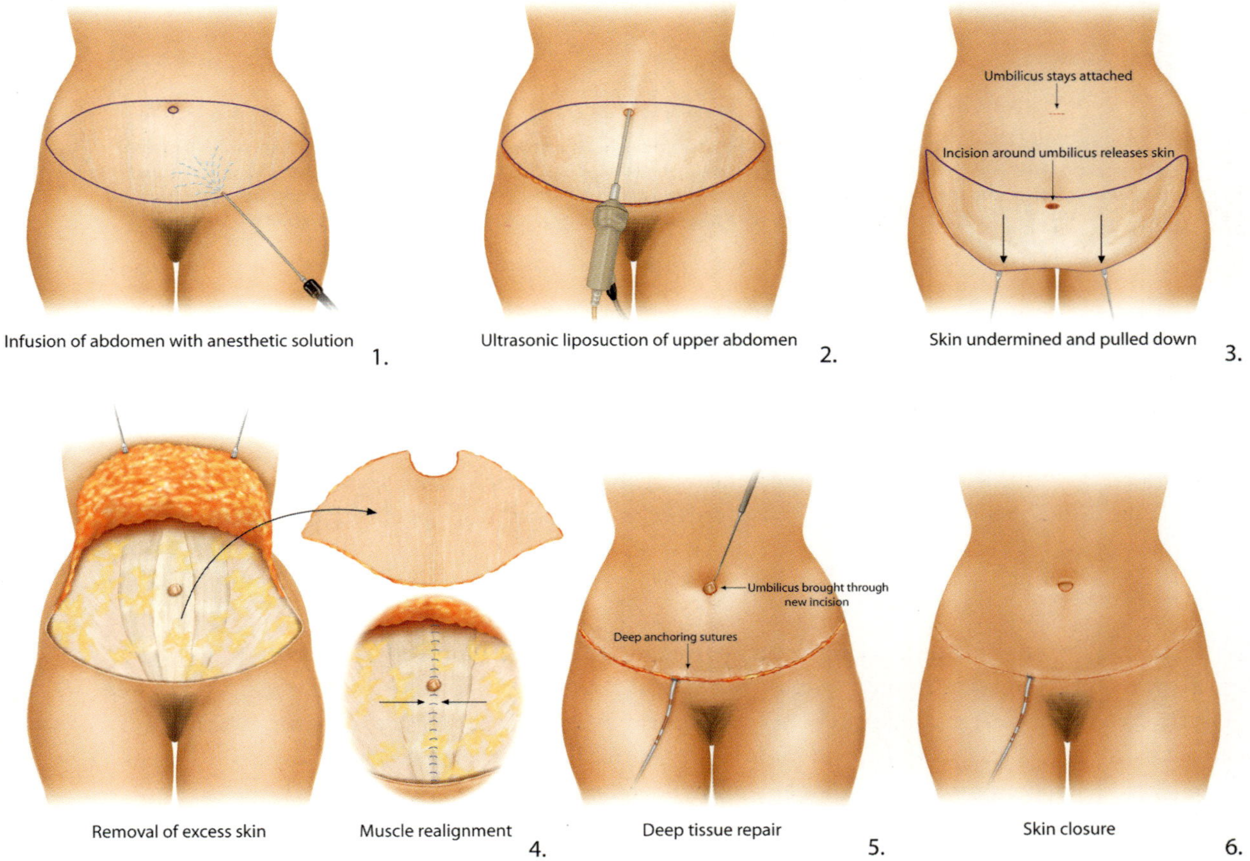

Abdominoplasty. *(Above left)* ***Preoperative markings show the low placement of the lower abdominal incision, within the bikini line, and the upper boundary just above the level of the umbilicus. The area is pre-injected with a local anesthetic solution.*** *(Above, middle)* ***Ultrasonic liposuction is performed in the upper abdomen. There is no need to treat the lower abdomen because this fat is removed with the excess skin, although the pubic area is frequently treated to remove any excess unwanted pubic bulge.*** *(Above, right)* ***The skin flap has been undermined, preserving the umbilicus, which remains attached to the abdominal wall. The skin is pulled down and the excess tissue is trimmed and discarded.*** *(Below, left)* ***The abdominal wall is exposed. The vertically-oriented rectus muscles are repaired in the midline using two layers of running sutures.*** *(Below, middle)* ***A new hole is made for the umbilicus, which is pulled through and sutured. The deep anchoring sutures are placed to prevent upward scar migration and minimize scar tension.*** *(Below, right).* ***The incision is closed in layers. A single drain exits along the incision line.***

Repair of Abdominal Wall – Lateral View

Abdominoplasty

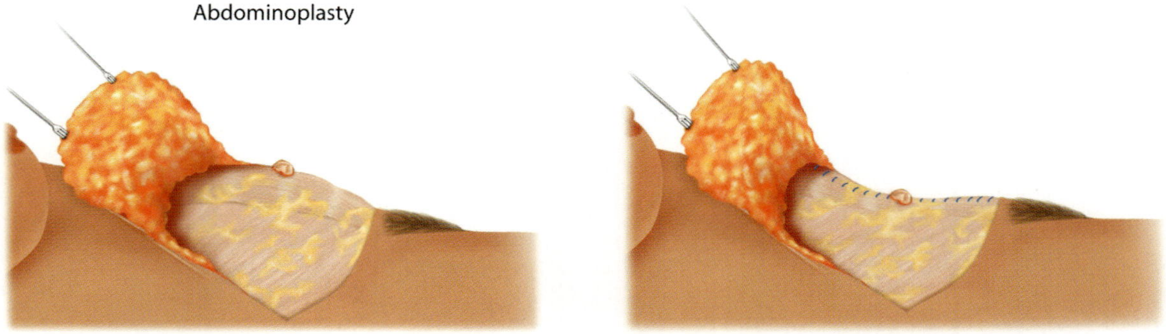

Before muscle repair 1. After muscle repair 2.

These two illustrations depict the patient as seen from a side view on the operating table.** (Left) **The abdominal wall is distended, having been stretched by pregnancy or weight gain.** (Right) **The muscle repair realigns the two rectus muscles in the midline, correcting the protuberance. This muscle repair is an advantage of the tummy tuck procedure over liposuction alone in patients with distended tummies caused by weakening of the abdominal wall.

Endoscopic Surgery

When endoscopic procedures were introduced in the 1990s, plastic surgeons tried this approach on the abdomen to determine whether an effective abdominoplasty could be performed using smaller incisions, with endoscopic tightening of the muscles. However, this approach did not prove practical because the skin remained stretched out. The skin did not contract sufficiently. It was clear that removal of excess skin was needed in most patients. Unlike the forehead lift (See *Ideal Facelift*), which was forever changed by endoscopic technique, abdominoplasty did not prove to be a worthwhile application of endoscopy.

The Incision

The incision for a tummy tuck is long, running from hip to hip. The incision needs to be long enough to allow removal of a wide apron of excess skin. The shorter the incision, the less skin may be removed. Patients readily understand that it is better to make the incision a little longer and remove extra skin, than to leave unsightly puckering at either end. It is important for the incision to be low. A common surgical error is to place the incision too high, so that it is above the bikini line. Some patients who have had previous abdominoplasties complain about a high-riding scar that is hard to hide (See P.M., Complications). It may be possible to lower the scar at a subsequent procedure, but obviously this is best avoided.

Patients are concerned about such a lengthy incision before surgery. However, after surgery, they do not mind the scar as long as it is kept low, within the bikini line. The trade-off—a much improved abdominal appearance for a scar within the bikini line—is a favorable one.

Why don't all plastic surgeons place the incision low, hidden within the bikini line?

It is easier for the surgeon to place the incision higher and bring the skin edges together with less tension. It is more challenging for the surgeon to keep the incision low.

The difficulty in placing the incision low is that the upper margin of the skin to be removed is fixed at the level of the belly button (if a vertical scar is to be avoided). By placing the incision lower, more skin will need to be removed between the incision and the level of the belly button. The wider this distance is, the farther the upper skin flap needs to come down to meet it (See Intraoperative Photographs). It may not be possible to bring the skin edges together with the patient lying flat on the operating table. The operating table needs to be capable of bending in the middle to provide flexion of the hips, and allow wound closure without excessive tension. As might be expected, the lower the incision, the tighter the repair, and the more the patient will be stooped over after surgery.

Without an operating table that has the capability of elevating the upper body and lower body simultaneously, putting the patient in a hips-flexed position, it can be difficult to close the wound without tension, so the surgeon is tempted to keep the incision higher.

Temporary Stooped Posture after Surgery

A low incision is not usually a problem in a patient with a large apron of extra skin. It is more difficult in a thin patient with less loose skin. Of course, a thin patient with minimal skin laxity to start with is more likely to wear a bikini and wants her scar as low as possible. She needs to know that it may take a week or two before she will be able to stand completely erect. However, women invariably accept being a little more stooped over at first if this means the incision can be kept lower, within the bikini line.

One of the benefits of an abdominoplasty is the removal of old abdominal scars, particularly vertical scars that may cause an unsightly cleavage, giving the abdomen the unwelcome appearance of buttocks.

Gentle Curved Incision Looks Best

In the past, abdominoplasty incisions have been made in the shape of a W (I used to do this), in the shape of a bicycle handlebars, or a straight line. However, the most appealing scar is a gentle concave curve like a saucer. This scar runs along a natural transition zone, within the natural creases demarcating the lower end of the torso, up and over the pubic area. Other patterns, particularly an inverted-T, are not natural (a "T" is not found in nature and should be avoided on the body and breast) and call attention to themselves, detracting from the aesthetics of the surgical result.

Most surgeons mark the incision with the patient in a standing position before surgery. "Photo panties" are used for reference, along with the natural creases within the bikini line (the "inguinal creases"). The incision courses below any existing scars from previous C-sections, hysterectomies, or other surgery. This way, any existing lower abdominal scar is removed along with the extra skin. Typically, the new scar ends up at about the same level as an old C-section scar, because it is pulled up a little by tension from above. For patients with an existing C-section scar, the trade-off in scarring is limited to the extra length of the abdominoplasty scar beyond what they had already from the C-section scar, plus the scar around the belly button.

One of the benefits of an abdominoplasty is the removal of old abdominal scars, particularly vertical scars that may cause an unsightly cleavage, giving the abdomen the unwelcome appearance of buttocks. Abdominal cleavage is never good (See L.P., Patient Photographs). These old scars are contained in the extra skin, which is discarded.

Deep Sutures to Anchor the Flap

It is important for the surgeon to anchor the abdominal flap with deep sutures. These anchoring sutures help to prevent upward pulling on the pubic skin, which could displace pubic hair upward onto the abdomen. The less exposed pubic hair, the better.

Closure of the deep connective tissue layer ("fascia") also helps to preserve a flat skin contour. Failure to perform an adequate deep tissue repair could create a depression along the scarline, made more visible by a ledge just above it (See P.M., Complications).

In fact, often "ugly" scars are unattractive because they have a crease associated with them. This crease can usually be avoided by repairing the wound meticulously in layers; the fascial repair supports the skin repair and helps to keep it from sinking down. This deep tissue repair also takes most of the tension off the skin closure, reducing wound tension, and optimizing the scar quality (See Intraoperative Photographs).

Experienced surgeons use these maneuvers to keep the scar low and inconspicuous, avoid upward traction on the hair-bearing pubic skin, and avoid a vertical scar. These technical points help deliver the best cosmetic result possible. Seasoned surgeons recognize the importance of attention to details. Although each point individually may seem insignificant, taken together they can make the difference between a mediocre result and a superb one.

Muscle Repair

One of the most satisfying components of an abdominoplasty is the muscle repair. Pregnancy and weight gain stretch the abdominal wall. The two "rectus abdominis" muscles, which are oriented vertically in the abdomen, are stretched apart. The muscles become bowed in the middle, often separated by several inches at the level of the umbilicus (See Intraoperative Photographs). Exercise cannot bring these muscles back together. They can only be realigned surgically. This is done by sewing the muscle borders together, up and down the abdomen like a zipper. Actually, the fascial envelopes that contain the muscles are sewn together, not the muscles themselves, because muscles are too elastic and don't hold sutures well. After surgery, and after the swelling has gone down, the borders of the muscle can now be seen, moved in closer to the midline. This repair replaces the muscles in their original position, where they were before being stretched apart by pregnancy or weight gain. It is an anatomic restoration. It is gratifying for the surgeon and nurses to see the muscles come together and the abdomen flatten dramatically in surgery. It is not hard to imagine already that the patient is going to be very pleased afterward.

The muscle repair helps flatten the abdomen and correct excessive protuberance.

Muscular realignment also improves the mechanical advantage of the abdominal muscles, alleviating back pain that is caused by muscle imbalance in some patients (including Patient C.B., Patient Photographs). Some patients report improved bowel function.

The muscle repair helps flatten the abdomen and correct excessive protuberance. However, it is important to recognize that the abdomen is not totally flat on profile, even in lean, muscular individuals. A slight convexity is pleasing to the eye. Like other areas of the human body (with the exception of the contour under the chin), total flatness is not natural and not required.

Anesthesia

Traditionally, abdominoplasty has been performed under general anesthesia, including paralysis, intubation, and ventilation—the maximum degree of anesthesia. However, this operation may be performed under total intravenous sedation, using an LMA™ and propofol infusion, just like liposuction and other cosmetic procedures. Muscle relaxants are avoided. This modified type of general anesthesia avoids possible problems sometimes caused by traditional general anesthesia.

Once the patient is asleep, the abdomen is infused with a dilute solution containing Marcaine® (bupivicane), a long-acting local anesthetic, and epinephrine to reduce blood loss. By injecting the abdomen this way and then allowing time for the epinephrine to constrict the small blood vessels, there is a remarkable reduction in bleeding at surgery. Patient comfort is enhanced with the use of Marcaine, which continues to work for many hours after surgery. This local anesthetic also reduces the amount of anesthetic needed during surgery, so that the patient recovers faster afterward.

Plastic surgeons may be used to having the patient paralyzed when performing the abdominal muscle repair. However, with the use of an infusion of local anesthetic there is no need for this extra degree of anesthesia. The patient benefits from a reduced risk, and there is no compromise of the surgical repair.

Surgery Center

While abdominoplasties have been traditionally done in a hospital setting with an overnight stay, they are being done more commonly today in ambulatory surgery centers, for healthy patients without medical conditions. This switch to out-patient surgery was made possible by advances in technique and anesthesia to reduce surgery times, reduce blood loss, improve pain management, and shorten the recovery times. Today we recognize the importance of early ambulation to help prevent blood clots in the legs. Also, treatment in an out-patient surgical setting helps contain costs and make the surgery more affordable.

Avoiding hospital admission also eliminates the risk of a hospital-acquired ("nosocomial") infection, which can be serious because of the increasing prevalence of bacteria that have developed resistance to multiple antibiotics (for example, MRSA) in the hospital setting.

Miniabdominoplasty

Patients sometimes ask about a mini-tummy tuck. They know that there is a long scar with a regular tummy tuck and they wonder if a mini-tummy tuck might offer the best combination of results and limited scarring.

How is a mini-tummy tuck different from a regular tummy tuck? In a regular tummy tuck, or "full abdominoplasty," the umbilicus is released from the surrounding abdominal skin and then reintroduced through a new hole once the skin drape has been pulled down (See Illustration and Intraoperative Photographs in this section). By contrast, in a mini-tummy tuck, the umbilicus is not released. It stays attached to the surrounding abdominal skin and can be pulled down because of skin tension from below. A much smaller ellipse of skin is removed from the lower abdomen. The scar is shorter and ends up looking like an extended C-section scar. A mini-tummy tuck provides no tightening of the skin of the upper abdomen because the umbilicus remains anchored, preventing any tightening of the skin above it. It may be possible to tighten the muscles of the lower abdomen, but it is difficult to tighten the muscles above the level of the umbilicus because there is limited exposure of the upper abdomen in surgery.

A mini-tummy tuck is really just a removal of extra lower abdominal skin (See Patient V.H., below). It does not treat the upper abdomen. If the patient is concerned about loose skin above the belly button, or a roll that borders the belly button, and most are, she is not a suitable candidate for a mini-tummy tuck. I perform very few miniabdominoplasties, about one for every 100 regular tummy tucks.

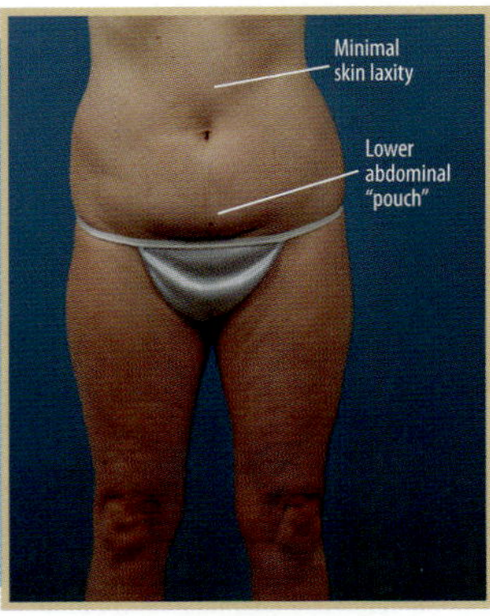

before

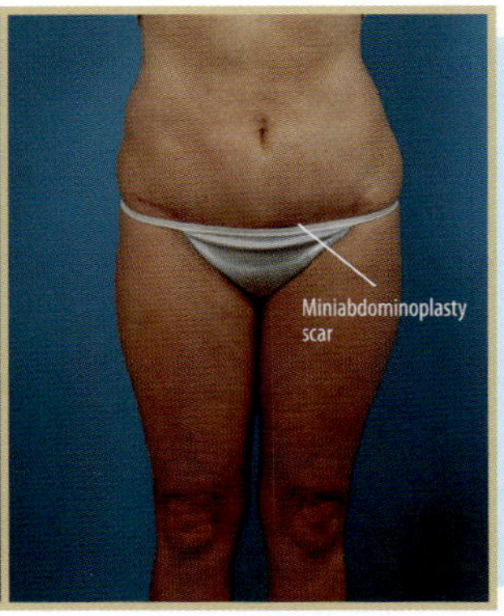

3½ months after

Miniabdominoplasty and ultrasonic liposuction of abdomen, flanks, and inner thighs.

Comments: This patient simply wanted to eliminate the excess skin of her lower tummy. She was not concerned about skin laxity above her belly button. She had simultaneous liposuction.

V.H., age 47, manager

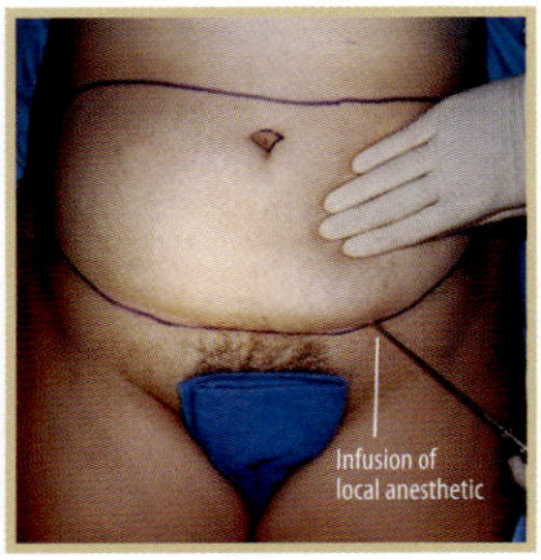

Intraoperative Photographs – Abdominoplasty

1. The abdominoplasty incision has been marked before surgery. The abdomen is infused with a solution containing a long-acting local anesthetic—Marcaine®—and epinephrine.

2. Ultrasonic liposuction is performed on the upper abdomen to remove extra fat in this area. Blood vessels and nerves are preserved as much as possible to optimize circulation and sensation of the flap.

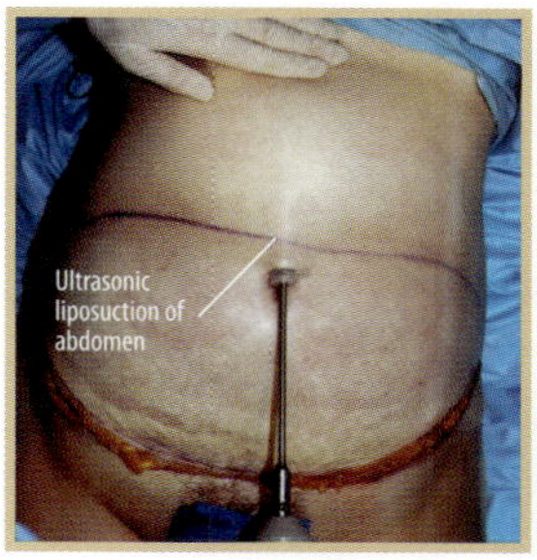

3. The flap is undermined all the way up to the level of the ribcage and then pulled down. The blanching of the flap is caused by epinephrine, which reduces bleeding during surgery. All the skin between the umbilicus and the lower incision will be removed.

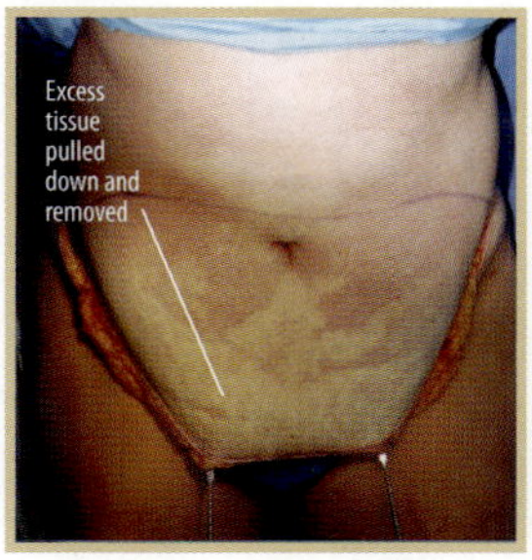

4. The extra skin and fat has been trimmed away. The site of the umbilicus, which is temporarily hidden, is marked. The muscle has been sutured together in the midline (*not shown*), tightening the muscle wall. The deep layer of tissue (fascia) has been repaired, and a drain has been inserted.

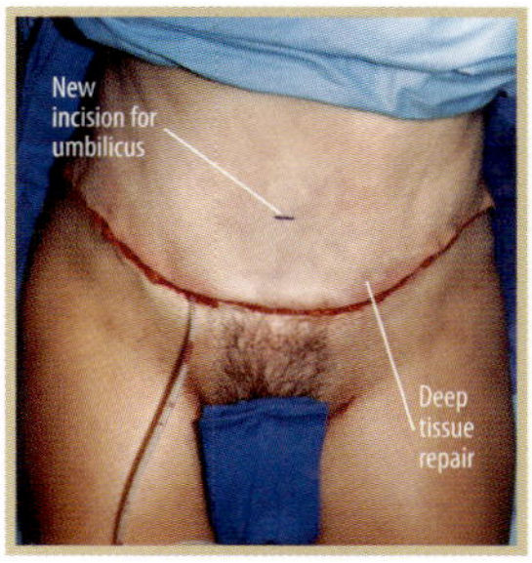

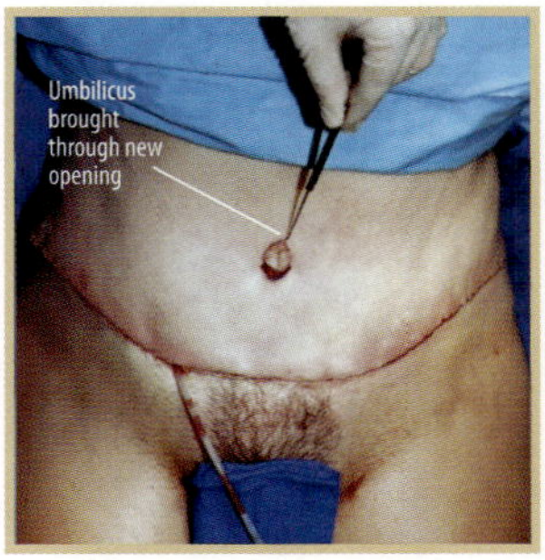

5. The abdominoplasty incision has been sutured.

6. The umbilicus is brought through a new opening and is about to be sutured in position.

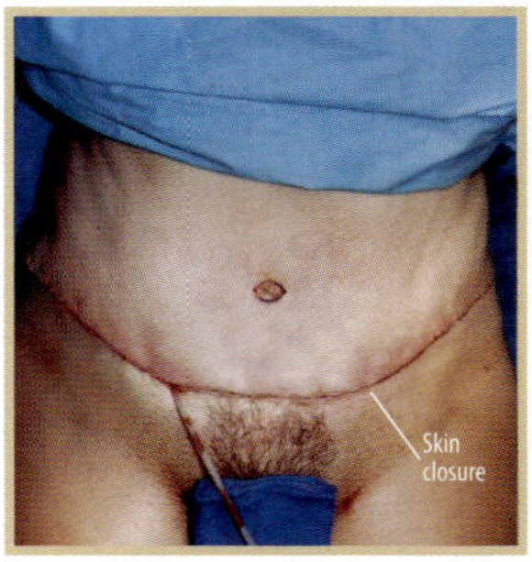

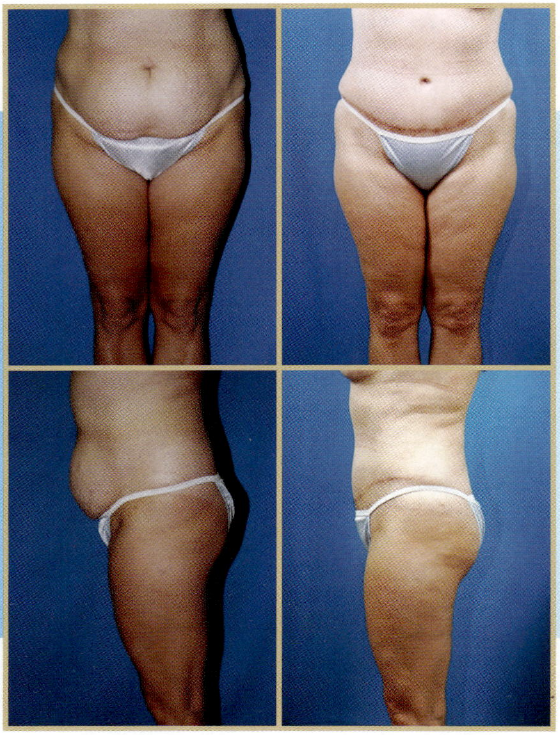

before *9 months after*

Abdominoplasty, ultrasonic liposuction of lower body, arms, and axillae, left breast scar revision, and submental lipectomy.

Comments: This patient's intraoperative photographs (*previous page*) show the sequence of the surgery. She is seen in the office the day after surgery. She is able to walk without assistance in a slightly stooped position. The abdominal dressing has been removed. The Steri-Strips are left in place along the abdominal wound. She is careful to sit with her hips flexed (back elevated and knees flexed). She will return in three days for removal of the drain.

Height: 5'3"
Weight before: 149 lbs.
BMI: 25.9
Children: 3
Liposuction volume: 2,000 cc
Flap weight: 5 lbs.
Dress size before: 12
Dress size after: 10
L.B., age 46, automobile inspector

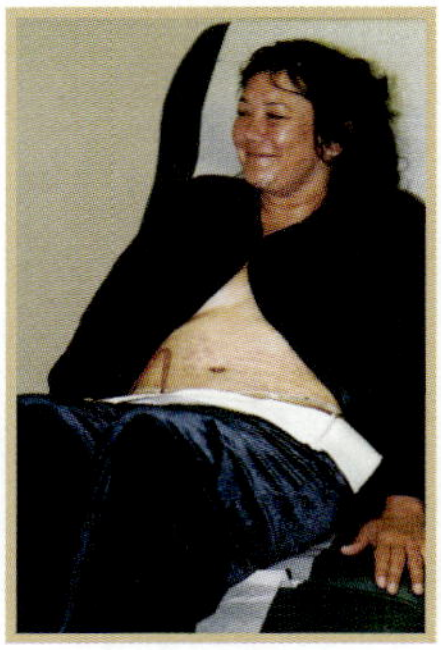

1 day after

Intraoperative Photographs – Muscle Repair

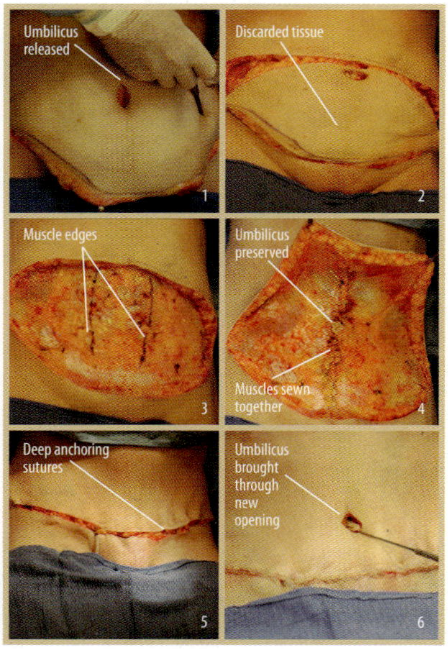

Abdominoplasty, ultrasonic liposuction of flanks, fat injection of buttocks, breast lift, and replacement of implants.

1. The abdominal flap is elevated and an incision is made around the umbilicus to release the skin around it. The umbilicus itself stays attached to the abdominal wall.

2. The excess abdominal tissue is excised.

3. The vertical markings (*blue*) show how far apart the muscles have been separated.

4. The muscles are realigned with two rows of running sutures.

5. Deep anchoring sutures are used to avoid any upward migration of the incision, avoid any contour depression, and to minimize skin tension.

6. The umbilicus is brought through the new skin opening.

Comments: This patient had an abdominoplasty (See preceding Intraoperative Photographs) and simultaneous breast surgery—the "mommy makeover." The combination of the breast lift and abdominoplasty enhances the appearance of her torso.

Height: 5′1″
Weight before: 104 lbs.
BMI: 19.4
Children: 2
Liposuction volume: 600 cc
Flap weight: 1 lb.
K.P., age 40

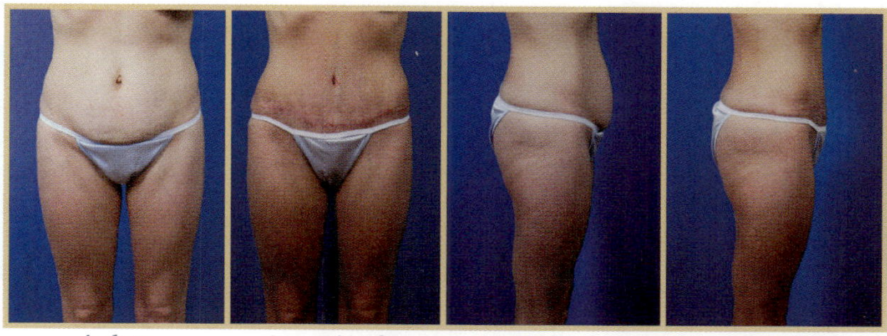

before *2 months after* *before* *2 months after*

Photographs and Testimonials

Women are presented first, followed by men. Patients are grouped by ethnicity and presented by age, youngest to oldest.

Females

Abdominoplasty – African-American

Abdominoplasty.

Comments: This patient was a competitive sprinter in college. Now she had a severe abdominal deformity after three pregnancies. She elected not to have liposuction simultaneously, but returned later for liposuction. She said her back pain disappeared after her tummy tuck. Note the reduction in the curvature of her spine ("lumbar lordosis") after surgery.

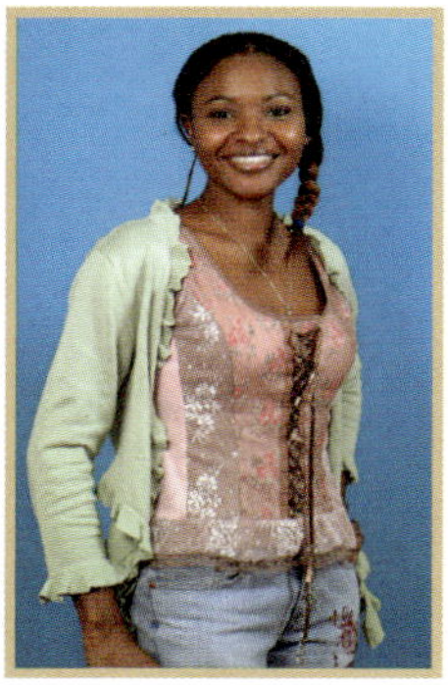

16 months after

Height: 5′5″
Weight before: 139 lbs.
BMI: 22.7
Children: 3
Weight after: 128 lbs.
Flap weight: 2.75 lbs.
Dress size before: 8
Dress size after: 6
C.B., age 32, systems analyst

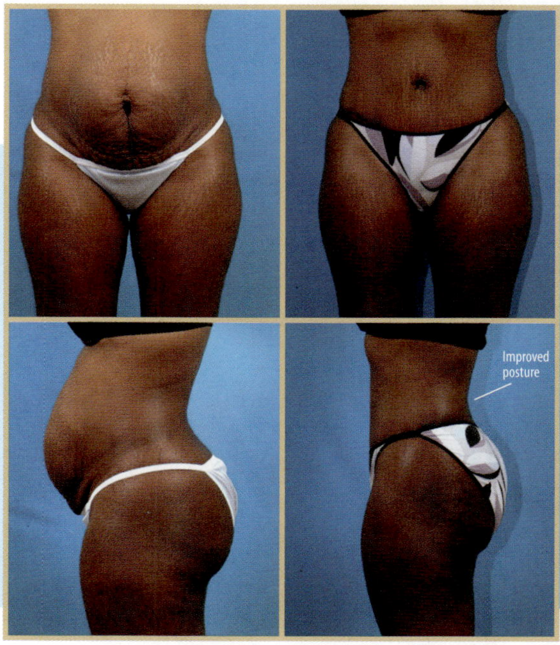

before *3 months after*

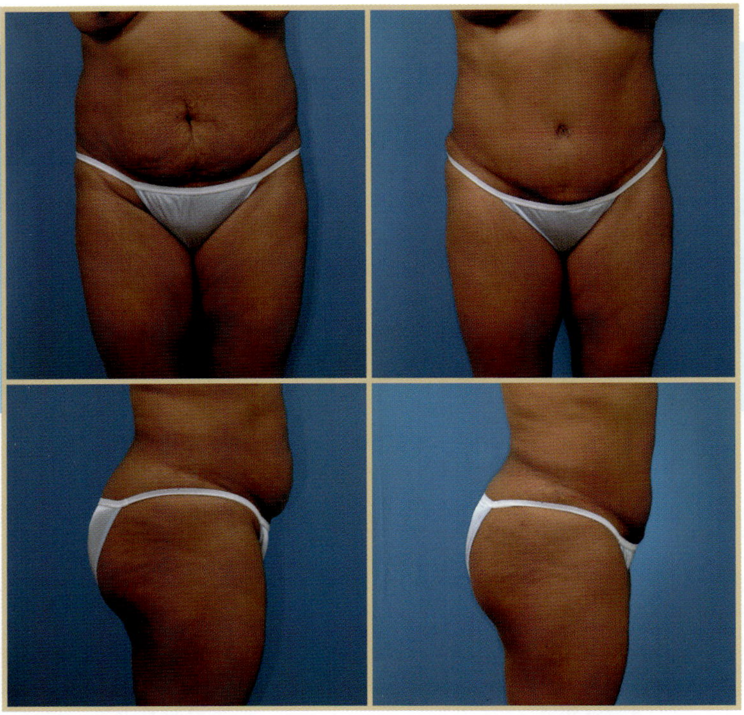

before *3 months after*

Abdominoplasty, ultrasonic liposuction of abdomen, flanks, inner thighs, arms, and axillae, breast lift and implants.

Comments: After surgery, this African-American patient admitted that she stood in front of the mirror for two hours admiring herself and had to call in late for work! She thanked me for her "new body."

Height: 5'4"
Weight before: 170.5 lbs.
BMI: 28.8
Children: 2
Weight after: 160 lbs.
Liposuction volume: 1,125 cc
Flap weight: 3 lbs.
Dress size before: 12/14
Dress size after: 8/10
R.I., age 39, office manager

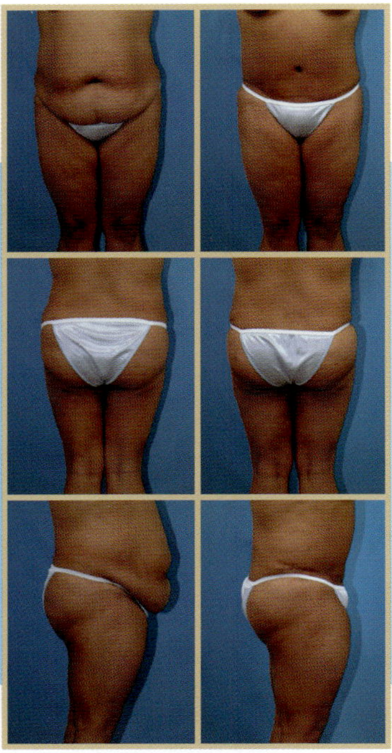

before *6 months after*

Abdominoplasty – Native American

Abdominoplasty, ultrasonic liposuction of lower body, arms, and axillae, and breast augmentation.

Comments: This patient was a full-blooded Seminole Indian, no doubt the only one I'll ever treat. Her abdominal deformity was so severe that she needed to lift up her tummy with her hands so I could mark her before surgery! She told me the surgery was less painful that she had imagined. She and her husband were excited when I took the dressing off the day after surgery and she was able to see the change in her tummy. She also said her back pain cleared up after surgery.

Height: 5'0"
Weight before: 157 lbs.
BMI: 30.1
Children: 2
Weight after: 141.5 lbs.
Liposuction volume: 1,400 cc
Flap weight: 8 lbs.
Dress size before: 12/14
Dress size after: 8
N.T., age 32, auto sales office worker

Healing of Abdominoplasty Scar

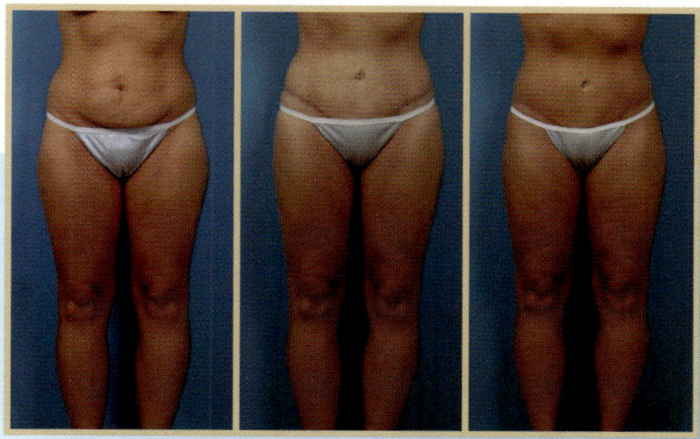

before *3 months after* *20 months after*

Abdominoplasty, ultrasonic liposuction of lower body including calves, arms, and axillae, breast lift and implants, submental lipectomy, and excision of accessory nipple, left abdomen.

Comments: This 28-year-old nurse had two children, ages three and six months, both delivered by cesarean section. She was not planning to have any more children. Her pregnancies had distended her abdomen, and she wanted to have this corrected. She would not wear shorts because of her thick calves. Liposuction was performed simultaneously. Two months after surgery she had dropped from a size eight to a size four and was comfortable wearing shorts for the first time since she was a child. This sequence of photographs shows the gradual improvement in the appearance of the abdominoplasty scar, which is kept low, within the bikini line.

Height: 5′3″
Weight before: 132 lbs.
BMI: 22.9
Children: 2
Weight after: 130 lbs.
Liposuction volume: 2,550 cc
Flap weight: 2.25 lbs.
Dress size before: 8
Dress size after: 4
B.M., age 28/29/30, registered nurse

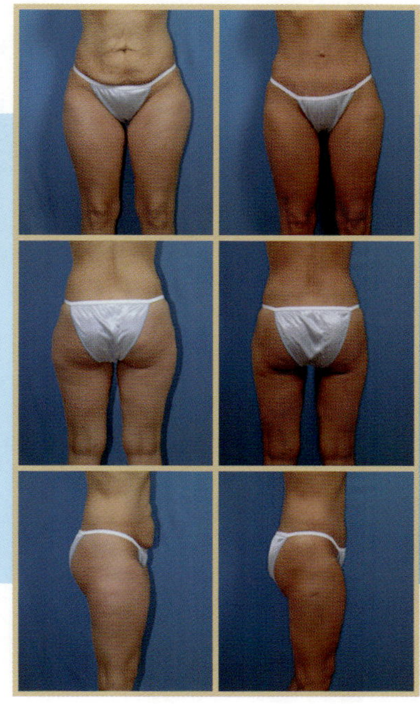

before *4½ months after*

Abdominoplasty and ultrasonic liposuction of lower body.

Comments: This patient had a very physical job working on an automobile assembly line, so she took a month off work. When asked if she was glad that she had the surgery, her response was, "absolutely." She said she dropped form a size five/six to a size four.

Height: 5′4″
Weight before: 116.5 lbs.
BMI: 19.7 lbs.
Children: 2
Weight after: 115.5 lbs.
Liposuction volume: 1,725 cc
Flap weight: 2 lbs.
Dress size before: 5/6
Dress size after: 4
S.R., age 32, auto assembly

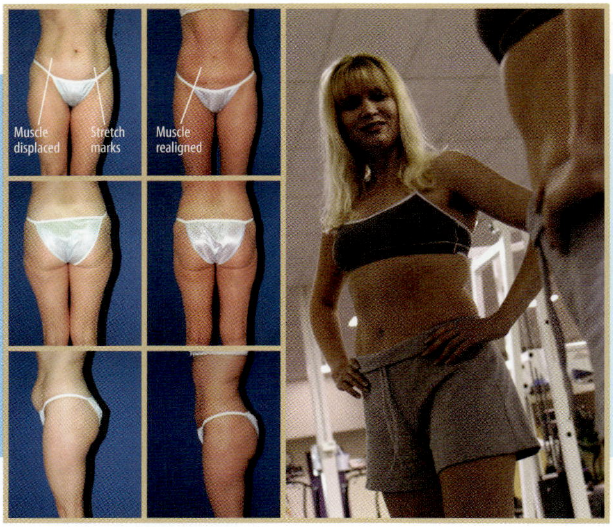

before *15 months after* *L.F.*

Abdominoplasty and ultrasonic liposuction of abdomen, flanks, and thighs.

Testimonial: "I always had a stomach, even before having five kids. I did thousands of crunches, leg raises, and used an exercise machine. I could feel that I had good muscles underneath, but you couldn't tell because my muscles were hidden under my pouch. I would wear clothes to hide my stomach, like pleated pants. It was affecting my self-esteem. I researched my options thoroughly before deciding to have surgery.

I love my results. It's beyond what I thought it would accomplish. Now I have a flat stomach and almost all my stretch marks are gone. My abdominal muscles are no longer hidden. I put more into my workouts.

I have a whole new wardrobe. It's awesome! I'm even wearing half-tops. My daughter told me to cover up—she thought I was showing too much. But she doesn't know how happy I am that I don't have to hide anything anymore."

Height: 5′ 4″
Weight before: 124 lbs.
BMI: 21.0

Children: 5
Liposuction volume: 1,325 cc
L.F., age 34, technical skills consultant

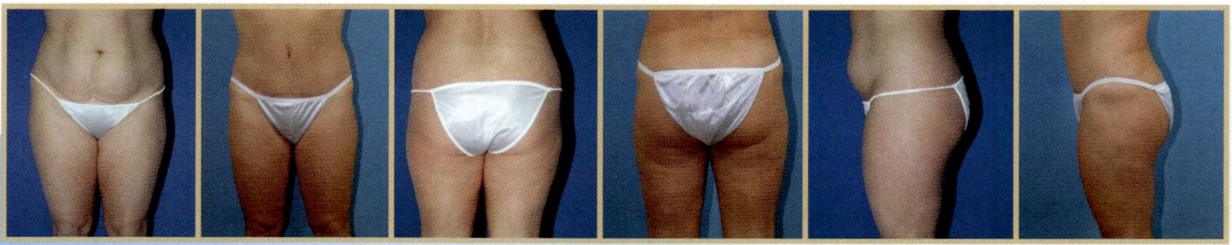
before *5 years after* *before* *5 years after* *before* *5 years after*

Abdominoplasty and ultrasonic liposuction of lower body and arms. Touchup, 3 years later: inner thighs and flanks.

Comments: This patient had an ugly scar from an emergency cesarean section. This scar was removed along with the extra skin of the lower abdomen, between the belly button and the pubic area. She had a breast reduction three years after her abdominoplasty (two years before these "after" photos). The belly button was oriented vertically. The orientation is a matter of personal preference. Today, the horizontal orientation is preferred by most patients.

Height: 5′1″
Weight before: 152 lbs.
BMI: 28.3

Children: 2
Weight after: 147 lbs.
Liposuction volume: 3,550 cc, touchup: 650 cc

Dress size before: 10
Dress size after: 8
A.D., age 35/40, hair stylist

Abdominoplasty and liposuction of lower body, arms, and axillae. Touchup, 6 months later: abdomen, thighs, knees, and arms.

Comments: This patient's skin has responded well to liposuction. The skin tone of her thighs appears better in the "after" photographs, despite the fact that over four years have elapsed since her procedure. Shortly after surgery, she told me she bought a bathing suit for the first time in 12 years!

Height: 5′ 7″
Weight before: 155 lbs.
BMI: 23.9
Weight after: 162 lbs.
Liposuction volume: 4,400 cc, touchup: 650 cc
Dress size before: 12
Dress size after: 8
P.B., age 35/39, supervisor

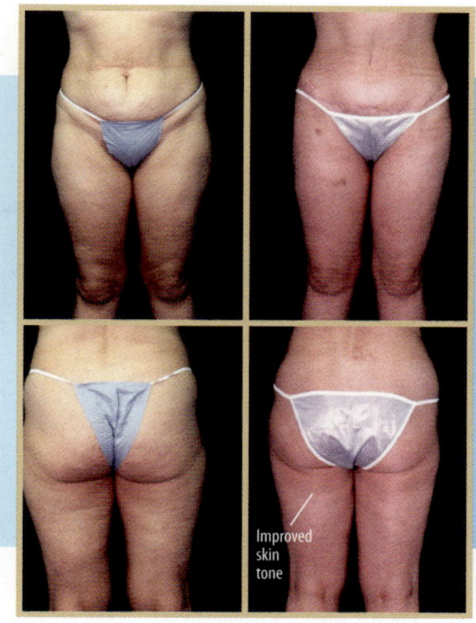

before *4½ years after*

Abdominoplasty, ultrasonic liposuction of abdomen, flanks, arms, and axillae, excision of skin lesion of left leg, and scar revision, left flank.

Comments: This patient said that the result exceeded her expectations. Not one to sit back and take it easy after surgery, she went scuba diving for great white sharks in a submerged cage (not included as a recommended activity on our Care after Surgery instructions). Fortunately, the sharks did not mess up any of my work. She is now contemplating having a breast augmentation and lift. She remarked, "Once you do one thing, you feel like doing others."

Height: 5′9″
Weight before: 169.5 lbs.
BMI: 24.6
Children: 2
Weight after: 166 lbs.
Liposuction volume: 1,500 cc
Flap weight: 5 lbs.
Dress size before: 12
Dress size after: 10
L.S., age 37/38, medical sales

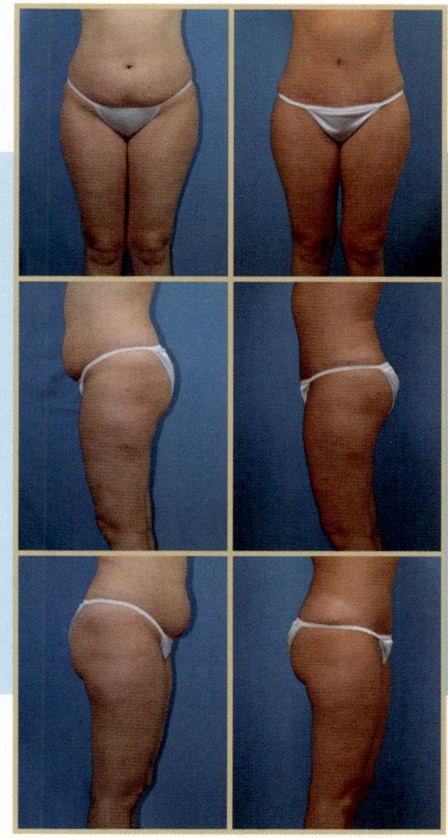

before *1 year after*

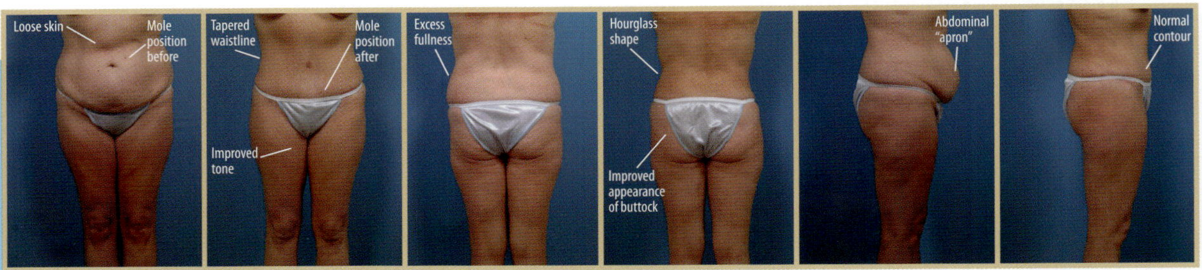

before *6 months after* *before* *6 months after* *before* *6 months after*

Abdominoplasty, ultrasonic liposuction of abdomen, flanks, inner thighs, arms, and axillae, and excision of multiple skin lesions of trunk.

Comments: This patient was 5'0" and weighed only 119 pounds, but her post-pregnancy deformity contributed to an unflattering body shape that made her look overweight. This undeserved body shape was corrected with an abdominoplasty and liposuction. In the "after" picture she weighed 113 pounds. Her drop in weight corresponds almost exactly to the weight loss expected from surgery—about four pounds for the tissue removed by the tummy tuck and another three pounds from liposuction (two pounds per 1,000 cc).

Height: 5'0"
Weight before: 119 lbs.
BMI: 22.8
Children: 1
Weight after: 113 lbs.

Liposuction volume: 1,700 cc
Flap weight: 4.25 pounds
Dress size before: 8
Dress size after: 4
R.K., age 44, teacher

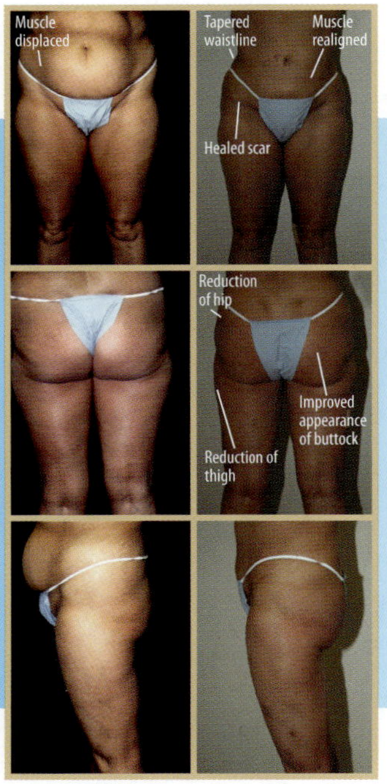

before *9 months after*

Abdominoplasty and liposuction of lower body. Touchup, 6 months later: lower abdomen and leg vein injections.

Testimonial: "After my two children were born, I had a pouch that wouldn't go away. Diet and exercise didn't do a thing for it. I'm thrilled with my tummy tuck. I now wear my shirts tucked into my jeans. It's really changed my personality. I have more self-confidence. For me, surgery was the answer."

Comments: After surgery, this patient has a more flattering hourglass figure. The effect of the muscle repair is visible on her frontal photographs. Her buttocks appear more rounded on the posterior photographs, a favorable illusion created by liposuction of the flanks. Her leg veins were treated subsequently, accounting for the bruising of her thighs.

Height: 5' 7"
Weight before: 170 lbs.
BMI: 26.2
Children: 2
Liposuction volume: 3,775 cc, touchup: 390 cc
A.S., age 44, hair stylist

Abdominoplasty, ultrasonic liposuction of lower body, arms, and axillae. Touchup, 3½ years later: lower body.

Comments: This patient had her body contouring surgery first, then facial rejuvenation. She wondered what more could be done to improve the skin laxity of her flanks. I explained that this skin laxity is caused by aging, with progressive loss of skin tone, and cannot be corrected by liposuction alone.

Height: 5′7″
Weight before: 162 lbs.
BMI: 25.0
Children: 2
Weight after: 152.5 lbs.
Liposuction volume: 2,700 cc, touchup: 2,250 cc
Dress size before: 12
Dress size after: 10
C.S., age 53/56, teacher

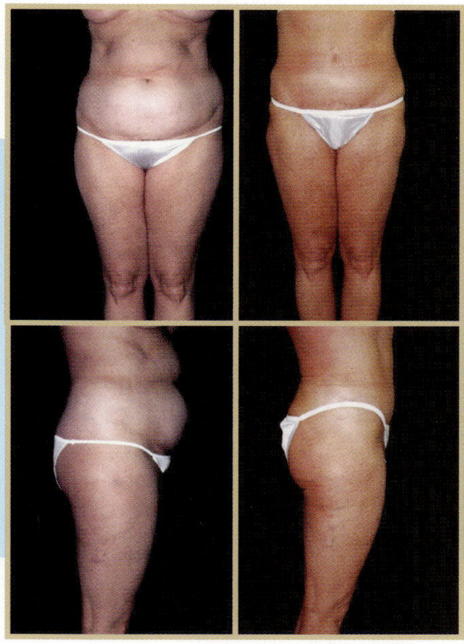

before *4 years after*

Abdominoplasty – Bodybuilder

Abdominoplasty and ultrasonic liposuction of lower body, arms, and axillae.

Comments: This patient of Hispanic and white ancestry was a competitive bodybuilder at age 54. However, her abdominal deformity was a limitation for her and proved difficult to conceal. The abdominoplasty scar was placed in such a way as to be hidden within her bikini.

Height: 5′0″
Weight before: 116.5 lbs.
BMI: 22.3
Children: 2
Weight after: 113 lbs.
Liposuction volume: 1,400 cc
Flap weight: 1.75 lbs.
Dress size before: 5
Dress size after: 1
C.B., age 54, manager

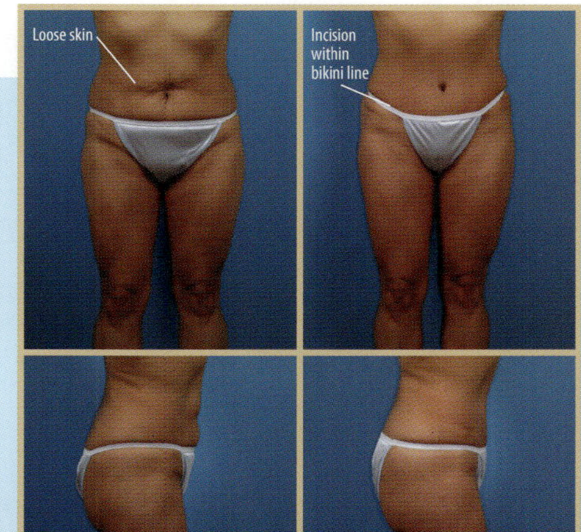

before *3 months after*

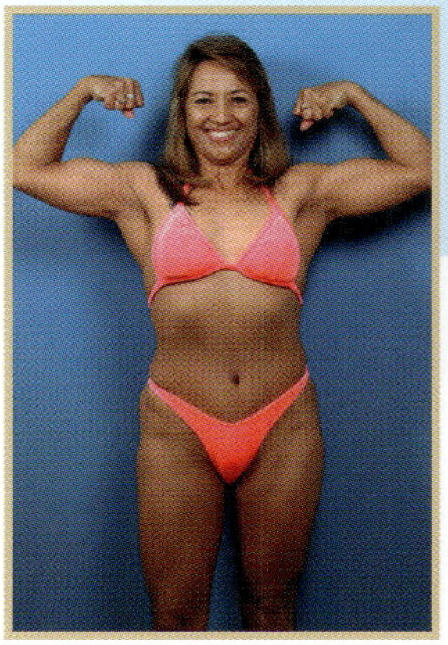

C.B.

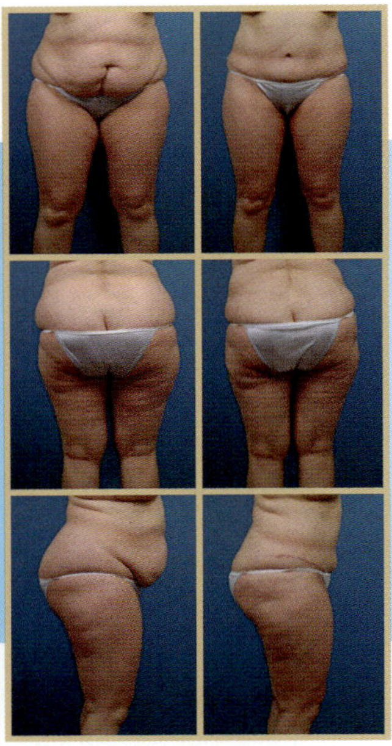

before *6 months after*

Abdominoplasty, ultrasonic liposuction of lower body, arms, and axillae, submental lipectomy, and excision of skin lesion of left inner thigh.

Comments: This patient had an ugly old vertical cesarean section scar, and a much better-healed old scar from her gall bladder removal, before this was done using the laparoscope. She returned to all of her usual activities and work two weeks after surgery. One month after surgery, she had dropped two sizes.

Height: 5′6½″
Weight before: 225.5 lbs.
BMI: 34.7
Children: 4
Weight after: 198 lbs.
Liposuction volume: 4,600 cc
Flap weight: 7 lbs.
Dress size before: 18
Dress size after: 14
L.P., age 58, C.E.O.

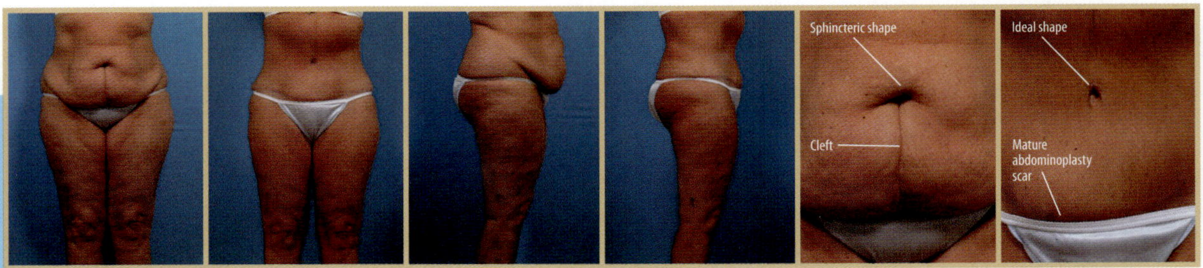

before *3 months after* *before* *3 months after* *before* *1 year after*

Abdominoplasty and ultrasonic liposuction of lower body.

Comments: This woman had hidden her tummy her entire adult life. After surgery, she told me she felt more comfortable meeting new people, was more confident, and had not felt this way since before having her children (her oldest was 42). She bought some "hip hugger" jeans for the first time, no longer wore a long T-shirt to cover her tummy, tucked in her tops, and did not mind showing off her belly button.

Height: 5′4″
Weight before: 168 lbs.
BMI: 28.4
Children: 3
Weight after: 160.5 lbs.
Liposuction volume: 2,950 cc
Flap weight: 6 lbs.
Dress size before: 14
Dress size after: 10
J.G., age 63, retired

Abdominoplasty – Hispanic

Abdominoplasty and liposuction of lower body.

Testimonial: "I have four children and had three C-sections. With each pregnancy, I began to develop a pouch that would never quite go back to what it used to be. When I was in high school, I weighed 98 pounds. With my first pregnancy, in my ninth month, I was over 170 pounds. Between children I dieted and did everything I could but I never lost that pouch. I wanted to look good but I never could. I would wear a girdle and deprive myself trying to look better, but I never could.

So after my fourth child, I decided that I needed something else. We moved to this area and I began looking into what could be done. I told my two sisters about Dr. Swanson and my older sister decided to have it done. She had it first and I took care of her. Then she took care of me.

Since I'd had three C-sections, I knew what it was like to have trouble bending over and moving around for the first few days after surgery. The staff was very supportive during my recovery so it was fine. I'm glad I did it. When I stand up, it's a straight line. I look better, therefore I feel better. Because I feel better about myself, I look better. It's a circle. My husband loves how I look. He loves it when I buy a dress that fits my body instead of me trying to cover up a flaw. It's just been great. My husband got excited helping me buy a dress. One size fits all my body. I dropped from a size 16 to a 10.

I think patients should be given a worst-case scenario and then it won't be that bad. I knew what abdominal surgery was like, but for someone who'd never had it, you're going to feel some pain—though not much—and you're going to need help getting up and getting to the bathroom the first couple of days. You're going to have to take time to let your body heal. You'll see an improvement everyday until you can stand up straight again. For a while you'll be hunched over. Try not to laugh or it'll hurt. It's uncomfortable, but not that bad. Not as bad as those three C-sections. Take it easy, be nice to yourself, rest, and within a few weeks you'll be fine."

Height: 5' 3"
Weight before: 148 lbs.
BMI: 25.7
Children: 4
Liposuction volume: 5,375 cc
Dress size before: 16/18
Dress size after: 10
M.U., age 42, secretary

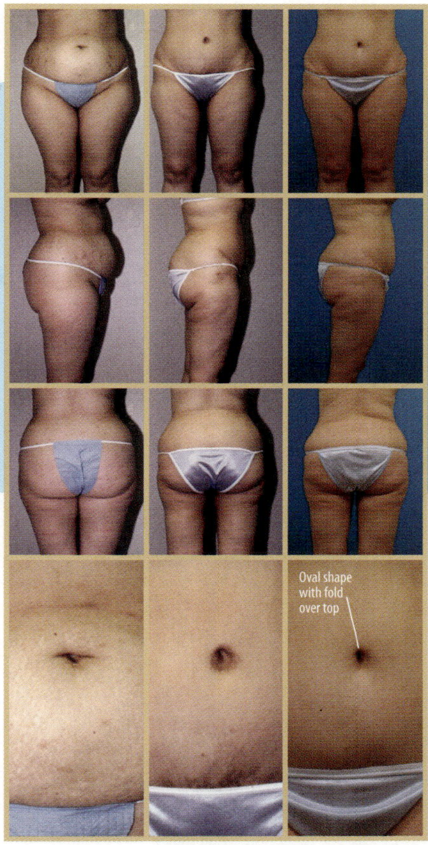

before *5 months after* *9 years after*

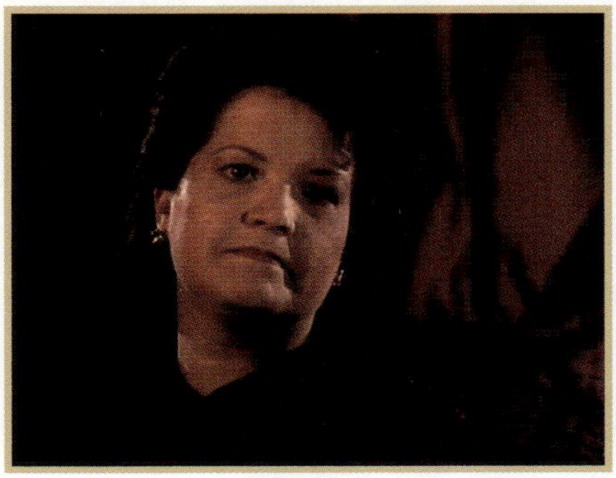

M.U.

Abdominoplasty and Breast Augmentation

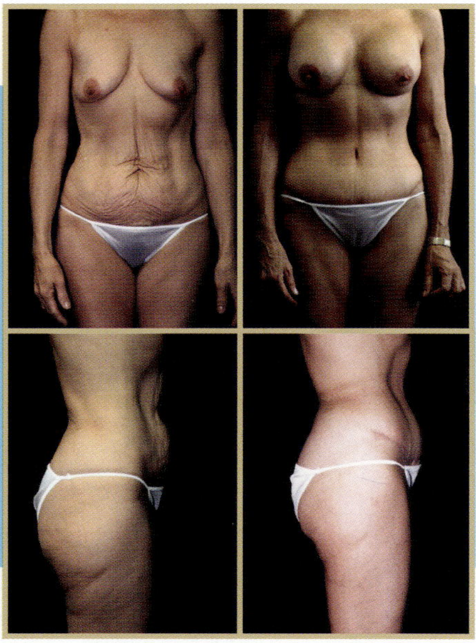

before 2 months after

Abdominoplasty (no liposuction) and breast augmentation.

Testimonial: "I had five children who really did a number on my abdomen. I'd also lost volume in my breasts. I'd been working out and never really had a problem controlling my weight. It seemed the more I worked out, the worse I looked. I knew I needed a little help. I decided to have a tummy tuck and a breast augmentation. I feel like a new person."

Height: 5′ 3″
Weight: 114 lbs.
BMI: 19.8
Children: 5
N.M., age 50, business owner

"Mommy Makeover"

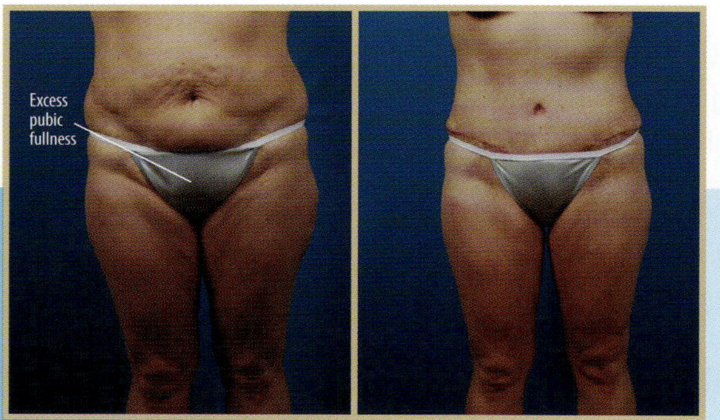

before 6 weeks after

Secondary (redo) abdominoplasty, ultrasonic liposuction of lower body and axillae, fat injection of buttocks, breast lift and implants, fat injection of lips, and submental lipectomy.

Testimonial (e-mail): "I am very pleased! Being able to see the before-and-after photographs really puts things into perspective. I just can't put into words how good I feel. It has affected every part of my being, the way I hold my head, walk and even the way I think. When I walk past a mirror now and catch a glimpse, I really do feel voluptuous.

I am one happy girl. Last Friday, I had to make a quick presentation at the basketball game for the cell phone company I work for. For the first time in my life, I was not nervous getting up in front of people. I felt/looked like a million bucks. My ex-husband tells me I 'look hot.' My kids say, 'Wow, Mom, you look so good.' My daughter told her new boyfriend, 'Wait until you meet my Mom, she's a hottie.' The wisdom of a 39-year-old and the body of a 29-year-old—what could be better? The confidence is pouring from me! :)"

Comments: This patient had a tummy tuck elsewhere eight years previously. The absence of a scar around the umbilicus suggests this was a mini-tummy tuck. She thought she looked "dumpy." She was concerned about her persistent stretch marks and pubic fullness. She had a "double bubble" of fullness of the lower abdomen and pubic area—women do not like a bulge in the pubic area (no "package," please!).

In addition to the redo tummy tuck and liposuction, she underwent a breast lift and implants, completing a "mommy makeover." After surgery, her contour deformity is corrected. Her torso appears longer, and she looks leaner and taller. The psychological benefit, as recounted in her e-mail, is profound.

Height: 4'11"
Weight: 128 lbs.
BMI: 25.5
Children: 2
Liposuction volume: 1,845 cc
Flap weight: 2 lbs.
J.B., age 39, customer service rep.

Male Abdominoplasty

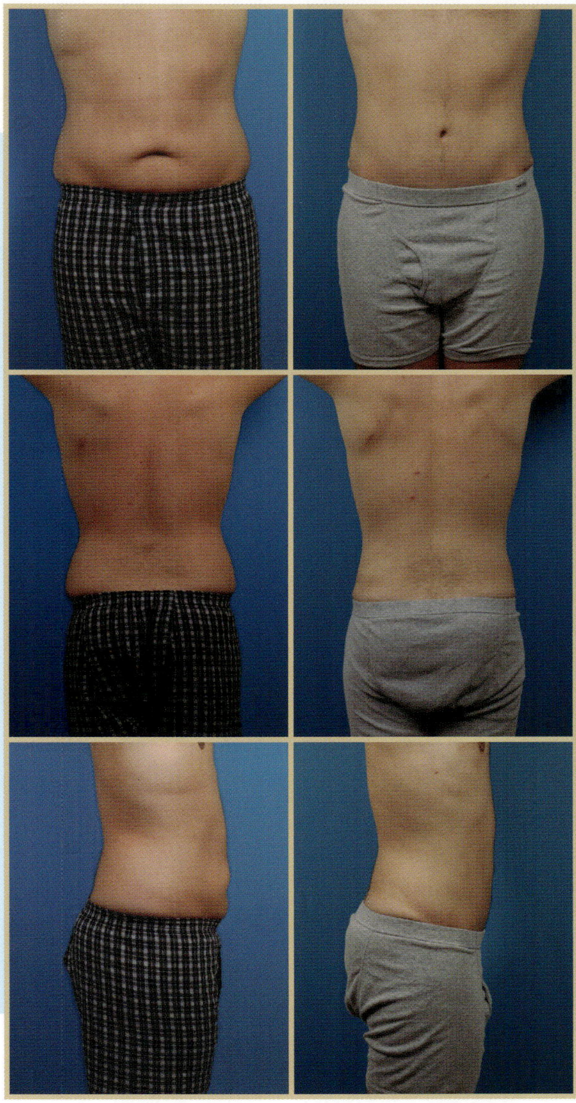

before 2½ years after

Abdominoplasty and ultrasonic liposuction of abdomen, flanks, inner thighs, and axillae. Touchup, 2 years later: flanks.

Comments: This young patient had skin laxity of the lower abdomen and conspicuous love handles after losing about 70 pounds. He had the surgery before starting college and successfully kept the extra weight off.

Height: 5'6"
Weight before: 178 lbs.
BMI: 28.3
Weight after: 181 lbs.
Liposuction volume: 1,200 cc, touchup: 450 cc
Flap weight: 4 lbs.
C.M., age 20/22, student

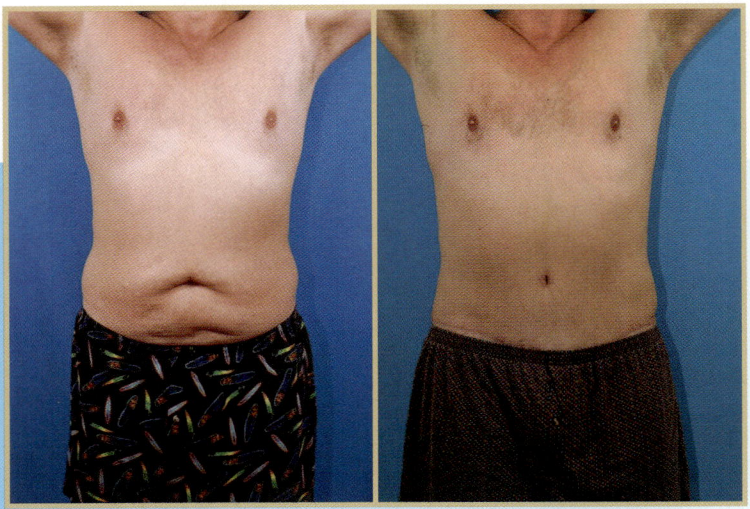

before *5 months after*

Height: 6'0"
Weight before: 217 lbs.
BMI: 28.8
Weight after: 211 lbs.
Liposuction volume: 550 cc
Flap weight: 4 lbs.
Waist before: 38
Waist after: 36
W.A., age 49, federal agent

Abdominoplasty, touchup ultrasonic liposuction of flanks and abdomen, ultrasonic liposuction of axillae, and excision of skin lesion of upper back.

Comments: This patient had previous liposuction after losing about 30 pounds. His skin tone was poor. He drove himself to his appointment four days after surgery (to have the drain removed) and was walking already in a fully upright position. He commented that the result was better than he had hoped for.

What to Expect after Surgery

Our Survey Says

Pain (1-10)	7.5	Exercise again (days)	45
Pain killers (days)	8.6	Sleep comfortably (days)	23
Need assistance (days)	6.3	Result (1-10)	9.0
Driving (days)	12	Improved self-esteem	91%
Time off work (days)	16	Do it again	97%
"Back to normal" (days)	43		

141 Patients

Other Questions

Back pain		Bowel function	
Better	33%	Better	21%
The same	66%	The same	73%
Worse	1%	Worse	6%

Abdominoplasty compared with a C-section (19 patients)

Pain		Recovery	
Better	21%	Better	16%
The same	32%	The same	26%
Worse	47%	Worse	58%

Abdominoplasty compared with a hysterectomy (10 patients)

Pain		Recovery	
Better	40%	Better	30%
The same	20%	The same	20%
Worse	40%	Worse	50%

Recovery

Patients in the recovery room after surgery are often already gratified by the change in their abdominal contour. Like breast augmentation, this immediate positive feedback offsets some of the physical discomfort. The local anesthetic is still working, and will continue to work for several hours.

Sometimes a urinary ("Foley") catheter is used during surgery, particularly if the operation is lengthy (5-6 hours), which might be the case if combination procedures are done, such as liposuction and a simultaneous breast lift and implants. The catheter is typically removed at the end of surgery before the patient wakes up.

The nurse provides assistance when patients get up to walk and go to the bathroom. Patients are in a stooped position, made necessary by the tightness of the abdominal repair. Most patients remain in the recovery room for about an hour. The nurse helps them get dressed and gives instructions to the caretaker, including how to care for the drain, which is not difficult.

The Drain

The drain accumulates bloody fluid after surgery. This fluid is mainly tissue fluid with a small amount of blood. It is quite dilute, so patients do not need to worry that they are losing a lot of blood when they see the bulb fill. The bulb is emptied when it is about a third or half full. If it gets too full, it loses suction. The bulb should always be collapsed—an indication it is working to produce suction.

Keeping the Hips Flexed

Patients need to keep their hips flexed to avoid too much tension on the wound closure. They tend to do this automatically. I tell caretakers (usually husbands) to help support the legs when patients swivel into the car because it is hard for patients to lift their legs up without assistance.

At home, a recliner works well because it provides elevation of the upper body and flexion of the hips. Patients can also use a bed, but will need to put pillows under their back, shoulders and head, and also one under their knees to maintain a flexed position at the hips. Some patients purchase a foam wedge and use it for their upper body. They will need some help at first getting in and out of bed and up to go to the bathroom.

Up Walking Right Away

Patients will likely urinate several times during the night after surgery. This is normal. After all, fluids were administered in surgery both through the I.V. line and by injection into the tissues. The kidneys work to remove this fluid during the first 24 hours after surgery. These short trips to the bathroom are helpful because they make patients use their legs. Early ambulation avoids prolonged immobilization, reducing the risk of blood clots. As a further precaution, we recommend that patients flex their ankles 20 times every hour after surgery while awake.

Follow-Up

Usually I see patients the day after surgery. This early follow-up visit ensures that they are mobile and getting up and around. The dressing is removed at this visit. The nurse takes the garment down part-way to do this. The wounds are inspected and then redressed with gauze along the incision line. Also, a layer of gauze is placed between the drain and the skin. This layer of cushioning prevents undue pressure on the skin from the drain. Otherwise, the drain might leave an indentation or even a scar. Patients are instructed to start bathing the day after surgery, or at the latest, the second day after surgery. They can get into a bathtub or use a shower. They need some assistance the first couple of times. While they are bathing, the garment may be washed, but not placed in a heated dryer. The adhesive bandages come off the day after surgery, or earlier if they are saturated. The semi-transparent adhesive tapes ("Steri-Strips™") are left intact along the incision lines. These will come off after about a week. The smaller ones at the liposuction sites can be removed in a few days.

I see patients three or four days after surgery to remove the drain. Patients imagine that this must be painful. In fact, drain removal is not particularly painful—less uncomfortable than removal of the dressing the day after surgery—and it usually takes just a few seconds. The drain site seals on its own in a few days. A gauze dressing is applied to absorb any fluid that continues to drain.

Sutures

The abdominoplasty sutures dissolve on their own. The belly button sutures usually come out two weeks after surgery. The skin is still numb, so this does not hurt.

Numbness

Patients often report temporary discomfort of their lower back after surgery. This may be due to liposuction used to treat the flank areas, and possibly the stooped posture after surgery. The tummy feels uncomfortably tight. The skin of the lower abdomen is numb because sensory nerve branches are traumatized or divided in performing the tummy tuck. It takes months for the feeling to gradually return, starting with the sides of the tummy. The last area to recover feeling is the area below the umbilicus, which can take up to two years. Persistent numbness is possible, but not of much concern to patients, who are very gratified by the appearance of their tummy.

The Scar

The downside of a full abdominoplasty is the long incision. However, the extra inches at the lateral ends usually heal the best because this portion of the incision has the least tension, and the incision may be kept within the bikini line, hidden in the natural inguinal crease. It turns out that this scar is usually not a concern for patients after surgery.

A full abdominoplasty requires a scar that goes around the umbilicus. This is because a large flap of skin is mobilized and needs to be freed of its attachment at the umbilicus. While the umbilical scar can heal very nicely and be inconspicuous, in some patients the scar widens and is noticeable. The umbilical scar may be revised later on, once the tension has diminished, to make it less conspicuous. Some patients form hypertrophic scars, and this can be a bothersome complication. Fortunately, the rewards in improved body contour are almost always a worthwhile trade-off, even when scarring is more noticeable. With time, scars tend to improve. They are raised and reddened at first, but they gradually soften, flatten, and fade (See B.M., Healing of Abdominoplasty Scar). This can take over a year.

Dog Ears

This term refers to puckering at the end of any surgical incision. Dog ears occur after abdominoplasties with some regularity, even for experienced surgeons. Whenever a surgeon removes extra skin, usually with an elliptical incision, there is a pucker at the end of the incision that develops when the skin edges are brought together, caused by tissue bunching beyond the end of the incision. This is a geometric reality. Dog ears may be avoided by making the incision longer and more tapered. The more tapered the end of the incision, the less tissue redundancy there will be when the edges are brought together. However, this is at the expense of a longer scar.

It turns out that puckering of human skin tends to improve with time. Unlike cloth fabric, human skin is a dynamic tissue capable of contraction. Small dog ears usually flatten out eventually. The surgeon's job is to make the incision just long enough to avoid a dog ear, while keeping it as short as possible. It is always possible to come back and remove an extra little pucker in the skin if necessary under local anesthesia in the office. Sometimes extra fat persists in this area as well, and this fat may be removed with a touchup liposuction or simply excised with the extra skin. There is minimal downtime after such a touchup procedure.

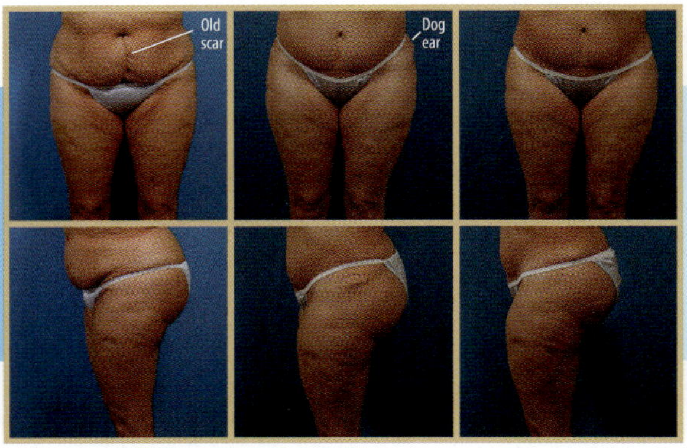

before *15 months after* *16 months after*

Abdominoplasty, ultrasonic liposuction of abdomen, flanks, arms, and axillae, upper blepharoplasties and facial fat injection. Revision of dog ear of left hip under local anesthesia, 15 months later.

Comments: This patient had an old vertical scar and contour deformity of the lower abdomen, which were corrected with a tummy tuck and liposuction. A persistent dog ear of the left flank was revised in the office under local anesthesia. She is seen on the date of this revision (*middle*) and one month later (*right*).

Height: 5'5"
Weight before: 170.5 lbs.
BMI: 27.9
Children: 1
Weight after: 161.5 lbs.
Liposuction volume: 1,625 cc
Flap weight: 7 lb.
Dress size before: 16
Dress size after: 10
P.A., age 59/60, horse trainer

Ideal Umbilicus

No doubt it would be possible to devote an entire book to the aesthetics of the belly button. Today, the appearance of the umbilicus has taken on greater importance than it did in the past, as the midriff is now more exposed and the belly button has become a frequent site for piercing.

A small, oval umbilicus with a skin fold over the top part is the goal. Ideally, the scar is concealed in a natural fold or tucked inside the perimeter of the umbilicus, although this is not always possible, especially in very lean patients.

It is important for the surgeon to avoid having the umbilicus point upward after surgery, which looks unnatural. This problem can occur when the new umbilicus position is marked too high in surgery. Instead, the umbilicus should be oriented slightly down.

A large, wide umbilicus is undesirable. A wide umbilicus can develop in women after pregnancy, often in the presence of a widening ("diastasis") of the space between the rectus muscles. Repair of the muscle layer corrects this problem by tightening the umbilical opening (See K.P., Intraoperative Photographs).

It is possible to make the opening too small ("constricted"), which makes it difficult for patients to clean the belly button. A tight umbilicus can occasionally occur due to contraction of the scar encircling it. This problem can be treated with a release under local anesthesia in the office.

It is not unusual for the umbilical scar to widen, especially on the sides. This scar spreading may be related to tissue tension after surgery. If this happens, the umbilical scar may be revised as an office procedure. The widened scar tissue is simply excised. This revision is done at least several months after surgery, when the wound tension has been fully relieved. With less tension on the scar, there is less likelihood of recurrence. However, for some unfortunate patients, scar hypertrophy or even keloids (See C.B., Keloid) can be a recurrent problem and the umbilicus never looks as nice as we would like. A few patients resort to a tattoo to camouflage the scar. Remarkably, even these patients tend to be happy ones because they would not give up their improved tummy contour, even with this scar.

Umbilical Appearance after Abdominoplasty

The following are close-up views of the umbilicus. These patients' before-and-after photos may be found in the Patient Photographs – Female Abdominoplasty section.

Abdominoplasty, ultrasonic liposuction of lower body, arms, and axillae, and breast augmentation.

Comments: This Native American patient's umbilical scar is tucked inside where it is hidden. This is possible in patients with sufficient local subcutaneous fat, but can be more difficult in very lean patients.

N.T., age 32

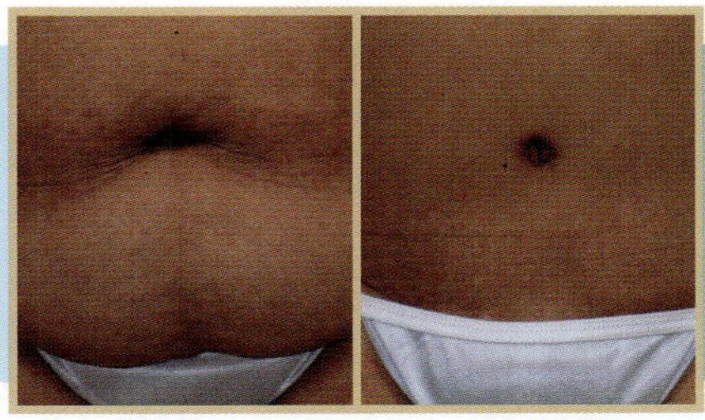

before *3 months after*

Abdominoplasty, ultrasonic liposuction of abdomen, flanks, inner thighs, arms, and axillae, breast lift and implants.

Comments: This African-American patient has a more attractive umbilicus after surgery. There is a tension-free flap of skin over the top. The redness of the scar has faded. There is some spreading of the scars along the sides that might be improved with a revision, but she was not concerned about this.

R.I., age 39/40

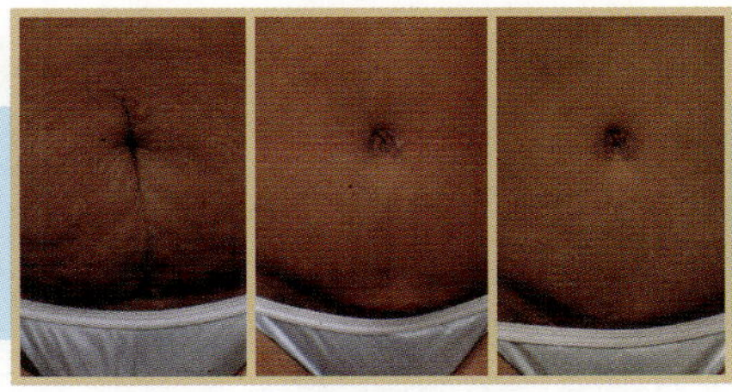

before *3 months after* *20 months after*

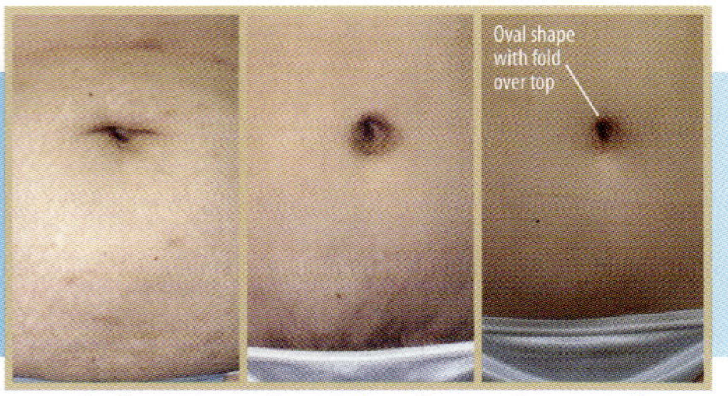

before *5 months after* *9 years after*

Abdominoplasty and liposuction of lower body.

Comments: Ideally, the umbilicus has a fold over the top and the scar is inconspicuous. This Hispanic patient's umbilicus looks better after her tummy tuck than it did before. She is seen five months and again nine years after her abdominoplasty.

M.U., age 42/51

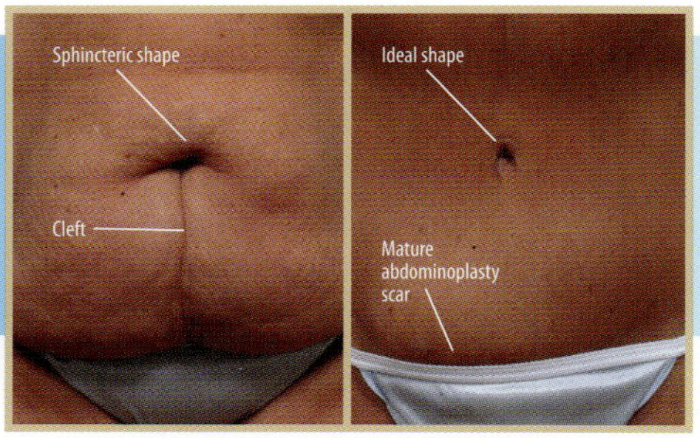

before *1 year after*

Abdominoplasty and ultrasonic liposuction of lower body.

Comments: This woman, who had three children, thought her belly button looked like the terminal end of the digestive tract (not her exact words), which is never a favorable comparison. Making matters worse, she also had a midline cleft, which patients sometimes say makes their abdomen "look like a butt." After surgery, her scar is inconspicuous and the sphincteric appearance has been eliminated. She has a bikini-worthy tummy.

J.G., age 63/64

Umbilical Orientation

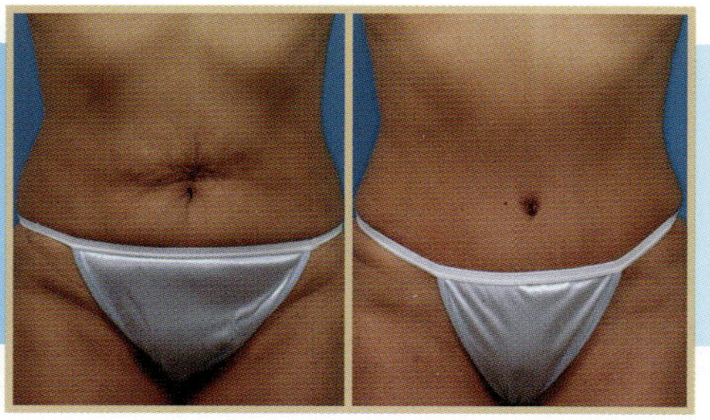

before *3 months after*

Abdominoplasty and ultrasonic liposuction of lower body, arms, and axillae.

Comments: Although the appearance of the tummy is improved, the umbilicus is oriented slightly upward. Ideally, it should be oriented slightly downward.

C.B., age 54

Keloid

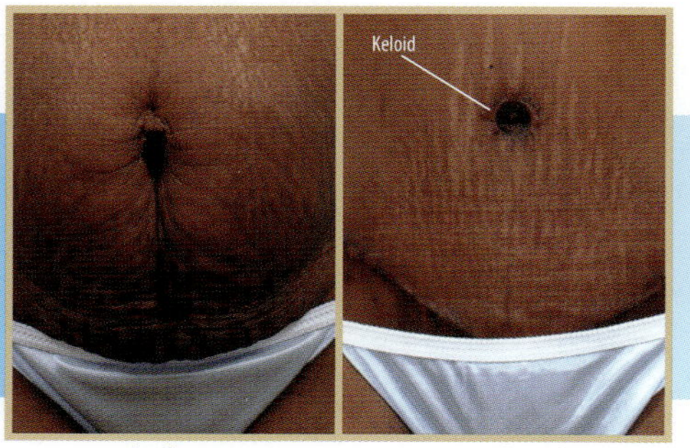

before *3 months after*

Abdominoplasty.

Comments: This patient developed a keloid after her abdominoplasty. This is a raised-up scar that can overreach the boundaries of the original incision and feel itchy. It was treated with steroid injections at the follow-up visits.

C.B., age 32

Revision of Umbilical Scar

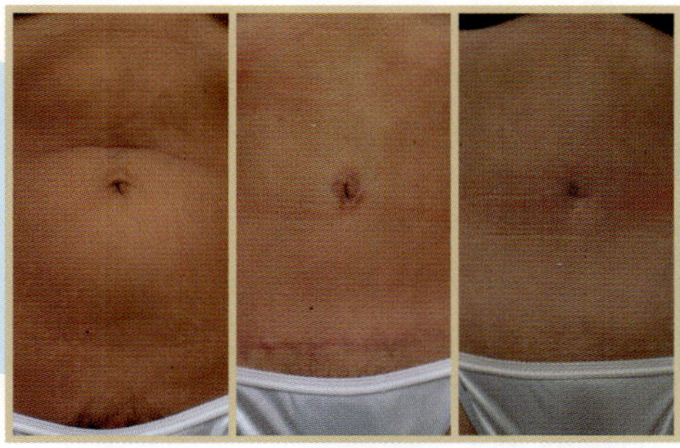

before *3 months after* *3 years after*

Abdominoplasty and ultrasonic liposuction of lower body. Umbilical scar revision, 8 months later.

Comments: This patient enjoyed boating during the summer and wearing a bikini. She is seen three months after surgery. Portions of the umbilical scar have become thicker and wider. The scar is still red. During the winter off-season, eight months after her tummy tuck, the scar was revised in the office under local anesthesia. Two years later, the scar has flattened and turned white ("matured") and is much less conspicuous. The abdominoplasty scar has also matured.

V.B., age 51/54

Complications

Infection

While infection is rare after liposuction, it happens from time to time after abdominoplasty. It presents with increasing redness ("cellulitis"), fever, and possibly a purulent drainage from the incision. A yellow, clear, or blood-tinged drainage is normal and to be expected. But a greenish or white drainage, or any foul-smelling drainage, is not. This indicates infection. Antibiotics are prescribed, and any purulent drainage is cultured. Infections typically respond to antibiotics, although drug-resistant strains of *Staphylococcus aureus* (MRSA) are becoming more prevalent.

Seroma

A fluid collection under the skin is called a seroma. If the swelling after surgery seems to be increasing rather than decreasing, this may be a sign that such a fluid collection has developed. Patients may reasonably wonder why the drain did not prevent such a problem. Should the drain simply be left in longer? It's a reasonable question. The problem is that the longer the drain is left in, the greater the risk of infection, which is why we prefer to remove the drain three or four days after surgery. The small risk of a seroma is balanced against the increasing risk of infection if the drain is left in longer.

If a seroma develops, it is treated by inserting a needle into the swollen area and draining off ("aspirating") the fluid. This maneuver immediately corrects the excess swelling, and patients are more comfortable. Fortunately, the needlesticks are not particularly painful because the skin is still numb. These aspirations, performed in the office, typically need to be repeated several times. Eventually the lymphatics start working again to absorb the fluid and external drainage is no longer necessary.

Surgeons find seromas a nuisance (as do our patients) and try to avoid them by preserving the loose ("areolar") connective tissue layer over the abdominal wall during the abdominoplasty. This is the layer of yellowish fat located just superficial to the muscle (See Intraoperative Photographs). The skin undermining is limited to just what is necessary to gain adequate release of the flap (limited undermining also helps preserve blood supply and sensation). I personally find it helpful to avoid the use of cautery during the dissection. Pretreatment with the Marcaine®/epinephrine solution reduces blood loss sufficiently to allow dissection using a scalpel. This technique limits tissue injury and inflammation that might otherwise cause more fluid release. The risk of seroma is minimized and, in my practice, is a rare occurrence after abdominoplasty.

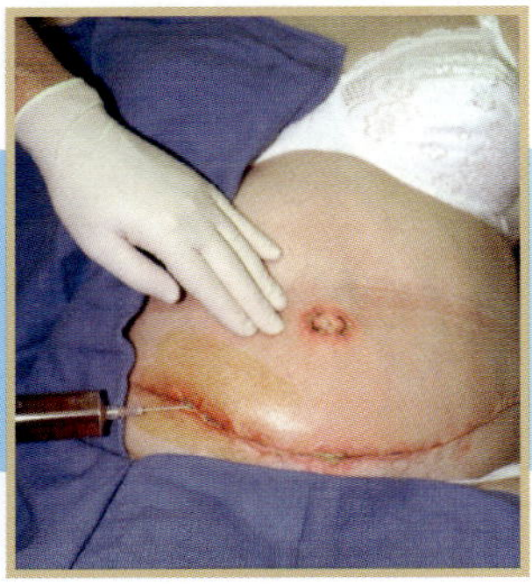

G.R., age 62, nurse

Abdominoplasty and ultrasonic liposuction of abdomen, flanks, inner thighs, knees, arms, and axillae.

Comments: This patient developed two complications—a seroma of the abdomen and cellulitis of the flank. A wound culture produced a scant growth of *Group D enterococci,* sensitive to the Cipro that she was prescribed. Her seroma was aspirated a total of 10 times over the course of one month. Despite this nuisance, she was still happy with her result and told me she'd received numerous compliments. She enjoyed tucking in her tops and wearing belts. She said she was fitting clothes she could never fit before.

Hematoma

A hematoma can occur after an abdominoplasty, possibly requiring a return to the operating room for evacuation, although this is very unusual. The drain helps to prevent such a collection from developing. Like any hematoma, prompt recognition and treatment is the key to a successful outcome.

Deep Venous Thrombosis

As discussed previously (Liposuction – How It's Done), a blood clot in the deep vein of the thigh (deep venous thrombosis) is a serious and potentially life-threatening complication of surgery. The risk of a DVT is that a clot may break off, travel to the lungs, and cause a pulmonary embolus, which can be fatal.

The risk of a DVT is increased by immobilization of the lower extremities. It can even occur in people after long plane flights. The risk may be reduced by avoiding paralysis (which reduces the sympathetic tone to the veins), the use of sequential compression devices in surgery, reduced operating times, and early ambulation. My patients are turned from side to side during surgery while I inject local anesthetic solution and during liposuction, so they do not stay in the same position too long. The prone position, which causes pressure at the hips, is avoided entirely.

Even if these precautions are taken, a DVT can still develop. It can even occur without surgery. Some surgeons advocate the use of blood thinners (heparin or Lovenox®) immediately before surgery, but this intervention has to be balanced against the risk of easier bleeding after surgery.

Abdominoplasty and ultrasonic liposuction of lower body.

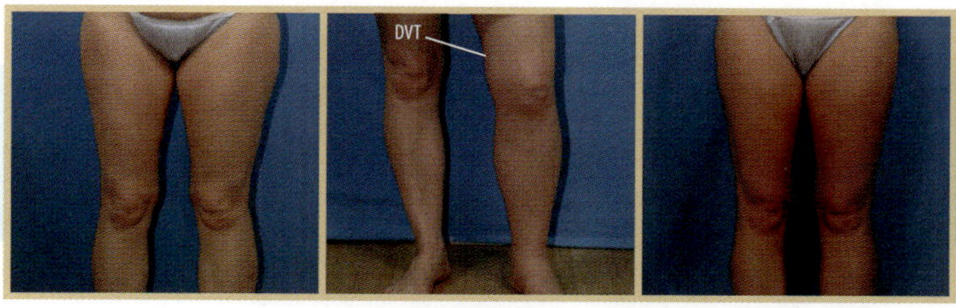

before *2 weeks after* *3 months after*

Comments: This patient called me nine days after surgery to report that her left leg had started to swell. This occurred on a Saturday morning. I saw her immediately in my office, diagnosed a DVT of the left lower extremity, and arranged hospital admission. A Doppler study confirmed the diagnosis, detecting a large blood clot extending up the left femoral vein. An enhanced CT scan of the chest was negative. She was anticoagulated with heparin and then placed on Coumadin®. She stayed in the hospital for one week. She is seen in follow-up at my office two weeks after surgery. Her left leg is still swollen. At the time of her three-month postoperative visit, the swelling has completely resolved.

K.J., age 39, student

Skin Loss

Skin loss typically occurs where the skin circulation is most at risk—usually the central portion of the upper abdominal skin flap, corresponding to the area of skin most removed from its blood supply. Old scars can act as barriers to skin circulation, further reducing blood supply.

Smoking causes constriction of the small blood vessels. In an area where the circulation is already partially interrupted by surgery, this constriction of small vessels can make the difference between tissue survival and loss. Cessation of smoking greatly reduces the risk of this complication. We recommend that patients quit smoking at least two weeks before surgery and continue to refrain from smoking for two weeks after surgery.

Abdominoplasty and ultrasonic liposuction of abdomen, flanks, and inner thighs.

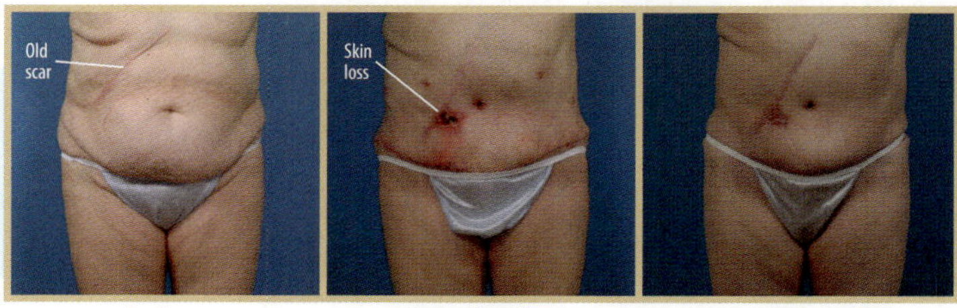

before *2 weeks after* *3 months after*

Comments: This 63-year-old nonsmoker recently had a breast reduction. She returned for a tummy tuck and liposuction. She had an old scar across her right upper abdomen, from removal of her gall bladder 35 years ago. Prior to surgery, we discussed the fact that this scar would compromise circulation to the abdominal skin and possibly cause some skin loss, which is exactly what happened. The patient was not overly concerned because she knew about this risk in advance. The wound gradually healed on its own, and the patient had no regrets.

L.M., age 63, retired

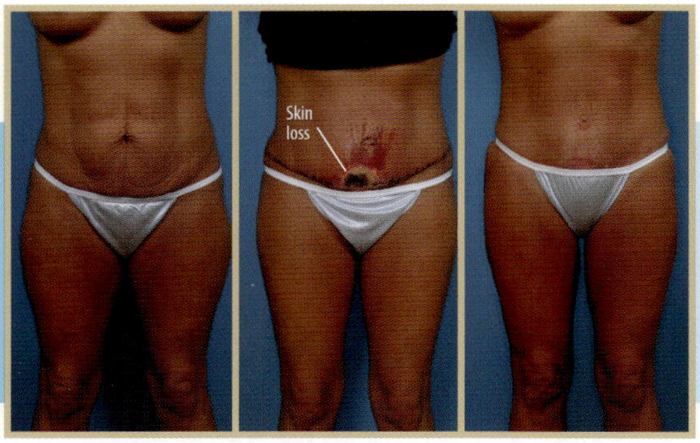

before *2 weeks after* *3 months after*

Abdominoplasty and ultrasonic liposuction of lower body.

Comments: This 50-year-old smoker did not follow advice to stop smoking. Her daughter scolded her and told her she'd better stop "or you won't look good in a bikini, Mom!" Once she stopped smoking, the wound started to heal quickly and was completely healed two months after surgery. She has some increased scar tissue along the midportion of the incision. This excess scar tissue may be revised later to give a thinner scar, but with time the scar will continue to soften, and a revision may not be necessary.

R.G., age 50, painter

Excess Scarring

The central portion of the abdominoplasty scar may spread, depending on the patient's healing characteristics and wound tension. Any factor that interferes with wound healing, such as an infection or skin loss (See R.G., above) can predispose the patient to a wider, more conspicuous scar. After about six months, the tension has been relieved. At this point, the scar may be revised.

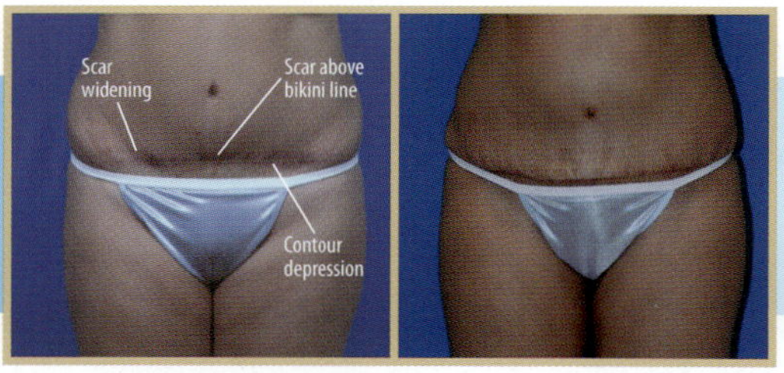

before *5 weeks after*

Revision of previous abdominoplasty, and ultrasonic liposuction of abdomen, flanks, and inner thighs.

Comments: This patient had a suboptimal linear scar from a previous tummy tuck performed elsewhere. The scar ran slightly above her bikini line and had widened. There was a contour depression associated with it. At surgery, the existing scar was revised, lowering its placement. A deep tissue repair corrected the depression and helped minimize skin tension, reducing the scar's propensity for spreading again. She was no longer self-conscious about her scar, which was easily concealed within her bikini line.

P.M., age 34

Care after Surgery

- Avoid straightening your hips fully. Walk in a stooped position to reduce tension on the abdomen.
- You can take stairs, but with assistance.

- At night, be sure to keep your hips flexed and sleep on your back ("supine"), not on your side. A recliner works well. Otherwise, use a bunch of pillows under your upper body and tuck one under your knees.
- The suction drain needs to be emptied when it is about one-third to one-half full. After emptying, be sure to squeeze the bulb when closing the valve. The bulb should stay collapsed, indicating that it is creating the suction needed to draw fluid off the abdomen. Don't be surprised if you have to empty it several times the night after surgery. This is normal. Although it looks like a lot of blood is coming out, it is mainly fluid (not much blood is needed to turn the fluid red). The drainage typically slows down after the first 24 hours.
- You should be getting up to urinate every three hours or so. Be sure to drink adequately to stay well hydrated. These trips to the bathroom are also helpful to get you up and moving. Early ambulation helps prevent blood clots from developing in your legs.
- Your tummy will feel very tight. This is normal.
- Sometimes there is blood-tinged drainage around the drain tube. Simply tuck some gauze in to absorb it and confirm that the suction drain is working. Be sure there are no kinks in the tubing and the bulb is collapsed.
- You can unzip the garment (if you are wearing a girdle) partly at the top if it is digging in to your sides. If the garment is uncomfortably tight in the inner thighs, you can cut the margin to relieve any uncomfortable constriction. Similarly, if the garment is too tight at the knees, it can be cut to release any tourniquet effect, although this is rarely necessary.
- Some bloody drainage into the dressing and through to the garment is normal after surgery. However, if this increases, or if the dressing becomes saturated, notify the office.
- At the time of your appointment the day after surgery, your dressing is removed. When you go home you can bathe later that day, or at the latest, the next day. You can immerse your tummy in the water. Just put the drain over the edge of the bathtub or hold it in the shower.
- Be careful when you take off the garment. You may feel light-headed at first. It is best to take off the garment and then sit for several minutes before standing. This allows your body some time to adjust to the new position. If you feel faint when standing, immediately lie down, even if this means lying down on the bathroom floor. It is much better to lie down than to fall down. The lightheadedness will go away. Don't try to fight the faint feeling. Give in and lie down. This lightheadedness can occur during the first few days after surgery. Later on, it is usually not a problem.
- Keep a layer of gauze between the drain tube and the skin when you have the garment on. This cushions the drain and avoids an indentation that could possibly leave a mark.
- Sometimes the tightness of the abdomen can cause heartburn. An antacid can help.
- Don't be surprised by swelling above the level of the garment. It is not possible to provide compression over the upper abdomen, because this might restrict breathing. Don't worry; this swelling will go down and you will not be left with a ledge over the top of the garment.

- Bruising usually occurs in the flanks and back because of the effects of gravity.
- Usually there is discomfort of the flanks and back caused by liposuction, which is typically performed simultaneously with the abdominoplasty.
- Wash the garment and then dry it in a no-heat dryer cycle. Keep the bottom of the garment at the knees partially zipped up, so the garment does not get completely tangled up in the wash.
- Avoid any activities that stress the abdominal muscles.
- Avoid taking too many pain killers. A side effect is nausea. It is very uncomfortable to vomit after a tummy tuck, so don't take more than two pain killers every four hours. You can take one-and-a-half pain killers or substitute a Tylenol® for the second pain killer. It is important to treat the pain, but don't exceed the prescribed dose.

  Tylenol may be used as an alternative to Vicodin® during the day. Patients should take either the prescribed pain killer (usually Vicodin) or Tylenol, but not both simultaneously to avoid too much acetaminophen (Vicodin contains the narcotic hydrocodone plus acetaminophen). This is a serious issue. Presently, acetaminophen toxicity is the leading cause of acute liver failure in the United States and, at the time of this writing, an FDA advisory panel is recommending reducing the maximum daily dose from 4,000 mg to 2,600 mg and limiting the amount in a pill to 325 mg (so that 500 mg extra-strength Tylenol would no longer be available).
- Most of the sutures dissolve. The belly button sutures are removed about two weeks after surgery. The Steri-Strips™ along the abdominoplasty incision are left on for about a week, but don't worry if some of them come off sooner. You can take the small bandages off the liposuction incisions when you first bathe after surgery (or sooner if any are saturated). Usually you do not need to replace these bandages, but if there is any drainage go ahead and put on another bandage.
- Sometimes patients report feeling or even hearing a "pop" from their abdomen. Just as they might imagine, this is caused by a suture popping. This can happen when the abdominal pressure increases, such as during vomiting, which is one reason we take steps to avoid nausea, including limiting the doses of narcotic pain killers after surgery. I use a double row of sutures to repair the abdominal muscles during surgery, so there is a backup. No need to worry.
- Constipation can be a problem after surgery, caused by a slowing of the normal muscular activity of the intestines. This is a side effect of narcotic pain killers such as Vicodin, which is another reason (besides reducing the potential for nausea) to gradually reduce the dose of this medication after surgery. Being active after surgery, up and moving around, helps too. You can take a mild laxative and/or stool softener. The constipation seldom requires a rectal suppository or enema.
- Expect swelling above the garment, where there is no compression, and along the lower abdomen. This swelling along the incision line can feel very firm. Gradually it softens. It can take several months for this swelling to completely go down and for the tissues to feel soft again.

- The pubic area ("perineum") is likely to be swollen and bruised after liposuction (if this area is treated) or just from fluid and blood settling into the area after an abdominoplasty. Even the labia, or scrotal area in men, can be swollen and bruised. Don't be alarmed by this. It is normal.

Frequently Asked Questions

Q: What can I do about my stretch marks?

A: Nonsurgical treatment is ineffective. Stretch marks on the lower abdomen can be eliminated with a tummy tuck. Stretch marks on the upper abdomen are moved down to the lower abdomen.

Q: Should I wait until I am done having children before having surgery?

A: It makes sense to wait until you are finished having children so that you don't stretch the skin again and possibly stretch out the muscle repair too. For women who are unsure about future pregnancies, a judgment call needs to be made—the advantages of having the results now, against the possibility of having to do another tightening procedure later on. Of course, limiting weight gain during pregnancy will help. The abdominoplasty itself does not affect your ability to get pregnant or cause any problem with expansion of tissues during pregnancy. Many of my patients have gone on later to have pregnancies, but very few return for revision of their tummy tucks.

Q: I've had previous abdominal surgery. What are the risks?

A: The abdominoplasty does not involve opening the abdominal cavity that contains the organs. Sometimes patients are concerned about adhesions—internal bands of scar tissue that can develop around organs and cause problems, such as bowel obstruction. Patients are reassured that, because the peritoneum is not entered, there is no risk of adhesions from an abdominoplasty.

Q: Do you use a pain pump?

A: Of course, this is not a "pain pump" (patients are having enough of that already) but a local anesthetic pump that delivers small amounts of local anesthetic into the surgical wound after surgery using a catheter and a pump. It sounds like a reasonable and humane measure to improve patient comfort. However, a study showed similar pain scores and use of prescription pain killers in patients treated with and without these pumps after abdominoplasty. Possible reasons for its ineffectiveness are a lack of penetration of the muscle fascia, and a compromised distribution in the wound due to gravity and suction drains used after surgery that may drain off the local anesthetic solution. These devices do not appear to be sufficiently beneficial to justify the added nuisance of looking after them, the expense, and occasional complications.

Q: I have a belly button hernia. Can it be repaired at the same time?

A: The umbilical hernia can be repaired at the same time as the abdominoplasty. Also, an excessively wide belly button can be tightened into a more attractive, smaller "innie."

Q: Do you do many tummy tucks on men?

A: Not as many as women, of course, because of the effects of pregnancy. However, any patient, male or female, who has lost weight or who has poor skin tone of the abdomen can benefit. One male patient of mine memorably told me after surgery, "Everything is better now."

Q: How much weight will I lose?

A: The weight of the abdominal tissue that is removed is typically in the range of 2-10 pounds, although I have removed as much as 15 pounds. Liposuction removes additional fat, usually several more pounds. This operation provides a major difference in body contour, much more than a similar amount of weight loss from dieting. Obviously, in patients who are overweight, optimal results can be expected only from a combination of weight loss from proper diet and exercise, and surgery to correct any abdominal deformity and body disproportion.

Q: How long before I can straighten up fully?

A: Your amount of stooping depends on the degree of existing skin laxity, how low the incision is placed, and how much skin is removed. Ironically, lean patients with less skin laxity (but still enough to be of concern), who want the scar as low as possible to keep it concealed, have the greatest abdominal tightness after surgery. These patients may require a couple of weeks to straighten fully. Most patients take about a week before they can stand fully straight.

Q: It feels very tight. Should I be careful to avoid pulling on the incision?

A: Yes, especially during the first week. Avoid pulling too much because this may place too much tension on the incision. After a week, you can stretch a little more. The key is to do a little more each day. Your body is a good guide and will tell you when to back off.

Q: When can I return to exercising?

A: You won't feel like exercising after surgery. You can start walking a mile or two in about two weeks and return to exercising fully a month after surgery. Abdominal exercises take longer, a minimum of six weeks.

Q: What are my alternatives to surgery?

A: If you have extra loose skin and weakening of the muscles from pregnancy or weight loss, an abdominoplasty is your best option. Liposuction is not a substitute—it does not remove the extra skin and does not repair the abdominal muscle laxity.

4 CHAPTER FOUR

Thigh and Buttock Lifts

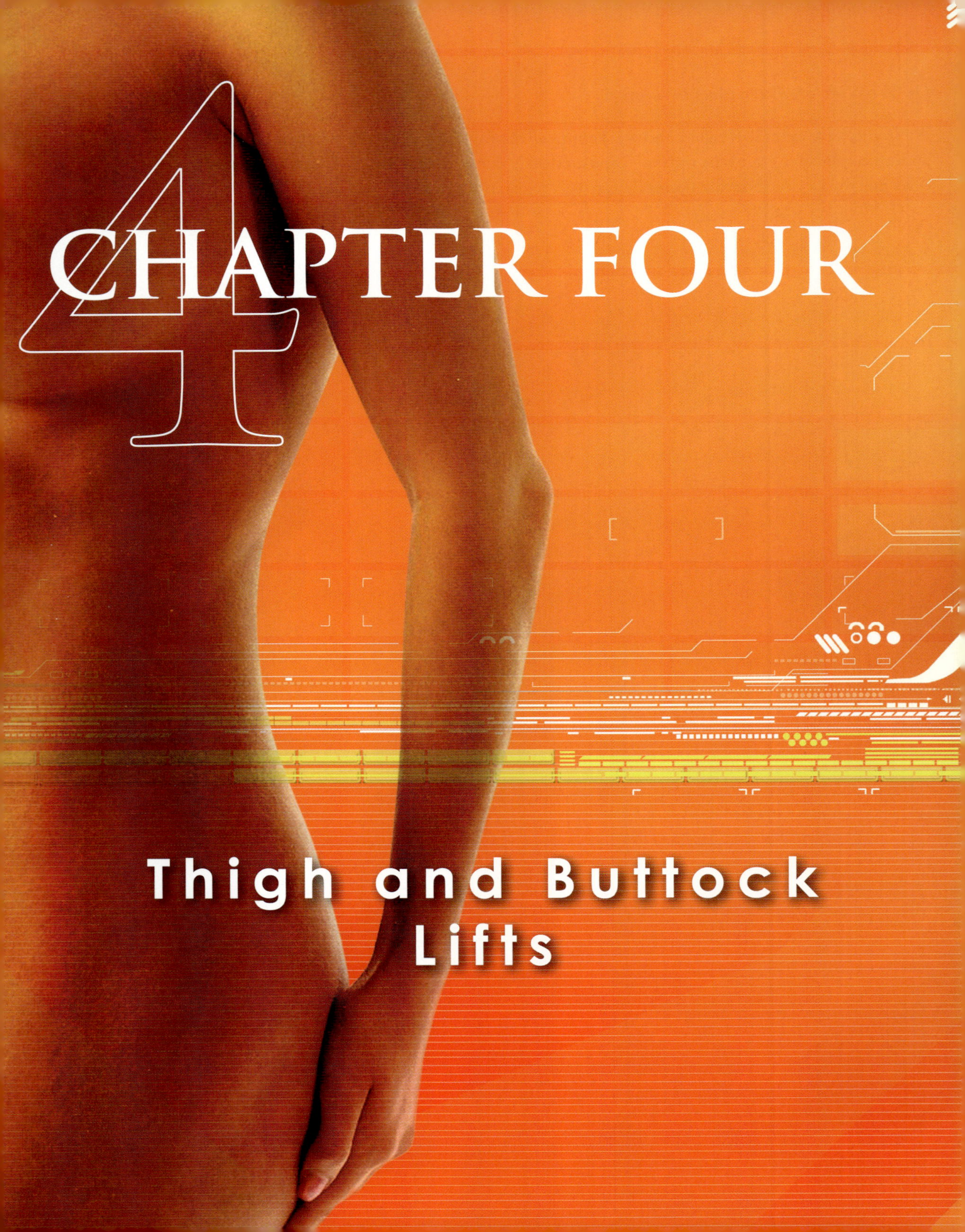

Introduction

Plastic surgeons consider the inner and outer thighs separately. The outer thighs may be lifted with the buttocks in an operation called an outer thigh lift. This may be done at the same time as an abdominoplasty. The combined procedure—outer thigh/buttock lift and abdominoplasty—is called a lower body lift. This operation is becoming more popular as more patients are losing large amounts of weight from dieting and after gastric bypasses or Lap-Band ("laparascopic adjustable banding") procedures.

The inner thighs have been a source of frustration for patients and plastic surgeons. The traditional technique for an inner thigh lift (also called a medial thigh lift) makes use of an incision that parallels the groin crease, on the skin of the upper inner thigh. Problems include limited effectiveness for the lower inner thigh (it only tightens the skin of the upper half of the inner thigh) and possible tension, which may pull across the groin, even pulling on the opening of the vagina.

This technique is very effective for removing extra skin that is distributed around the circumference of the thigh.

Recently, a different approach has been advocated—a longitudinal excision of excess skin from the inner thighs. This leaves a scar down the inseam of the thigh (See A.D., Patient Photographs), similar in concept to an arm lift. This technique is very effective for removing extra skin that is distributed around the circumference of the thigh. For patients with very loose skin, particularly after massive weight loss, the tradeoff is favorable. It has become my preferred technique for treatment of loose skin of the inner thigh.

This patient had inner thigh lifts performed one year previously. The vertical scar runs along the inseam of the inner thigh where it is not easily seen.

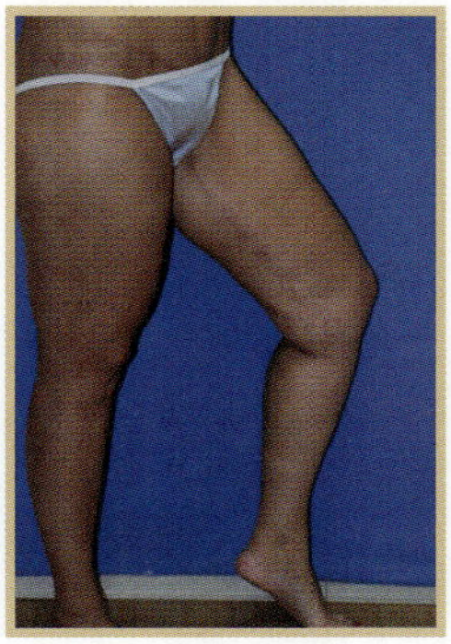

1 year after

How It's Done

The extra tissue to be removed is marked before surgery. In an outer thigh lift, the excess tissue is removed at the level of the waist. In the past, excisions have been tried lower on the thigh, at the level of the buttock crease (where the back of the thigh meets the buttock), but this placement leaves unnatural scars.

Plastic surgeons have learned it is better to place the scar up higher so as not to cause scarring in the normal ("inferior gluteal") crease under the buttock. The transition between buttock and thigh is ideally a smooth one, and scar-free. This higher placement, at the level of the hip, coincides with the level of the abdominoplasty scar. The excess skin and fat is removed, and the tissues of the outer thigh and buttock are elevated and sutured at this bikini-line level.

The buttocks may be injected with fat simultaneously, or some of the excess flank tissue may be preserved and transposed as a buried flap to augment the buttocks. This maneuver can be helpful for patients who have lost weight and have flat buttocks (See V.B., Intraoperative Photographs, Massive Weight Loss).

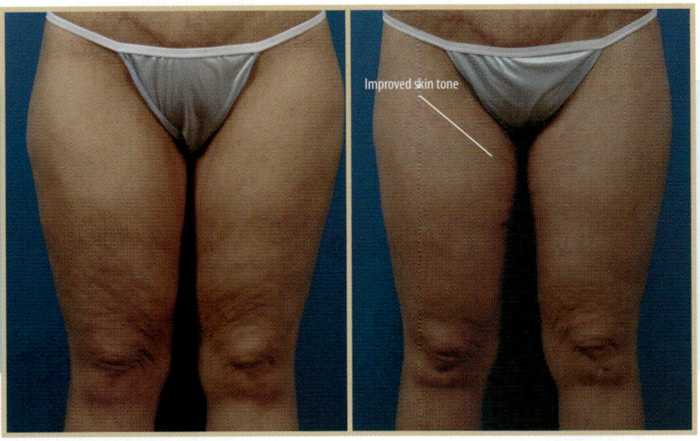

before *6 weeks after*

Inner thigh lifts and revision of outer thigh lifts.

Comments: This patient lost 150 pounds after a gastric bypass. She had a previous outer and inner thigh lift elsewhere in which the groin crease incision was used. This surgery did not adequately correct the circumferential skin excess of her thighs, especially the area above her knees. Accordingly, a longitudinal approach was used, providing a greater degree of skin tightening than the traditional incision in the groin crease. Her scar is inconspicuous, placed to coincide with the inseam of her thigh (See previous page).

Height: 5'7"
Weight: 144 lbs.
BMI: 22.2

Children: 2
Flap weights: right 42 grams, left 34 grams
A.D., age 33, registered nurse

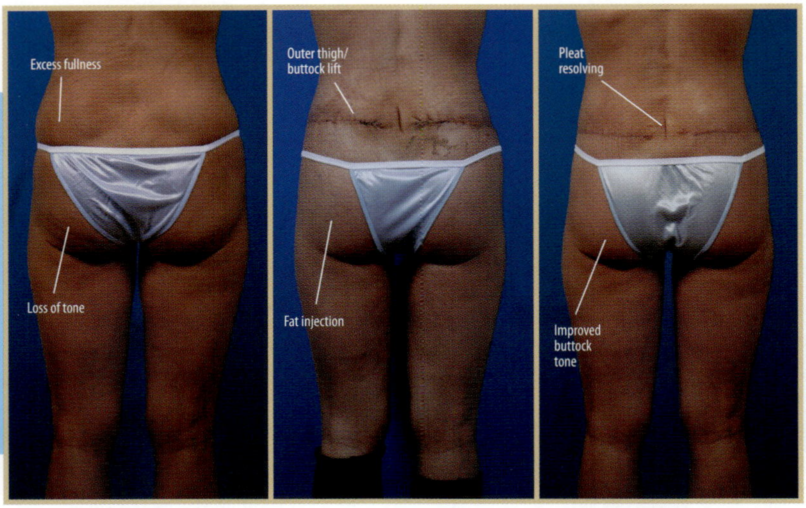

before *3 weeks after* *3 months after*

Outer thigh and buttock lifts, ultrasonic liposuction of abdomen, inner and outer thighs, and flanks, and fat injection of buttocks (80 cc per side).

Comments: This patient was concerned by sagging of her buttocks and thighs. She wanted to improve her tone and trim down her thighs and flanks. Remarkably, she drove herself to her appointment the day after surgery. She liked the tight feeling of her thighs and buttocks. Within a month she was working out again. The pleat of the middle of the back gradually settles down on its own. The incision is contained within her bikini lines, so it remains concealed.

Height: 5'10"
Weight before: 146 lbs.
BMI: 20.7

Children: 2
Liposuction volume: 675 cc
Flap weights: right 266 grams, left 272 grams
R.S., age 33, sales manager

Inner and outer thigh lifts, liposuction of abdomen, flanks, and thighs, and revision of abdominal scar.

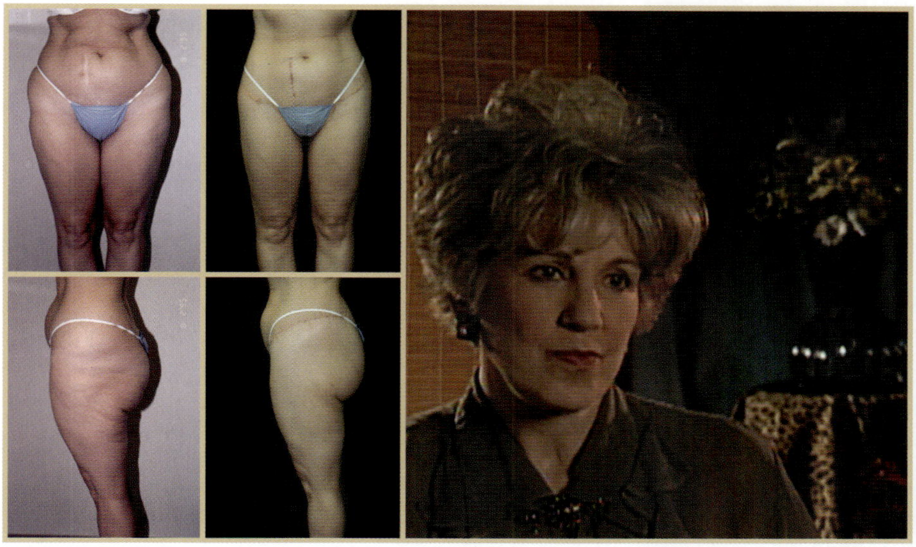

before *8 months after* *L.S.*

Testimonial: "All of my adult life I had trouble finding clothes to fit. If they would go over my hips they would be way too big in the waist. This made it very difficult to buy clothes, extremely difficult to wear slacks. I always wanted to be able to wear white slacks without bulges. I went through years of exercise, years of jogging, years of walking, years of dieting and still didn't get rid of what we call the saddlebag thighs. I was always embarrassed by my appearance in shorts. Now I can wear shorts and not feel self-conscious.

I would advise anyone considering any type of plastic surgery to not be shy about it, to not be hesitant about it. Don't be embarrassed because you feel like your thigh bulges are bigger than anybody else's. I know we all tend to see ourselves terribly when we obsess about these figure flaws. I would suggest to anybody considering it to just step right up there and ask about it. You won't be made to feel embarrassed. You will be treated with respect and dignity, and all your options will be laid out before you, and you can make your choice, you can make an informed decision and informed choice, and I would urge anybody considering plastic surgery to go for it.

The liposuction and thigh lift was my first cosmetic procedure with Dr. Swanson. I was so pleased with the results that I have since had two facial procedures. Now I feel like my rejuvenation is complete."

Height: 5'6"
Weight before: 148 lbs.
BMI: 23.5
Children: 1
Weight after: 152 lbs.
Liposuction volume: 4,050 cc
L.S., age 50/52, educator

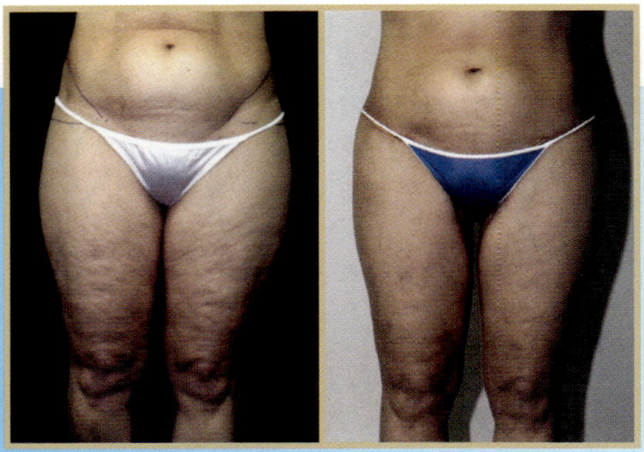

before 2 months after

Outer thighs lifts, inner thighs lifts, and liposuction of lower body.

Testimonial: "I had the lipo done because I couldn't wear shorts any more, not even to cut the grass. I was being very self-conscious about the way I looked. Also I had it done because years and years of exercising just didn't seem to help. Age, hereditary factors were creeping up faster than I could exercise. So I thought to look better in my clothes I had liposuction done.

When I put on my clothes, my jeans, shorts, I feel so much better. I feel confidence in myself. I feel like I look better. I feel great. I feel real happy about it. The bruises went away within a month. So did the swelling. I can't even find on my own body where he made the incisions.

If someone is thinking about having surgery, there must be a reason for them to think about it like myself. You must be uncomfortable about how you look or how you feel. I would say it is well-worth the money and then some. I'm glad I did it. I think it's a great way to look good. I'm glad it's out there. I'm glad it's available."

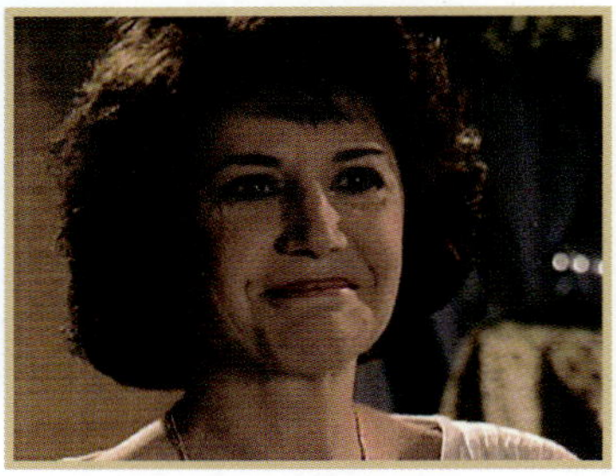

M.K.W.

Height: 5′2″
Weight before: 127 lbs.
BMI: 22.8
Liposuction volume: 2,300 cc
M.K.W., age 54, self-employed

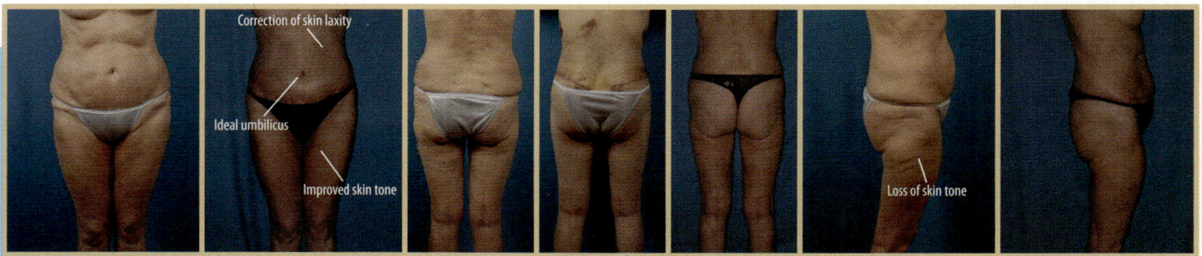

before 5½ months after before 8 days after 5½ months after before 5½ months after

Lower body lift (abdominoplasty and outer thigh/buttock lift), ultrasonic liposuction of abdomen, flanks, arms, and axillae, and fat injection of buttocks (100 cc per buttock).

Comments: This patient had a previous mini-tummy tuck and liposuction elsewhere. She was concerned about an extra roll of the upper abdomen, which she would grab to demonstrate. Also, she did not like her flank rolls. This procedure tightened the skin of the abdomen and improved the tone of her buttocks and thighs. Fat injection filled out her deficient lateral buttocks.

Height: 5′7″
Weight before: 131 lbs.
BMI: 20.2
Children: 3
Liposuction volume: 1,250 cc
Flap weight: 1 lb.
S.D., age 66/67, retired former model

What to Expect after Surgery

Fortunately, the discomfort after thigh and buttock lifts is not as severe as might be expected, particularly in view of the extent of the surgical dissections. Patient R.S. (See Patient Photographs) drove herself to her appointment the day after surgery (she did not have an abdominoplasty simultaneously). Patients do notice the tightness of the buttocks and thighs immediately after surgery and are gratified by this. They need to be careful not to stress the wounds by flexing the hips too much (a *little* flexion is needed after a simultaneous tummy tuck). My experience is that patients who have a lower body lift (abdominoplasty + outer thigh/ buttock lift) have a recovery experience that is not substantially different from an abdominoplasty alone. There is minimal extra discomfort from the outer thigh/buttock lift.

I do not routinely use drains when performing thigh and buttock lifts. I limit undermining and do not use cutting electrocautery, which I believe reduces the risk of seromas (fluid collections) after surgery. Nevertheless, seromas do occur and when they do, they need to be drained by inserting a needle in the office on multiple occasions. As the lymphatics regenerate, the fluid accumulation gradually diminishes and eventually stops.

Complications

Seroma

Seromas are relatively common (about one-third of patients) because large areas may be undermined, particularly when thigh lifts are done in combination with an abdominoplasty.

Infection

Any increased redness, purulent drainage, or fever can signal an infection. Any drainage is cultured, and antibiotics are prescribed.

Wound Opening (Dehiscence)

Tension is intentionally placed on the deep connective tissue layer (fascia) to correct the tissue sagging, which of course is the objective of surgery. The closure is subjected to stress from hip flexion. Occasionally, the wound may partially open. This is called a dehiscence. If the opening is small, it is allowed to heal in on its own. Larger openings require surgical closure.

Delayed Wound Healing

Skin loss along the incision line may result from compromised circulation. Old surgical scars can reduce skin circulation to the lower abdomen (See L.M., Abdominoplasty Complications). Smoking is another factor.

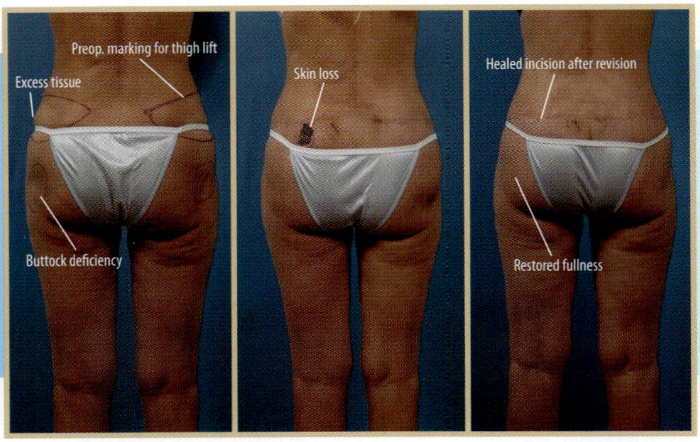

before *5 weeks after* *11 months after*

Outer thigh lifts and buttock augmentation with transposition flaps.

Comments: When this patient's dressing was removed the day after surgery, the adhesive from the tape took off a layer of skin. This was not just a superficial loss, but a full-thickness skin loss. The wound was allowed to heal on its own, taking advantage of the natural contraction of wound healing, which made the scar smaller and easier to revise. The scar was then removed along with additional skin on both sides. A positive effect of this secondary surgery was additional lift for the buttocks. Needless to say, adhesive tape was not used again on this patient.

Despite her complication, this patient came to a successful outcome. Her photos demonstrate the benefit of a combined outer thigh lift and flap transposition to fill out the buttocks, which tend to lose volume and tone with age. This patient's intraoperative photos showing the flap transposition are contained in the next section (Massive Weight Loss, Intraoperative Photographs). The "after" photos shown here, obtained 11 months after her original surgery, were taken just one month after her revision, so there is still some temporary pleating close to the midline.

V.B., age 53/54, director of weight loss clinic

Contour Deformity

If the deep connective tissue layer (deep fascia) is not adequately repaired, or comes loose after surgery, there may be a depression along the incision line that can be corrected with a subsequent surgical revision.

Scar Deformity

Like scars in other locations, the scar may spread and benefit from a later revision. Typically, at least six months are allowed for scar maturation prior to a scar revision. This time period allows the tissues to relax, reducing tension and optimizing the final scar appearance.

Asymmetry

Symmetry is the goal, but complete symmetry is impossible to achieve in practice. It is not unusual for patients to return for a touchup liposuction or revision of a scar to raise it or lower it, or simply to make it less conspicuous. Fortunately, small degrees of asymmetry in body contouring surgery are tolerable; very few patients are completely symmetrical to start with.

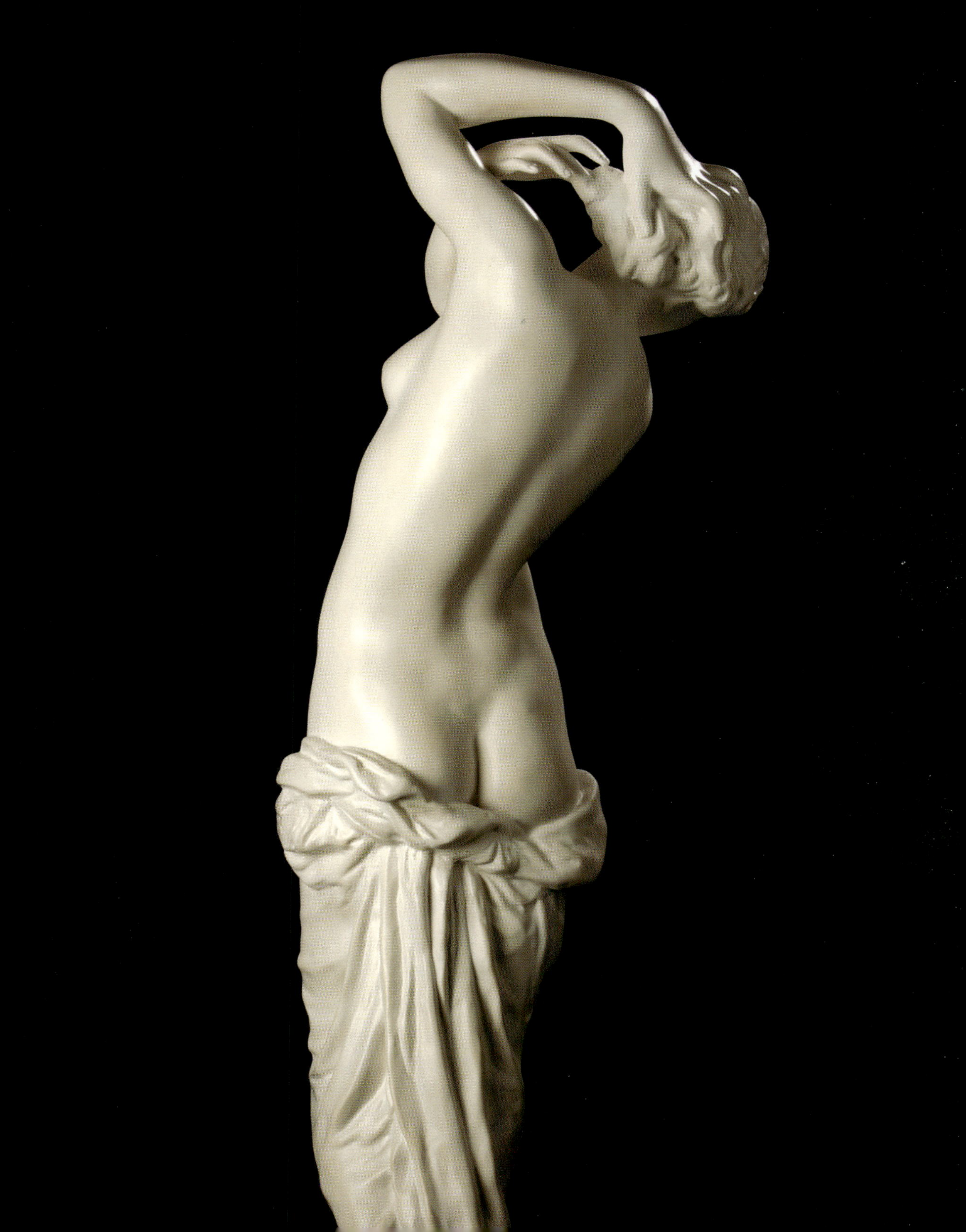

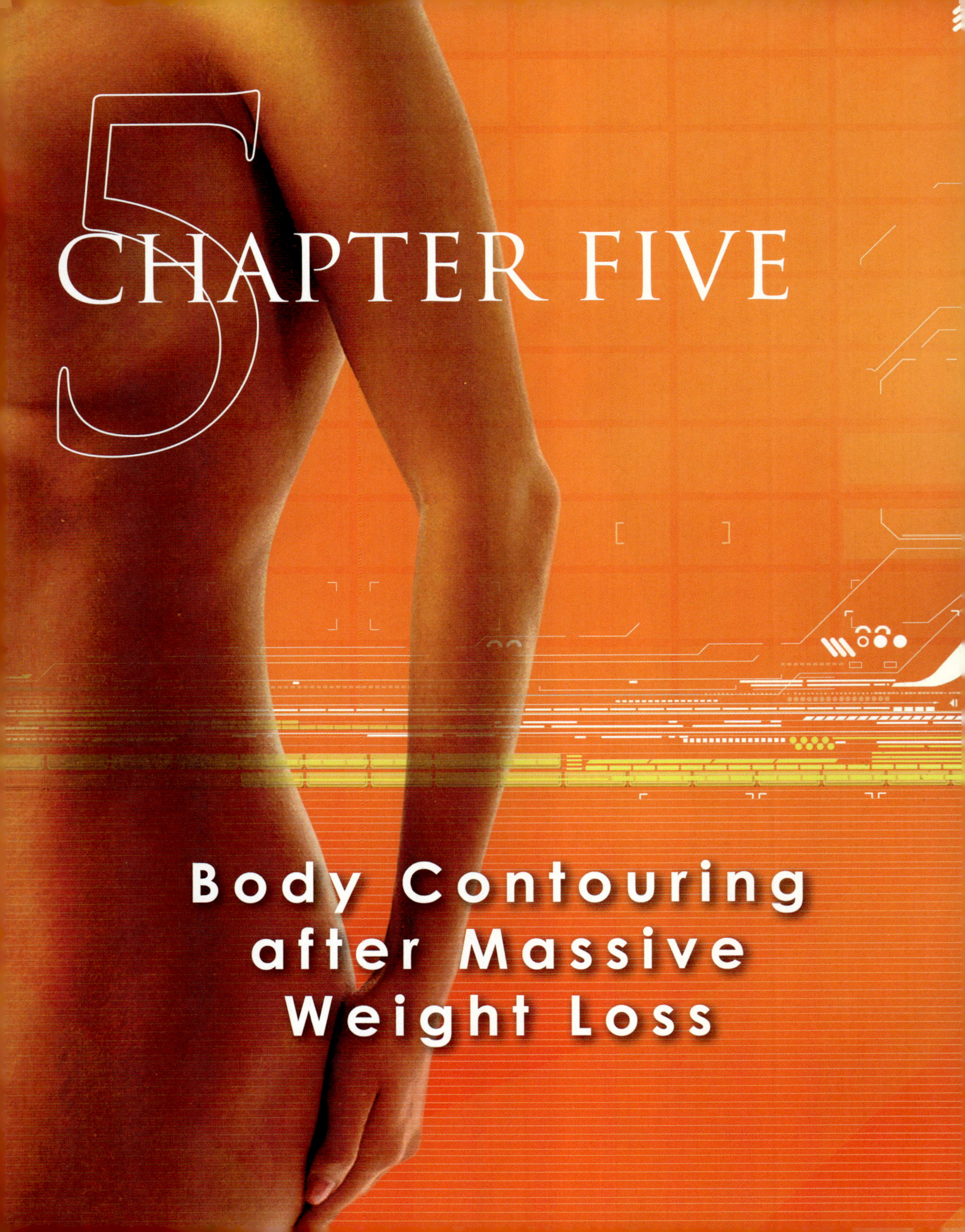

5 CHAPTER FIVE

Body Contouring after Massive Weight Loss

Introduction

Plastic surgeons are treating a growing number of patients after massive weight loss. This trend is likely due to the prevalence of obesity in America (now affecting one in three adults) and greater public awareness of this problem and the health consequences. Newer surgical remedies such as Lap-Band® (laparascopic adjustable banding) procedures have gained popularity.

After successfully losing a great deal of weight (75 pounds or more), patients are often disappointed to find that their tissues do not contract as much as they would like, leaving folds of redundant skin. The face, neck, arms, breasts, trunk, thighs, and knees may all be affected. The breasts deflate. The buttocks appear flattened. Advertisements for weight loss products don't generally show photographs of people who have lost a lot of weight in bathing suits.

It does seem unfair that patients who successfully lose large amounts of weight should have a whole new set of issues to deal with. The skin has lost its ability to contract to take up slack. Because loose skin is a major problem, they need excisional techniques that leave long scars. And because so many areas are affected, they usually require more than one operation. Patients accept the trade-off of scars for getting rid of loose folds of skin, which are more embarrassing than scars.

Patients accept the trade-off of scars for getting rid of loose folds of skin, which are more embarrassing than scars.

However, the results are never quite as good as the surgeon would like because of the compromised skin tone. Touchups are to be expected. Because numerous procedures are done, the risk of at least one complication is high. When all problems are counted—delayed wound healing, seromas, asymmetry, and scars that may benefit from revision—the likelihood of some kind of complication approaches 100%!

Sometimes insurance pays for bariatric surgery, such as a gastric bypass or Lap-Band procedure, because of the medical problems caused by obesity and the expense in treating such problems later. However, insurance does not typically pay for treatment of the skin deformities that result from massive weight loss. For patients that just paid for their bariatric surgery, or even those who were fortunate to have it covered by their insurance, the thought of paying much more for their plastic surgery can be disappointing. Indeed, obesity and its consequences are not to be underestimated.

A trusting patient-physician relationship is the key, along with the understanding that treatment will be ongoing over a period of months to years. With proper education, these patients can be very happy, and the results can indeed be life-changing (See S.S., Patient Photographs).

Nutritional Status

Patients who undergo Lap-Band surgery do not tend to have nutritional deficiencies because the absorptive capability of the digestive tract is preserved. The digestive tract remains intact. It is a purely restrictive procedure. A small gastric pouch and outlet are created, so that patients feel satisfied earlier. Absorption is preserved, and nutritional deficiency is unlikely. This is the most common bariatric procedure performed today and the safest.

By contrast, gastric bypass surgery, most commonly the Roux-en-Y procedure, not only reduces the stomach size, but also interferes with absorption of nutrients ("malabsorption"), by literally bypassing portions of the digestive tract. These patients are often anemic, as a result of reduced absorption of iron, vitamin B12, and folate, and need to supplement their diets accordingly. One-third of gastric bypass patients may remain iron-deficient, even with oral supplementation. Their hemoglobin levels are often below normal or borderline. In addition, they may be deficient in protein, vitamin A and C, selenium and zinc—all important nutrients for wound healing and immune function. These patients may have a more dramatic weight reduction than Lap-Band patients, but their nutrition is jeopardized.

Possible Hospital Admission

Combination procedures can increase surgical blood loss because of greater tissue resections. This needs to be considered in surgical planning. Patients need to be aware of the possible need for a blood transfusion.

Hospital admission is a possibility, especially for patients with low preoperative hemoglobin levels who may require a blood transfusion. As discussed above, after gastric bypass surgery, it is common for the hemoglobin level to remain below normal, due to reduced absorption of iron. Such borderline-anemic patients may be pre-treated with erythropoietin, a hormone that can boost the hemoglobin level by stimulating the production of red blood cells.

How It's Done

Surgery in Stages

A "battle plan" is developed at the first consultation. It is usually best to treat the patient's priorities first. An abdominoplasty is typically the first order of business. This is done with simultaneous liposuction. If the outer thighs and buttocks are saggy, a lower body lift is recommended, which is a tummy tuck and an outer thigh/buttock lift done at the same time. Sometimes an inner thigh lift is done as well, either at the first operation or a subsequent one. It is more common today to use a longitudinal incision down the inseam of the inner thigh, rather than an incision in the groin crease, to remove the greatest amount of excess skin and provide maximum circumferential tightening of the thigh.

Today we recognize the importance of augmenting the buttocks, which usually appear flat after major weight loss.

Today we recognize the importance of augmenting the buttocks, which usually appear flat after major weight loss. Fat injection may be done, or flaps raised at the time of the outer thigh lift may be transposed to fill out the buttocks (See Intraoperative Photographs, next page).

The second operation may be a breast lift. Usually implants are used to restore lost volume and provide upper pole fullness. This large topic is covered in the separate volume, *Ideal Breast*. Brachioplasties may be done simultaneously. It is not unusual to do a touchup liposuction or scar revision at the same time.

The third operation may involve some fine-tuning—more liposuction, revision of a scar, or tightening of a lift. A facelift may be considered, although most patients are more concerned about their body and defer this procedure for another time.

The sequence of procedures is individualized according to the patient's priorities. Most patients wish to get as much accomplished in one operation as is feasible. This is understandable. The surgeon needs to maximize efficiency to get as much done as possible while avoiding overly lengthy surgery or excessive blood loss.

Intraoperative Photographs

Outer thigh/buttock lift with simultaneous buttock augmentation using a pedicled flap. The excess tissue from her hip is used to fill her buttock. No tissue goes to waste. This patient's before-and-after photos are contained in the Thigh Lift section (See V.B., Thigh Lift Complications)

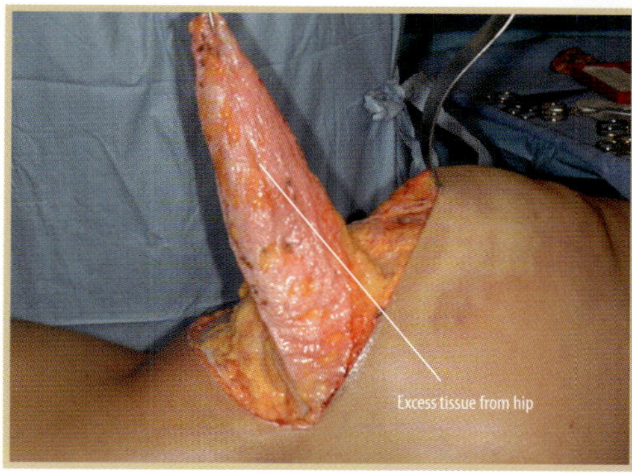

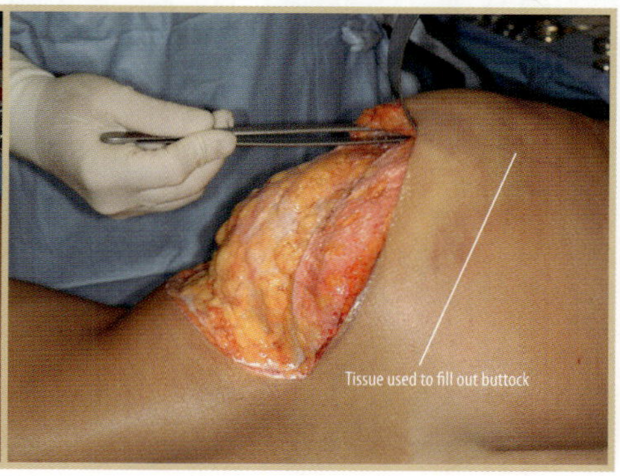

Patient Photographs

Females

Abdominoplasty and ultrasonic liposuction of abdomen, flanks, inner thighs, arms, and axillae.

Comments: This patient lost 100 pounds after a Lap-Band procedure performed three years previously. She was pleased that she could now see her belly button. She is still quite swollen, less than a month after surgery. Her outer thighs were relatively unaffected and were not treated. She plans to return for a breast lift and implants.

Height: 5'6"
Weight before: 185 lbs.
BMI: 29.4
Children: 1
Liposuction volume: 2,200 cc
Flap weight: 7 lbs.
A.J., age 36, manager

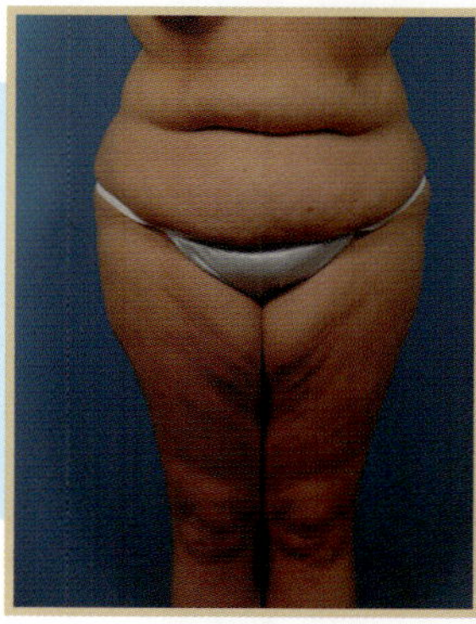

before

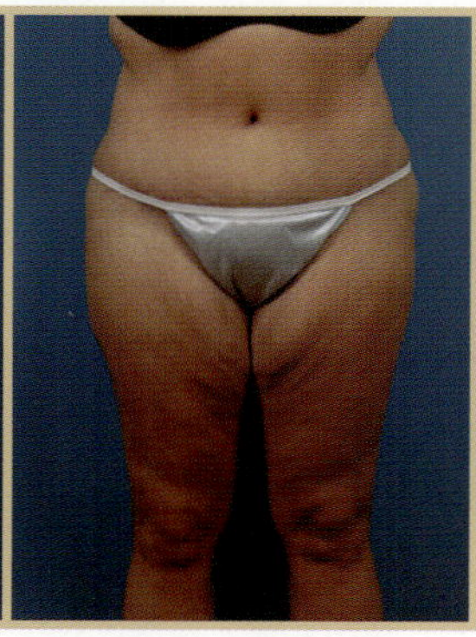

3½ weeks after

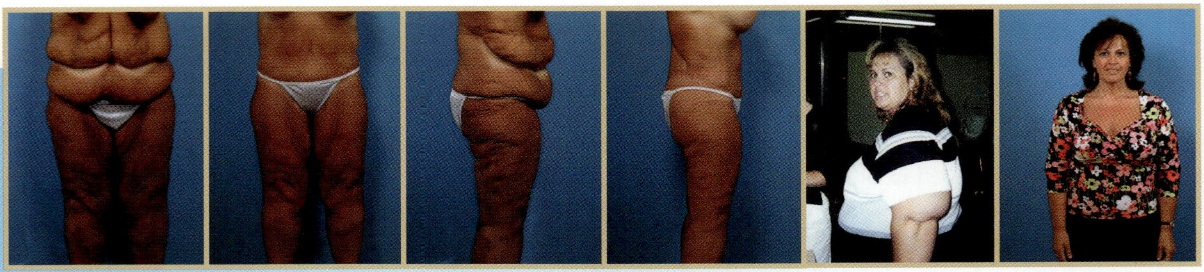

before *2 months after* *before* *2 months after* *before weight loss* *2 mos. after 2nd surgery*

Lower body lift and ultrasonic liposuction of inner thighs, knees, and medial calves. Second procedure, 3 weeks later: breast augmentation, breast lift, ultrasonic liposuction of arms, brachioplasties, and inner thigh lifts.

Comments: This 42-year-old single mother lost 150 pounds after a gastric bypass. Her surgery was performed in two stages, spaced three weeks apart. The photos were taken two months after her second operation. She returned later for removal of additional loose skin of the inner thighs using a longitudinal incision along her inseam. A confident person to start with, she reported a huge improvement in self-esteem. She had gotten married the last time I saw her in follow-up, and commented that her husband did not mind the scars, which he called a "road map to his favorite places."

Height: 5'5"
Weight before: 191 lbs.
BMI: 31.2
Children: 1
Weight after: 190 lbs.

Flap weight: 10 lbs. (abdominal)
Liposuction volume: 900 cc, touchup: 500 cc
Dress size before: 14/16
Dress size after: 8/10
S.S., age 42, analyst

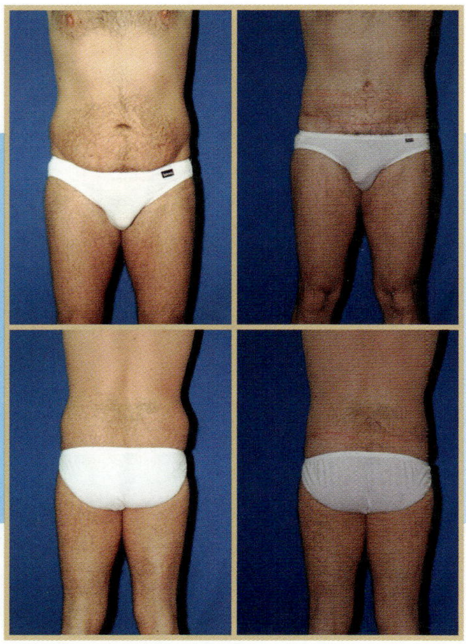

before *5 months after*

Males

Lower body lift (abdominoplasty, outer thigh and buttock lift) and ultrasonic liposuction of abdomen, flanks, and breasts.

Comments: This patient had lost about 70 pounds. A lower body lift was performed, using an incision that ran almost all the way around his trunk, elevating the buttocks and removing the excess abdominal skin. Liposuction was performed simultaneously. Note the improvement of his love handles. The scar is still red at this point, but will fade to white in time. He has some skin markings from the binder he was wearing when these pictures were taken.

Height: 6'0"
Weight before: 189 lbs.
BMI: 25.2
Liposuction volume: 1,150 cc
Flap weight: 4 lbs. (abdominal), 2 lbs. (excess flank tissue)
K.K., age 37, registered nurse

Abdominoplasty, inner thigh lifts, and ultrasonic liposuction of inner thighs, flanks, outer thighs, knees, axillae, and breasts.

Comments: The patient had a gastric bypass 30 years previously and subsequently lost about 200 pounds. He finally decided to have surgery after his wife had a tummy tuck. As expected, he has marked skin laxity of the abdomen and thighs. He also had an unusual (for men) gynecoid fat distribution, affecting the outer thighs, which were treated with liposuction. He was able to stand straight up in four days. He took only two weeks off work. After surgery, he commented that putting on clothing was much easier and he no longer experienced back pain. His memorable comment was, "Everything is better now."

Height: 6'0"
Weight before: 264 lbs.
BMI: 34.3
Weight after: 258 lbs.
Flap weight: 10 lbs.
Liposuction volume: 3,325 cc
Waist before: 45 in.
Waist after: 42 in.
H.B., age 61, health care administrator

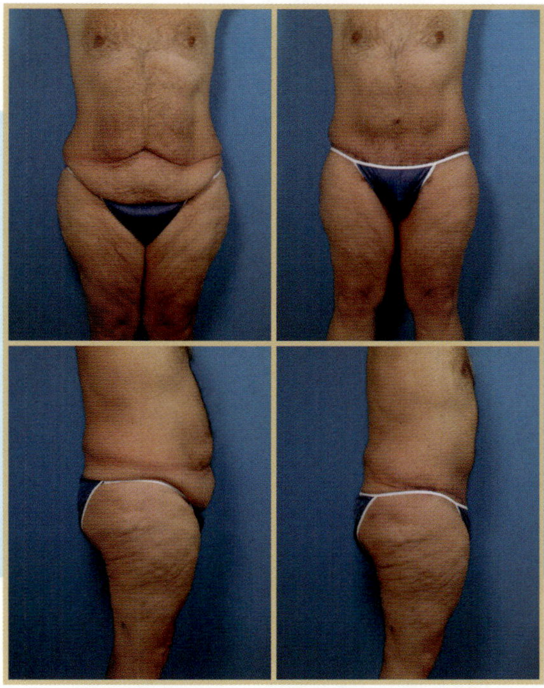

before *5 months after*

What to Expect after Surgery

Surgery after massive weight loss usually involves a combination of procedures—abdominoplasty, thigh and buttock lift, breast lift (usually with implants), brachioplasty, and liposuction. The reader is directed to these sections (and, for women, the separate volume, *Ideal Breast*) to learn what to expect after these procedures.

Complications

Surgery to treat deformities that result from major weight loss is a major undertaking, which is why the work is typically done in stages. There is a saying in surgery, "major surgery—major complications." Some surgeons have reported complication rates as high as 100%. Indeed, the complication rate depends on how you define a complication. Seromas are relatively common (about one-third of patients) because large areas may be undermined when thigh lifts are done in combination with an abdominoplasty.

Complications include infection, delayed wound healing, scar deformities, asymmetry, and contour deformities. The skin will never be as taut as it was before being stretched out by obesity. Scarring is significant. However, these patients are grateful for the improvement, and tend to value elimination of loose skin over scarring. Touchup procedures are common and should be regarded as part of the process.

Deep Venous Thrombosis

Deep venous thrombosis can occur after any long procedure, and the risk may be as high as 9% in patients undergoing body contouring surgery after massive weight loss, occurring almost exclusively in patients who remain obese (BMI>35). Sequential compression devices are used and patients ambulate as soon as they awaken in the recovery room.

Care after Surgery

Postoperative instructions are contained in the preceding Abdominoplasty and Thigh Lift sections.

Frequently Asked Questions

Q: How much weight can you take off?

A: Actually, the weight of the tissue removed at surgery is not as much as you might think, typically less than 10 pounds. However, large sections of skin are removed, and this can make a dramatic difference in appearance.

Q: How much surgery can be done at one time?

A: Patients usually want to have as much done at one time as possible to maximize their result and reduce trips to the operating room. However, it is rarely possible to achieve all the goals in one operation. Usually the priorities are treated first. Financial reality may mean that some things will just have to wait. The surgeon makes a judgment about what combination of procedures can be done in a reasonable time frame, without incurring excessive blood loss. My own practice is to limit the surgery time to about six hours. However, with efficient use of operating time and techniques to reduce blood loss, we can often accomplish quite a lot in this time (See Patient Photographs).

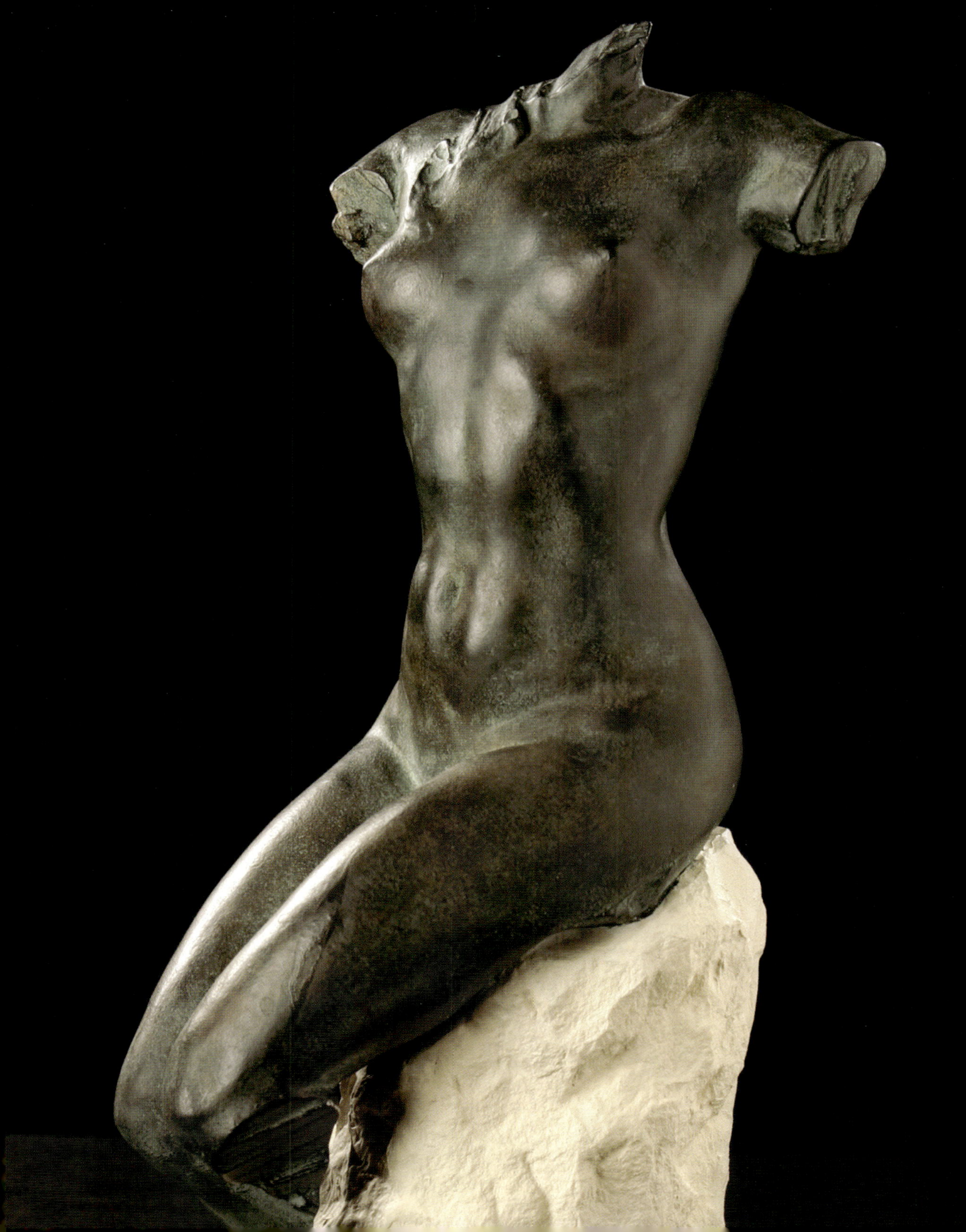

CHAPTER SIX

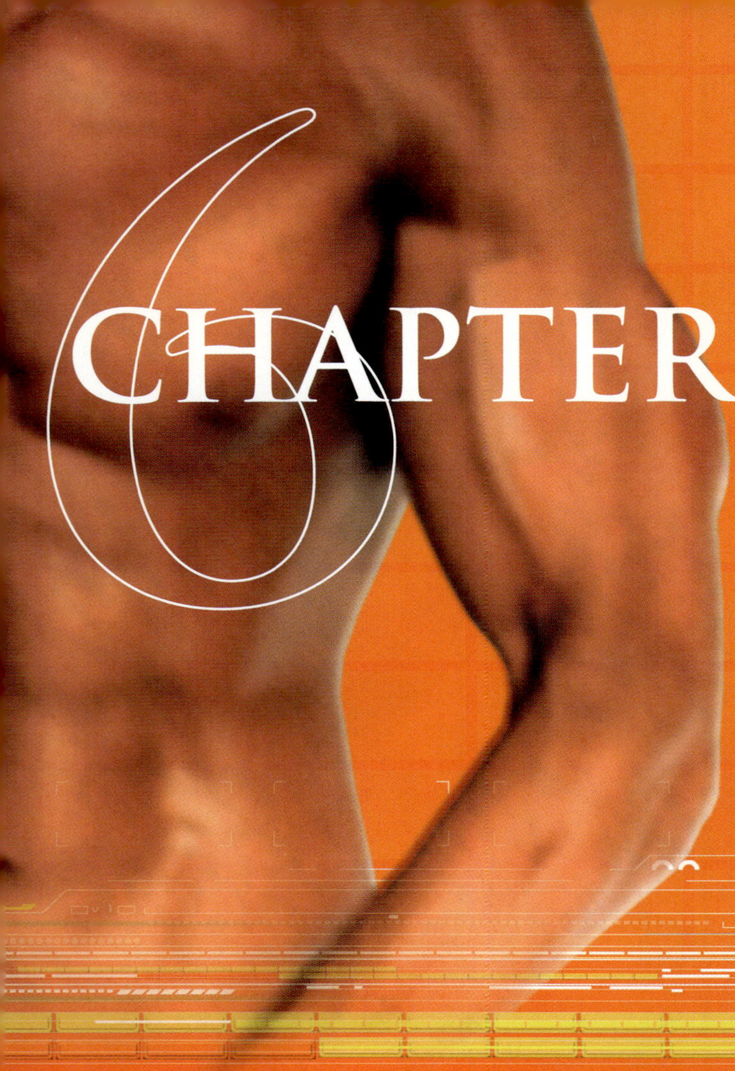

Breast Reduction in Men

Introduction

We tend to think of breast reduction as a female procedure, but many men also opt to have their breasts reduced. "Gynecomastia" is the term for enlargement of male breasts. It is a common condition, affecting about one-third of males overall, and an even larger percentage of adolescent boys and men over 65.

What Causes Breast Enlargement in Men?

Most of the time, there is no known cause. The problem is cosmetic. Men feel self-conscious without a shirt, and in severe cases, even with a shirt on. Gynecomastia can start with puberty, resolving on its own in most cases, or develop in older men as the balance of circulating testosterone and estrogen shifts toward the latter.

Men feel self-conscious without a shirt, and in severe cases, even with a shirt on.

Sometimes gynecomastia may be caused by a specific drug or medical problem. Chronic alcoholics and men who use anabolic steroids as part of a bodybuilding program are more likely to develop this condition. Certain hormonal abnormalities, inherited or acquired, usually involving either a deficiency of testosterone or excess of estrogen, can cause breast enlargement. Hyperthyroidism can cause it too. Marijuana and cancer chemotherapeutic agents can bring it on. Gynecomastia can also be a side effect of a number of heart and blood pressure medications. In rare cases it may be associated with an estrogen-producing testicular tumor. If one of these medical conditions is suspected, the patient is referred to another specialist for investigation. Usually insurance companies regard this condition as cosmetic.

Most commonly, there is no underlying hormonal imbalance and no medical cause. Gynecomastia is seen predominantly in two age groups: (1) young men, whose pubertal breast bud development did not go away, and (2) men aged 50 and over, when breast development can occur due to hormonal changes. Excess breast tissue is unresponsive to diet and exercise.

The problem is not trivial. Men have told me, "This makes me feel like I'm a woman," even one memorable heavily-tattooed patient of mine who competes as an ultimate fighter. Another patient, a successful trial attorney in his early 60s, told me after surgery, "For the first time in my life, I feel normal." He said he thought his breast problem had made him try to overcompensate by being aggressive professionally. One young man told me he faked hydrophobia as a teenager, even to the point of seeing a psychiatrist, so he would not have to take off his shirt for swimming classes in high school. Another told me no one had seen him without his shirt off since he was 15, *including his fiancée*. The psychological implications of this eminently correctable problem can be profound.

How It's Done

There are two treatments:

- **Liposuction.** Excess fat is suctioned from the breasts, a familiar technique.

- **Excision of Breast Tissue.** Breast tissue is excised using an incision along the lower margin of the areola for access. This operation has the awkward and unnecessarily alarming name "subcutaneous mastectomies." Often, liposuction is performed simultaneously to remove fatty tissue of the breast and its lateral extension below the armpit, and to smooth the contours.

Liposuction Alone

Liposuction alone may be used to treat breasts that are primarily fatty in consistency. Often liposuction of the breasts is performed at the same time as liposuction of the abdomen and flanks. In fact, one-third of men in my practice who have liposuction of the abdomen and flanks decide to have their breasts treated too. They say, "While I'm there, let's get it done." This breast tissue can be quite fibrous, and ultrasound helps to break down the fat component, facilitating its removal.

Liposuction is not very effective in removing breast tissue itself. Consequently, only about half of the overall breast volume (the fatty component) may be removed using liposuction on its own, and less in young men who have firmer breasts (i.e., more breast tissue, less fat). If a 50% reduction is acceptable to the patient, liposuction alone is the procedure of choice. This includes most older men whose priority is their abdomen and flanks, and some reduction of the breasts is a bonus. Men who want a more dramatic reduction, or whose excess breast tissue is a priority, need to consider another option—direct excision.

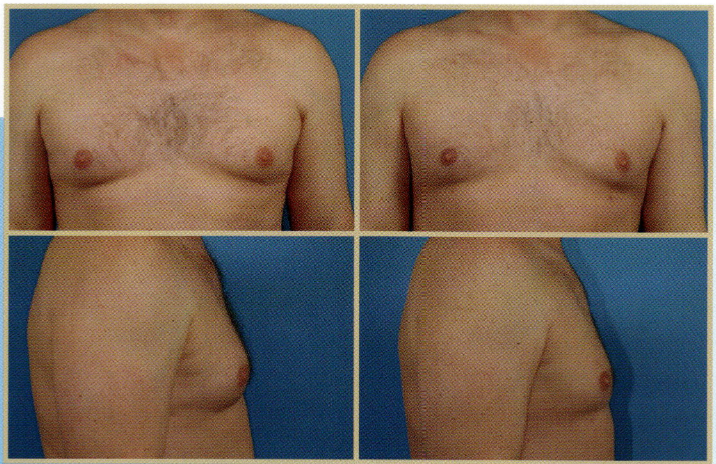

before *3 months after*

Ultrasonic liposuction of abdomen, flanks, breasts, and axillae, and submental lipectomy.

Comments: This patient was most concerned about unwanted fat around his waist and flanks. He decided to have his breasts treated ("while I'm there"). The before-and-after photos show a reduction of perhaps 50%. The short inframammary incisions, located just below the breasts are inconspicuous three months after surgery. These before-and-after photos demonstrate the degree of improvement to be expected after liposuction alone, without any additional excisional surgery (i.e., no cutting tissue, just liposuction). There is no periareolar scar.

Height: 6'0"
Weight: 230 lbs.
BMI: 31.2
Right breast liposuction volume: 200 cc
Left breast liposuction volume: 250 cc
J.B., age 41, sales

Male Breast Reduction (Excision of Breast Tissue)

Breast tissue itself is difficult to remove by liposuction alone because it is a denser tissue type than fat. Young men with firm breasts or patients who desire a dramatic change in profile (i.e., a flat chest) and bodybuilders who want to emphasize their pectoral muscles are better served by direct excision (subcutaneous mastectomies). Liposuction is usually done at the same time to remove the fatty component and also to treat the axillary areas where there is often a fat roll extending around the chest on either side.

Young men with firm breasts or bodybuilders who want to emphasize their pectoral muscles are better served by direct excision.

When breast tissue is excised, a longer incision is needed to allow enough room for the surgeon to insert scissors to cut out excess breast tissue. The "periareolar" incision follows the lower border of the areola, where it is well-concealed in this natural boundary. A separate small incision in the inframammary crease is used for simultaneous liposuction (this is the only incision used when liposuction is done alone). This inframammary incision serves dual purpose as an opening for the drain, which is secured with a suture at this site until it is removed a few days after surgery. The periareolar incision is closed in layers using deep absorbable sutures and a running Prolene nonabsorbable suture in the skin. This suture is removed about a week after surgery.

It is important to note that subcutaneous mastectomies remove breast tissue, not skin. If the breasts are particularly large and the skin loose (which may happen after massive weight loss), it may be necessary to remove skin at the same time as breast tissue. While this is done commonly in women as part of a breast reduction, skin removal is usually not required in men. Although the skin may not be as tight as we'd like, it contracts to some extent, and the result is usually acceptable and avoids the additional scarring that would result from a skin excisional procedure.

While breast reduction scars are concealed by a bikini top in women, breast scars are not so easily hidden in men when they go shirtless. Ideally, the surgery should allow a man to expose his chest without feeling self-conscious. Therefore, the scars need to be kept to a minimum so as not to exchange one cosmetic flaw for another.

Occasionally the surgeon has no choice—there is simply too much skin—and an operation resembling the female breast reduction (but without leaving much breast tissue behind, so the chest is almost flat) is undertaken. Patients are happy to be rid of the unwanted breast tissue and loose skin, but they may not be comfortable without a shirt because of the scars. Fortunately, a skin-excisional procedure is seldom needed in men, and when it is necessary, these men are very happy to be rid of their "man boobs"—the scars are an acceptable trade-off.

Intraoperative Photographs

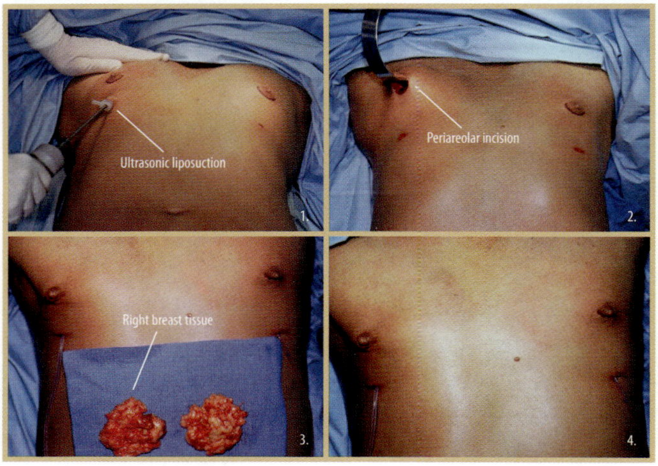

Comments: These photographs show the surgical steps used to remove breast tissue. *(Above, left)* The area is first treated with ultrasonic liposuction to remove fatty tissue. *(Above, right)* Periareolar incisions allow access for direct excision of excess breast tissue. *(Below, left)* The tissue removed is composed of firm glandular breast tissue (the white part) and yellowish fatty tissue mixed in. *(Below, right)* The incisions are closed. The liposuction incisions are used to secure the drains, which are removed in the office in three or four days.

Patient Photographs

Male Breast Reduction – Teenager

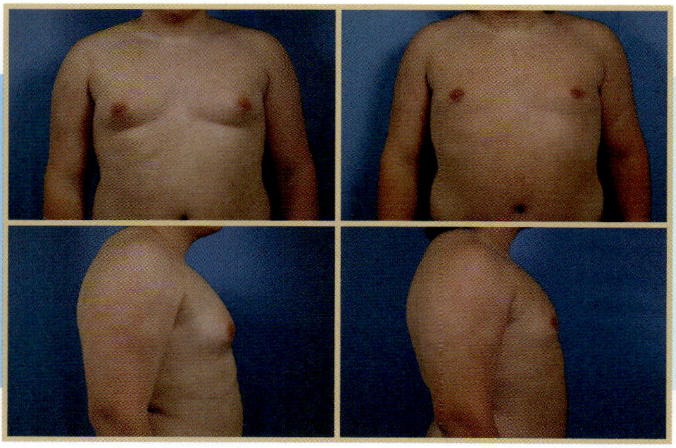

before ***2½ years after***

Subcutaneous mastectomies, ultrasonic liposuction of abdomen, flanks, breasts, and axillae, and submental lipectomy.

Comments: This 15-year-old's self-confidence improved after this unwanted breast tissue was eliminated. Pubertal gynecomastia is common. If it persists, it can have profound psychological ramifications.

Height: 5'10"
Weight: 221 lbs.
BMI: 31.3
Right breast: 87 grams
Left breast: 90 grams
Right breast liposuction volume: 175 cc
Left breast liposuction volume: 225 cc
J.B., age 15, student

Subcutaneous mastectomies and ultrasonic liposuction of breasts.

Comments: This 18-year-old Indian-American male was embarrassed by his breast tissue and would not take off his shirt in the summer. He was already pleased with his result, only 11 days after surgery.

Height: 5'9"
Weight: 158 lbs.
BMI: 22.9
Right breast: 47 grams
Left breast: 53 grams
Right breast liposuction volume: 175 cc
Left breast liposuction volume: 125 cc
R.P., age 18, student

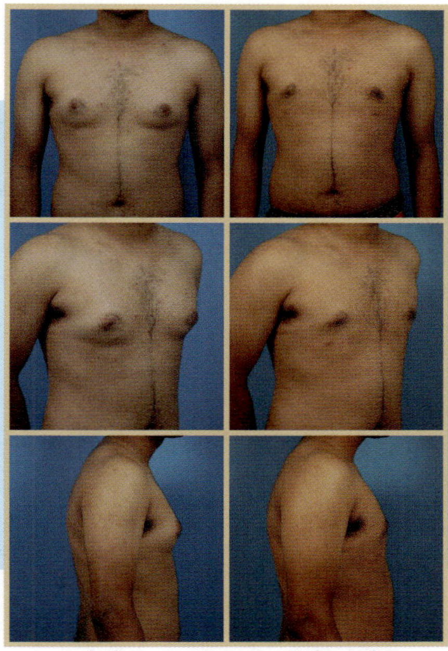

before *11 days after*

Male Breast Reduction – Twenties

Subcutaneous mastectomies, ultrasonic liposuction of breasts, abdomen, flanks, and axillae, and submental lipectomy.

Comments: This 28-year-old Pakistani-American physician had gynecomastia and fatty excess of the trunk. On the day after surgery, a hematoma was drained from the left breast. The improvement under the chin is also evident in these photographs. He said that he thought his attractiveness, on a scale of 1 -10, had increased from a 2/10 (not a flattering self-assessment by any means) to a 7/10. He had noticed a definite upswing in female interest. He was so pleased with the result, he said he would recommend this surgery for his patients. Notably, he was motivated to lose about 30 pounds. A hypertrophic scar at the left inframammary drain site was later revised.

Height: 5'6"
Weight before: 208 lbs.
BMI: 33.1
Weight after: 179 lbs.
Right breast: 75 grams
Left breast: 92 grams
Right breast liposuction volume: 200 cc
Left breast liposuction volume: 200 cc
I.H., age 28, physician

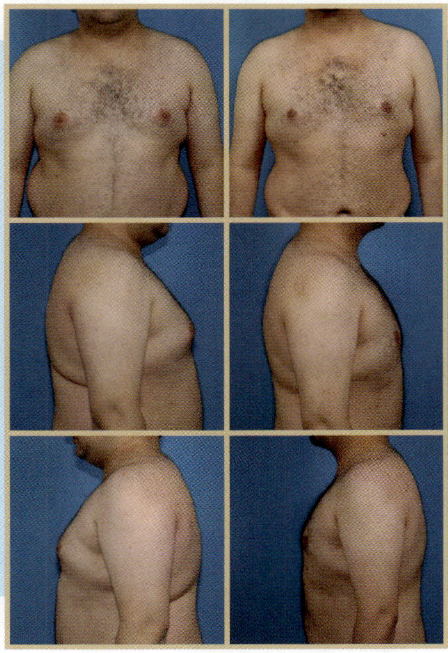

before *15 months after*

Male Breast Reduction – Thirties

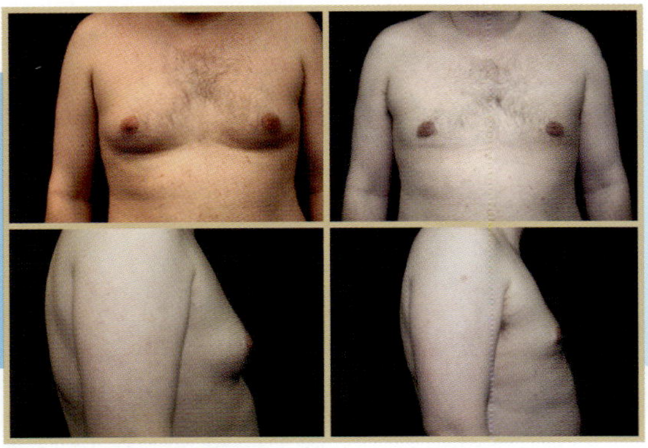

before *3 months after*

Subcutaneous mastectomies and ultrasonic liposuction of breasts.

Comments: This 37-year-old's breasts had always been a source of embarrassment to him and persisted despite weight loss.

Height: 6'2"
Weight before: 225 lbs.
BMI: 28.3
Right breast liposuction volume: 150 cc
Left breast liposuction volume: 200 cc
J.Y., age 36, production manager

Male Breast Reduction – Fitness Enthusiast

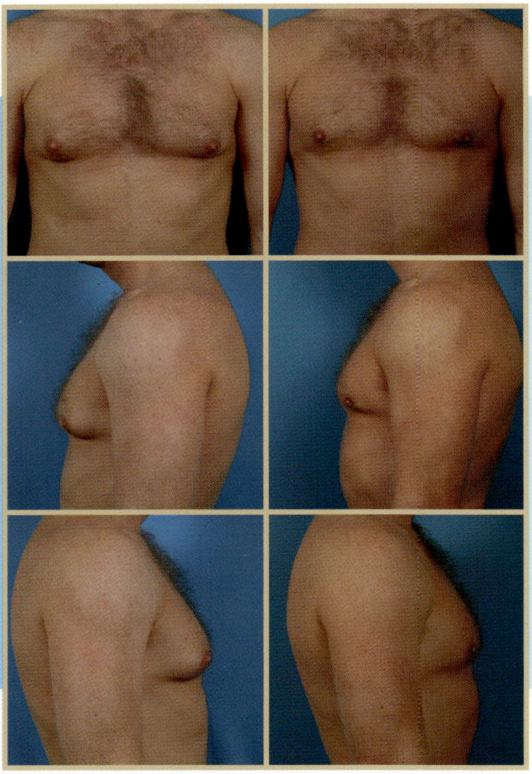

before *2½ years after*

Subcutaneous mastectomies and ultrasonic liposuction of breasts.

Comments: This 39-year-old triathlete was in excellent physical condition and very lean. His breast tissue was glandular, firm in consistency (i.e., minimal fat mixed in), and could not have been removed by liposuction alone. His periareolar incisions have healed nicely and are almost invisible. His pectoral muscle definition is more evident and his chest has a masculine appearance. Importantly, he has no telltale signs of surgery.

Height: 6'1"
Weight before: 175 lbs.
BMI: 24.0
Right breast: 25 grams
Left breast: 15 grams
Right breast liposuction volume: 150 cc
Left breast liposuction volume: 150 cc
C.C., age 39/41, attorney

Male Breast Reduction – Forties

Subcutaneous mastectomies, ultrasonic liposuction of abdomen, flanks, breasts, and axillae, submental lipectomy, and jawline augmentation.

Comments: This 40-year-old had a typical male-pattern fat distribution. His breasts made him self-conscious. After surgery, he was comfortable with his shirt off.

Height: 5'8"
Weight before: 170 lbs.
BMI: 25.5
Right breast: 52 grams
Left breast: 63 grams
Right breast liposuction volume: 200 cc
Left breast liposuction volume: 250 cc
J.G., age 40, V.P., educational resources

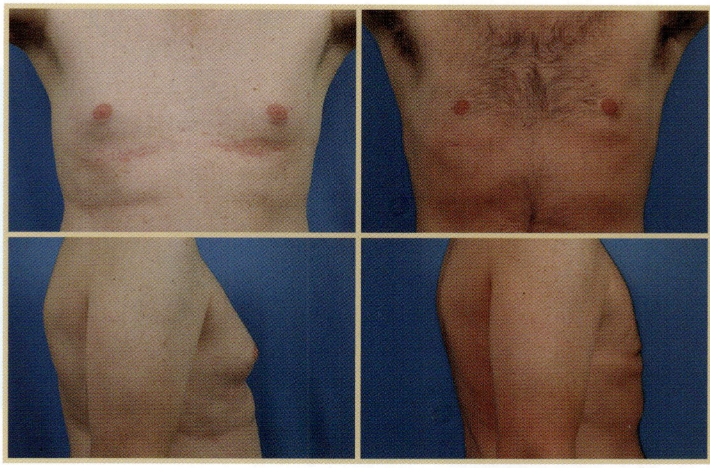

before *3 months after*

Secondary Male Breast Reduction

Secondary subcutaneous mastectomies, and ultrasonic liposuction of abdomen, flanks, and breasts.

Comments: This patient was 6'4" tall and had a very large frame. He had scoliosis (which accounts for his right shoulder being higher than the left). He had undergone previous surgery elsewhere for his gynecomastia. This redo procedure was undertaken to treat persistent excess breast tissue. Skin contraction afterward was remarkably good, so he did not require subsequent skin-tightening surgery, which would have left more visible scars.

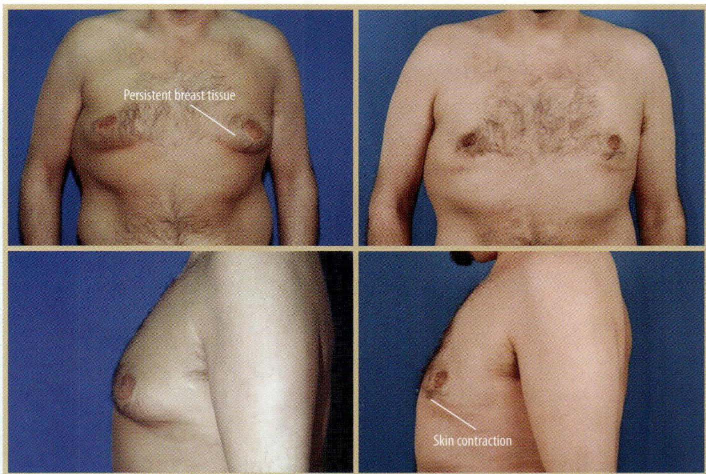

before *11 months after*

Height: 6'4"
Weight before: 236 lbs.
BMI: 28.7
Right breast liposuction volume: 225 cc
Left breast liposuction volume: 225 cc
E.W., age 37, landlord

What to Expect after Surgery

Men should expect about a 50% reduction in breast volume after liposuction alone (See J.B., Liposuction Alone). There is still breast tissue left behind. Only excisional surgery allows complete removal of the excess fat and breast tissue, and this was the procedure used in all other men presented in the preceding Patient Photographs section.

Men may return after liposuction for subcutaneous mastectomies if they want a more dramatic reduction, essentially a flat chest (there are no burnt bridges after liposuction), but it is obviously advantageous to get the job done in one procedure. Discriminating patients, for whom a flat chest is a priority (not just an add-on with liposuction of the trunk) elect to have the excisional procedure.

After Liposuction

Liposuction is not especially painful. There is some bruising and swelling, usually around the sides of the chest because the blood tracks around the sides due to gravity.

The scars from liposuction are small, one on each side, located in the natural inframammary crease under each breast. These incisions are closed with dissolving sutures.

After Excision

When breast tissue is cut out, a drain is used on each side and left in for three or four days. There is usually minimal discomfort, even after excisional surgery. In fact, the chest is numb at first. It takes a few months for the feeling to return to normal. The periareolar sutures are removed about a week after surgery.

Complications

Liposuction of the breasts is remarkably safe. Infection is very unusual, similar to liposuction of other areas of the body. Occasionally a hypertrophic scar may form (See I.H., Patient Photographs) that can be revised to make it less noticeable.

Because subcutaneous mastectomies involve sharp dissection of breast tissues and creation of a pocket (unfortunately named "dead space") where fluid can collect, a hematoma is a possibility. Any increased swelling, pain, and bruising on one side may signal a hematoma, which requires urgent surgical treatment—evacuation of the blood clot and cautery if there is a bleeding vessel.

Surface irregularities can occur. These may respond to a touchup liposuction or sometimes to fat injection to treat a depression. It is important to leave a cushion of breast tissue under the nipple to avoid a saucer-like depression, which can be difficult to correct. This problem is seen frequently in patients who have been treated by non-plastic surgeons, who may not be aware that overexcision produces this deformity. Even in lean males, there is a small amount of breast tissue that must be preserved.

Care after Surgery

- A small amount of bloody drainage on the dressing is normal.
- The dressing is removed on the day after surgery. You can then bathe and shower when you return home. There are semitransparent adhesive tapes (Steri-Strips™) on the incisions. These tapes usually stay on for several days. If one is starting to peel off, go ahead and trim it or remove it.
- Avoid strenuous activities for two weeks after surgery. Avoid any heavy lifting for two weeks. This helps prevent excessive swelling.
- Most patients are able to return to work within a week after surgery. If your work is physical you will require two weeks off.
- Strenuous exercise (examples: running, aerobics, tennis) should be avoided for three weeks. However, gentler exercise such as walking can be resumed one week after surgery. You may return to unrestricted activity one month after surgery. Your body will tell you—if your breasts are sore you are probably overdoing it.
- Once the tapes are removed, apply antibiotic ointment to the incisions, particularly any areas of crusting, twice daily. The crusts gradually come off on their own.
- Bruising is normal and usually goes away within a few weeks. It extends to the sides and abdomen because of gravity. Swelling is also to be expected and takes a month or two to resolve.
- Do not use aspirin or aspirin-containing products for at least two weeks before surgery and two weeks after surgery. They affect platelet function and may increase bleeding. Use acetaminophen (Tylenol®) instead. Acetaminophen does not affect platelet function.
- Notify the office immediately if one breast appears to be getting much larger than the other. This could signal a hematoma, which requires prompt surgical attention.
- After excisional surgery, you may wake up wearing a compression garment with Velcro straps on your chest. This can be replaced with a less cumbersome garment that provides gentle compression of the chest, such as a tight-fitting athletic shirt (Under Armour® is one brand). Usually this is done after the drains come out. The garment helps limit swelling, and most patients feel more comfortable wearing it. Most patients wear such a garment for 3-4 weeks and later while exercising.

Frequently Asked Questions

Q: What will I look like after surgery?

A: You do not see your final result right away, of course. It takes a few months for the swelling to fully go down. However, most patients notice a difference when the dressings come off the day after surgery, even with swelling. It takes about three months for the swelling to do down completely.

Q: Is it painful?

A: The surgery is not particularly painful. In fact, the breasts are numb after surgery. Gradually, the feeling returns.

Q: Are there any side effects from this surgery?

A: Skin response is variable and depends on your age, skin elasticity, weight loss, and the amount of breast tissue. There may be some loose skin causing skin folds afterward. It is possible to overresect breast tissue, leaving a concavity, although this is unusual if the operator is an experienced plastic surgeon. Contour irregularities sometimes develop, and a touchup procedure such as a touchup liposuction or fat injection may be needed later.

Q: How much work will I miss?

A: Most men are able to return to work within a week, some in just a few days if their job is not physical and they are no longer taking prescription pain killers. You need two weeks off if you have a physical job.

Q: Can this condition recur?

A: The fat and breast tissue that are removed at surgery are gone forever, and your breasts will always be less full than they would have been without the surgery. However, it is possible that the breast tissue that is left behind might enlarge ("hypertrophy") and require retreatment, but this is unusual in the absence of a medical condition, medications, or steroids that might stimulate breast tissue development.

Q: How long does the surgery take?

A: The actual surgery takes about 30 minutes for liposuction alone, or an hour-and-a-half for the combined procedure—subcutaneous mastectomies and liposuction.

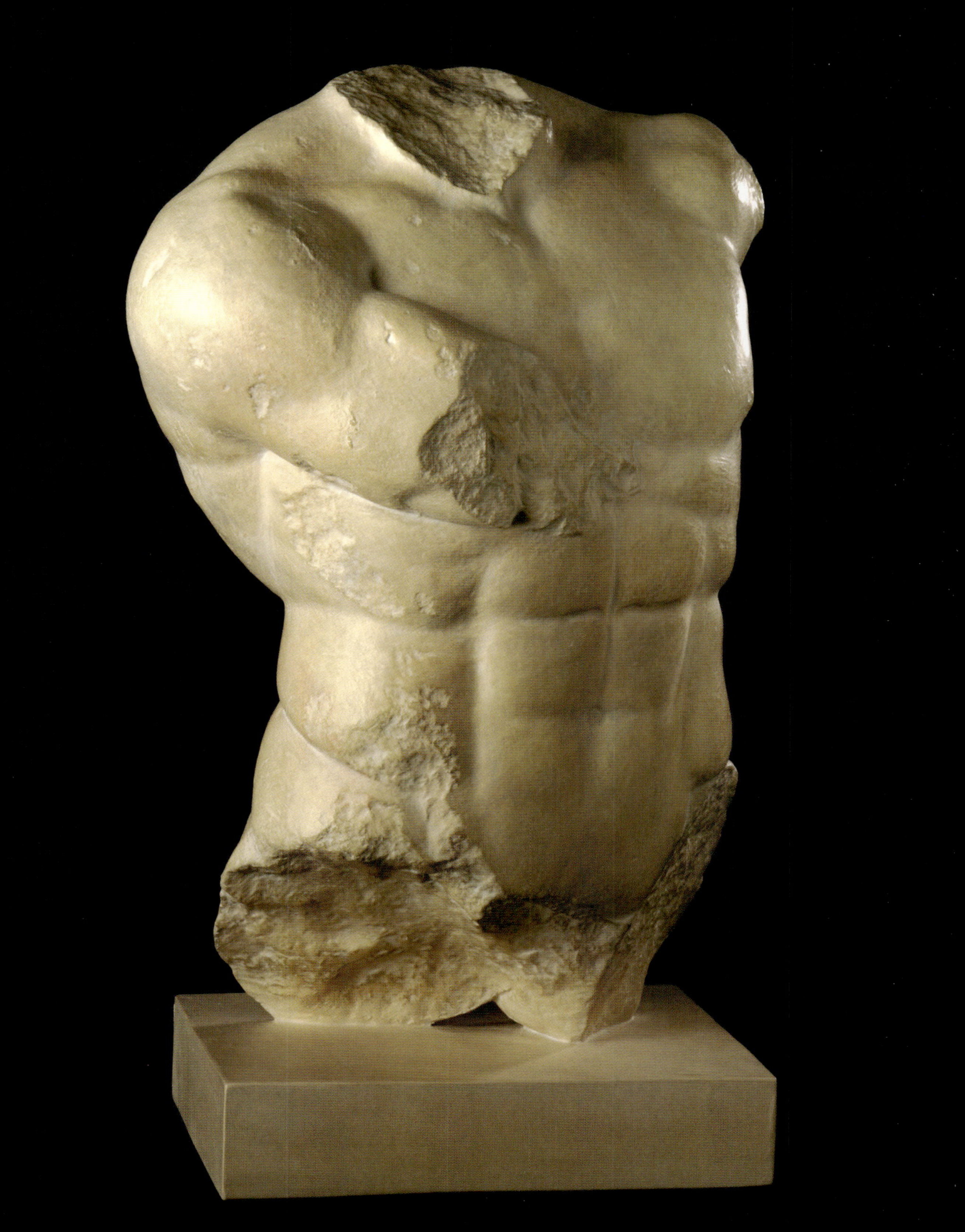

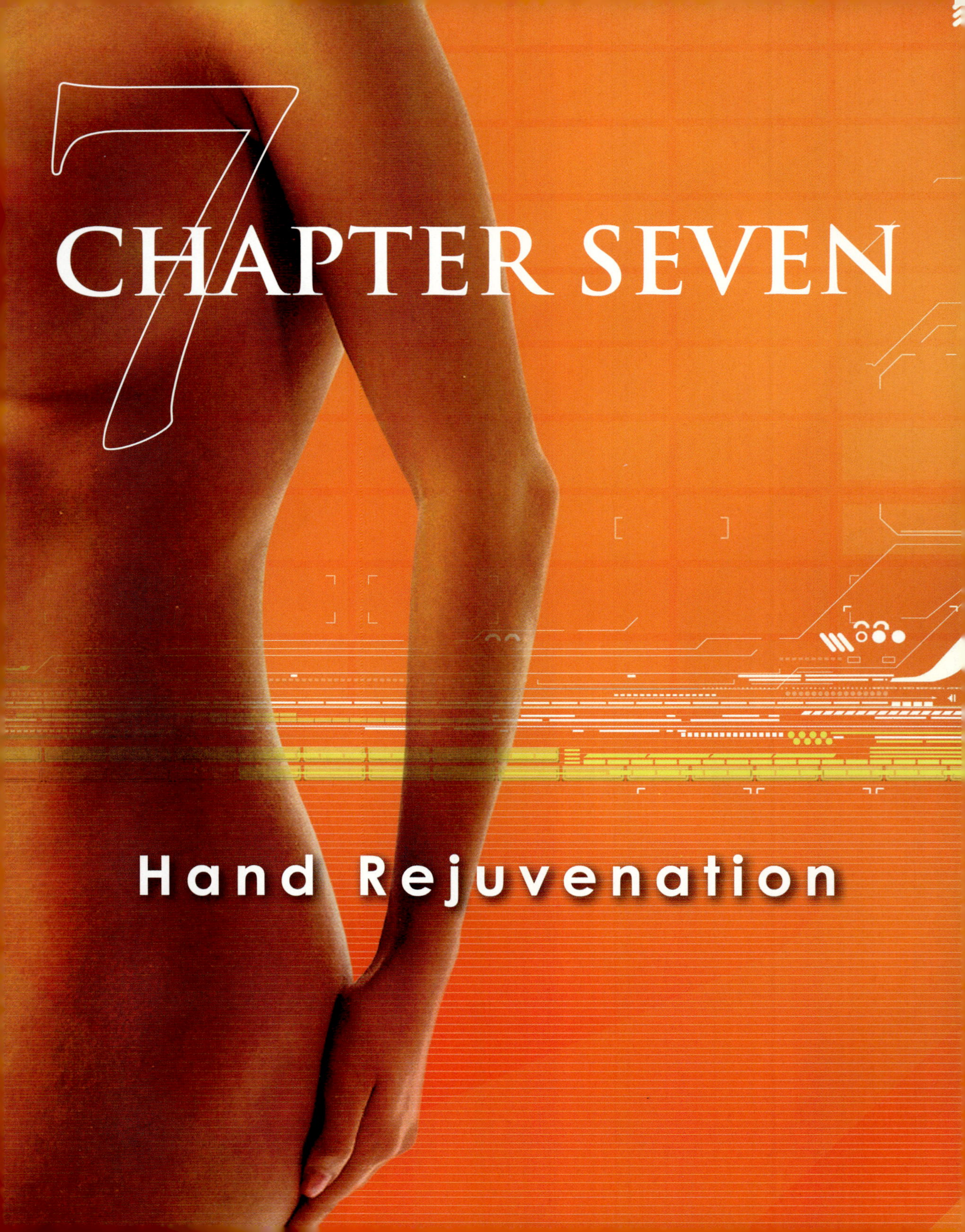

CHAPTER SEVEN

Hand Rejuvenation

Introduction

Hand rejuvenation is becoming more popular. Hands can be a giveaway for aging. Fat injection can help by providing a layer of cushioning between the skin and the underlying tendons and veins, making them less conspicuous. Laser resurfacing can be done simultaneously to treat brown spots.

How It's Done

Fat is obtained from a donor site, usually the tummy or outer thighs. The fat component is separated from the fluid either using a centrifuge or by using the LipiVage™ system that separates the fat as it is harvested. Using one or two incisions at the level of the wrist, the fat is injected over the back of the hand. A blunt cannula is used and care is taken not to puncture the veins. The fat is massaged gently to even it out.

Intraoperative Photographs

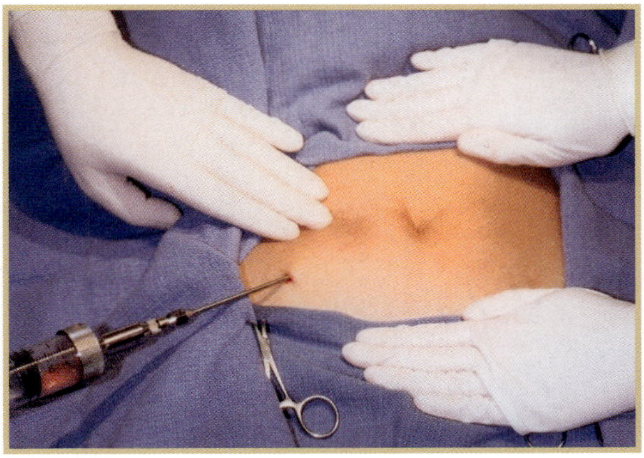

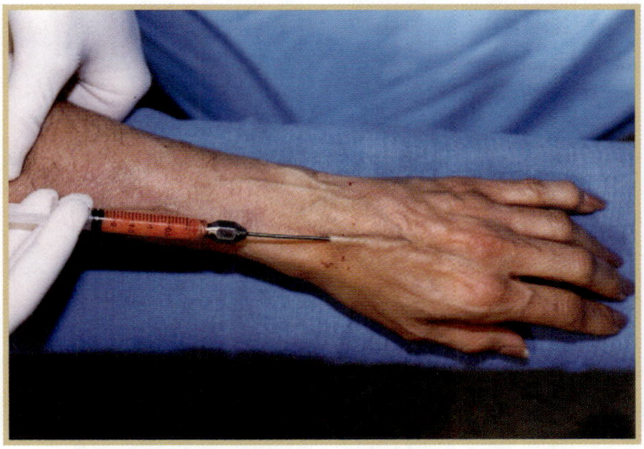

The hand is injected with fat. The tummy serves as the fat donor site.

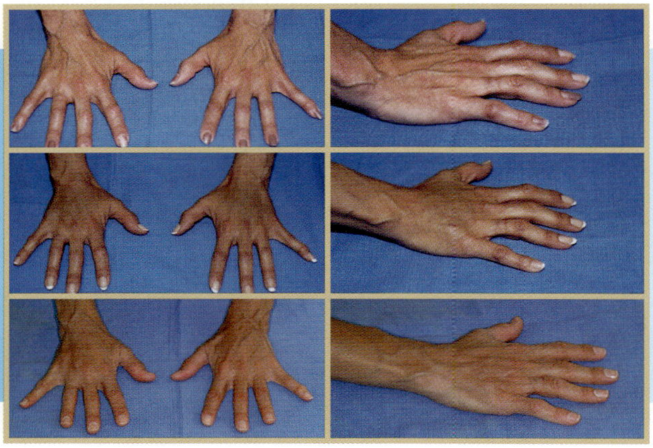

before

10 days after

3 years after

Fat injection of hands.

Comments: This patient was self-conscious about her hands. By filling in a cushion of fat, her veins are less prominent. She is seen 10 days and then three years after her original procedure. A touchup was done once, three months before the most recent photos were taken.

Injection volume: 7 cc per hand,
touchup: 6 cc per hand
D.C., age 45/48, teacher

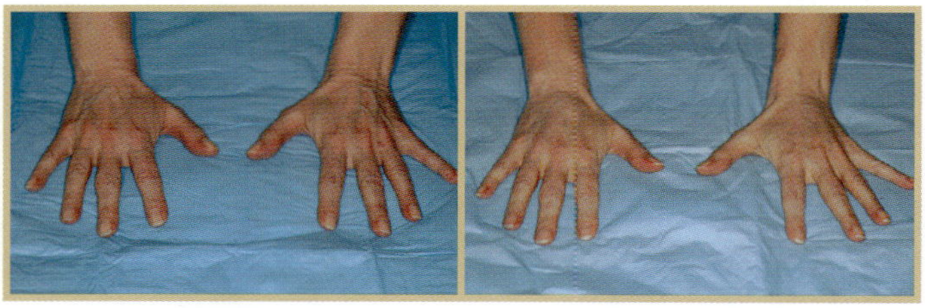

before | 3 months after

Fat injection of hands.

Comments: This patient had fat injection of her hands at the same time as her facelift and facial fat injection, which is commonly done to make the best use of the fat harvested at surgery, and to treat aging hands conveniently at the same time as facial rejuvenation.

Injection volume: 11 cc per hand
B.M., age 50, CPA

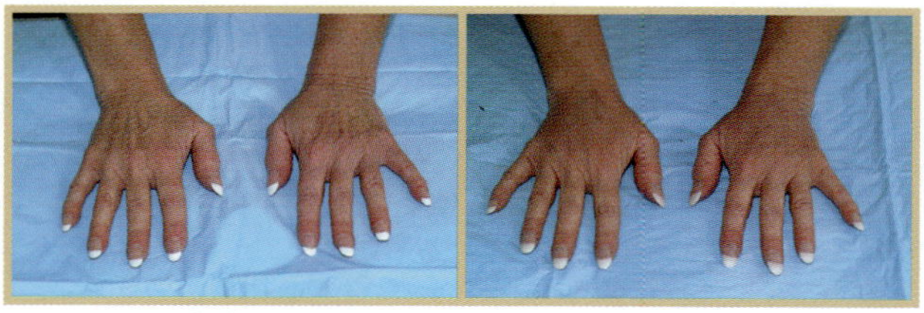

before | 1 month after

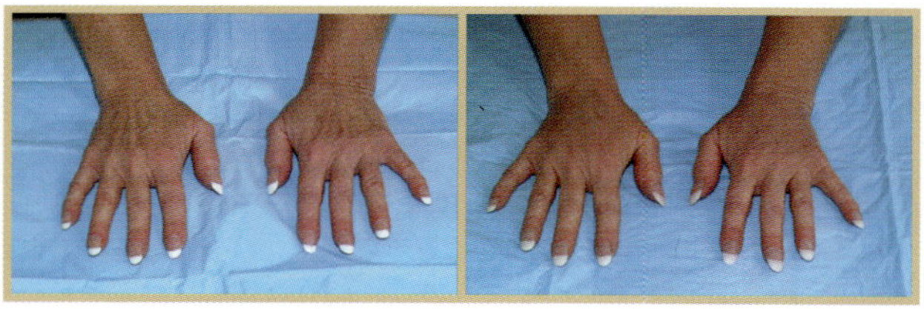

1 year after | 3½ years after

Fat injection and erbium laser resurfacing of hands.

Comments: This patient looked very youthful in her face but thought her hands gave away her age. She elected to have her hands treated simultaneously with facial laser resurfacing and fat injection of the lips. She returned to work as a hair stylist one week after this procedure. One year later, the injected fat has not absorbed. The effect is still evident three-and-a-half years later. She has not had any subsequent fat injections or hand laser treatment.

Injection volume: 11 cc per hand
B.W., age 55/56/58, hair stylist

Fat injection and erbium laser resurfacing of hands.

Comments: This patient has volume deficiency and brown spots from sun damage. Fat injection restored a cushion of soft tissue under the skin, and the erbium laser treated her brown spots.

Injection volume: 10 cc per hand
M.R., age 56, retired

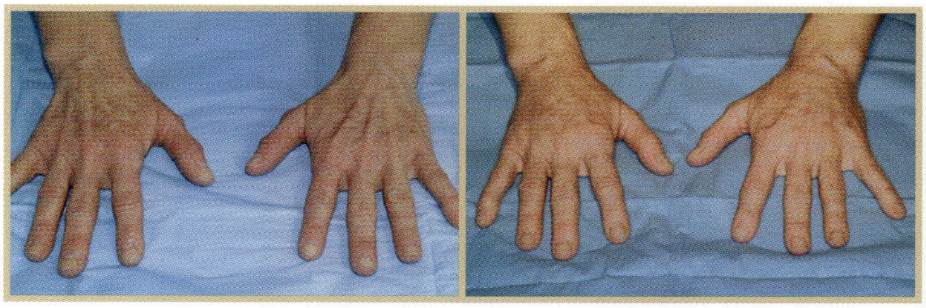

before *5 weeks after*

What to Expect after Surgery

Fat injection of the hands is not a painful procedure. Swelling and bruising are normal. It is best to avoid manual activities such as gardening for at least two weeks. Compressive gloves can be worn for comfort and to limit swelling.

Complications

Fat injection of the hands has proved to be a safe procedure. It is possible to do a touchup procedure later to optimize the result or to treat unevenness.

Care after Surgery

- You can wash your hands right away.
- The small sutures on the back of your wrists are removed in the office after a few days. Sometimes they come out on their own.
- Avoid sun exposure because this might cause hyperpigmentation.
- Minimize manual work the first two weeks after surgery.

Q: Is it painful?

A: No.

Q: Will this help my brown spots?

A: No. Laser resurfacing (usually the erbium laser) is used to treat brown spots. This may be done simultaneously with fat injection.

Q: Will I need to do it again?

A: Fat absorption is variable. You may want to have another treatment at a later time. Often the hands are treated simultaneously with facial procedures. The fat is used both in the face and hands to reduce signs of aging.

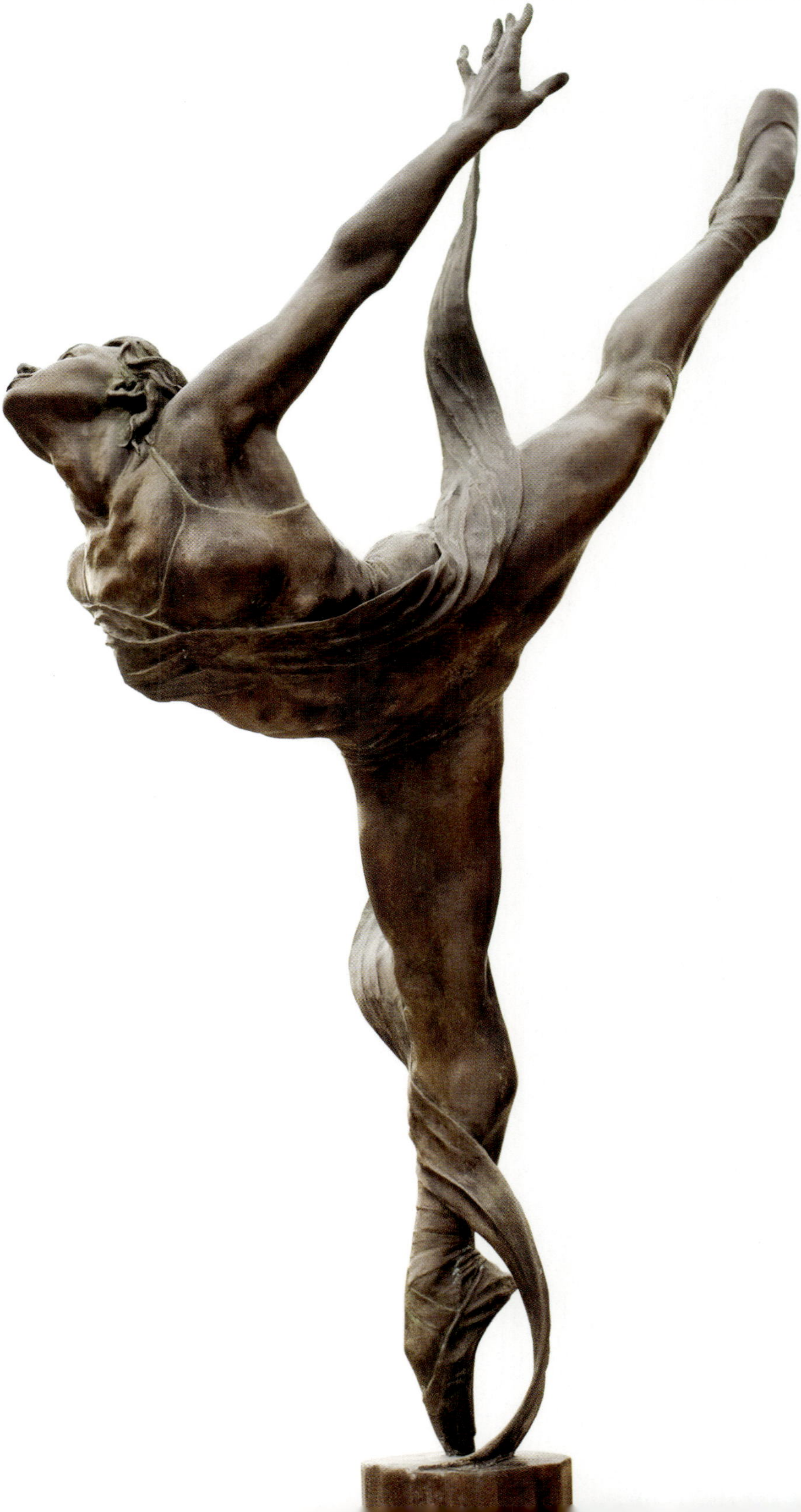

8 CHAPTER EIGHT

Calf Augmentation

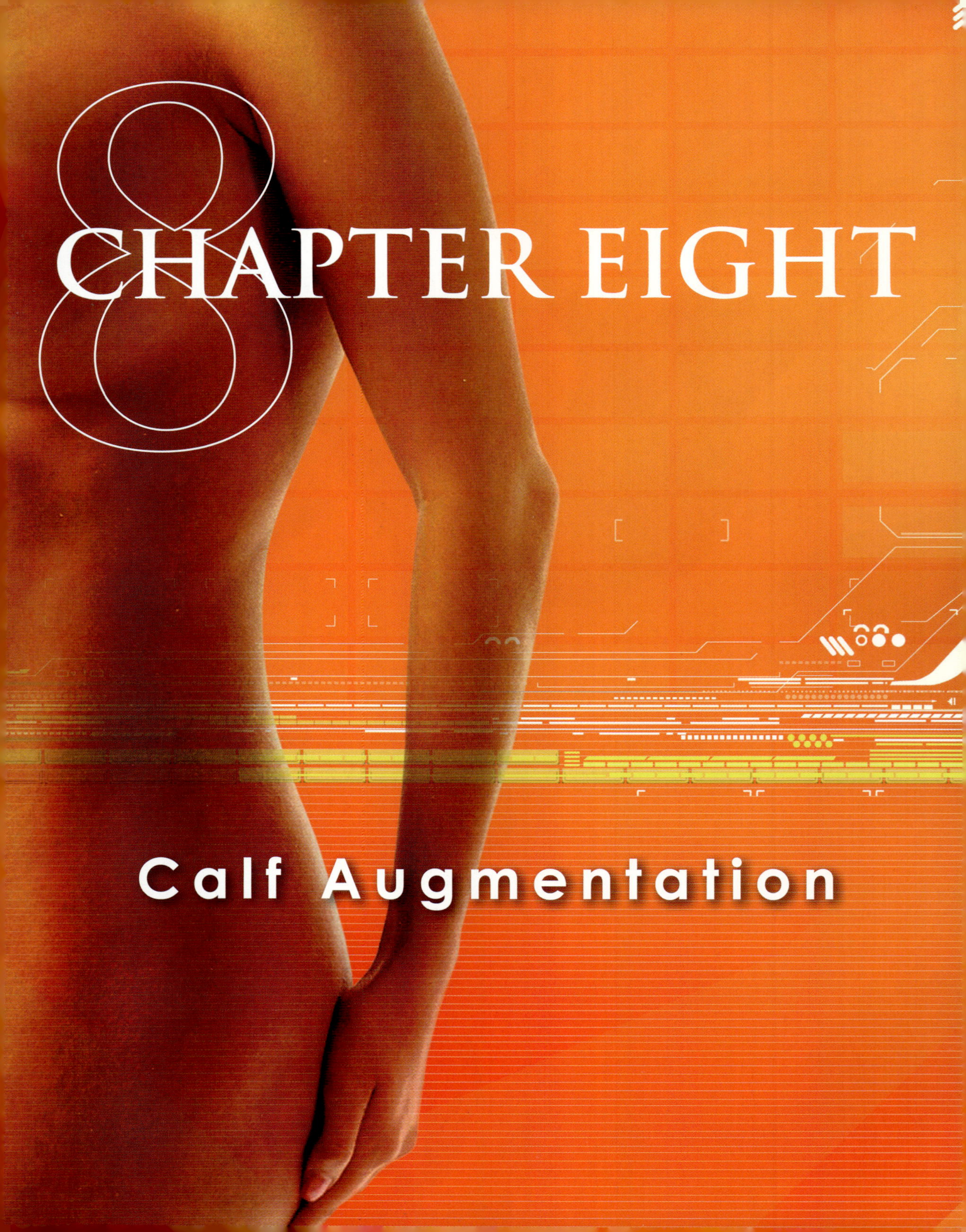

Introduction

Thin Calves

Many women and men have thin ("hypoplastic") calves. This condition is often inherited, but may also result from certain medical problems that affect muscle development, like polio in the past and some rare neuromuscular disorders. Women say that they have "chicken legs" and are reluctant to expose them. Although there is an apparent deficiency of calf muscle, no amount of exercise seems to bulk them up. Some patients are bodybuilders who have no trouble developing their quads but cannot seem to improve their calves.

One of my patients told me he wore three layers of socks drawn up over his calves to help camouflage his "stick legs." Despite working as a manager at a golf club, he would never wear shorts, even in the middle of summer!

Fortunately there is a solution—calf augmentation. This procedure helps balance proportions, so that the fullness of the calf may be in proportion to the fullness of the thigh.

Although there is an apparent deficiency of calf muscle, no amount of exercise seems to bulk them up.

How It's Done

A small incision is made in the crease behind the knee. A pocket is then made under the sheath that envelopes the muscle. A silicone implant is placed in this pocket. A size is chosen to provide the desired fullness without too much tension on the skin. While some surgeons place two implants in the calf at once, my preference is to use just one, placed in the posterior compartment where the deficiency is most obvious. If any additional augmentation is needed laterally, I prefer to use fat injection (See J.J., Patient Photographs) rather than a second implant. I believe this approach minimizes the risk of complications.

Because the implant is placed under the muscle sheath, it looks and feels natural. The implant is made of solid silicone and feels like rubber. A soft consistency ("durometer") is chosen to mimic the feel of the muscle.

Like a breast augmentation, the benefits are immediately apparent. Patients may go on to work out again in the gym, same as before, after about a month. Any increase in muscle size from exercise complements the result. The scar is relatively inconspicuous, located in the crease behind the knee.

Intraoperative Photographs

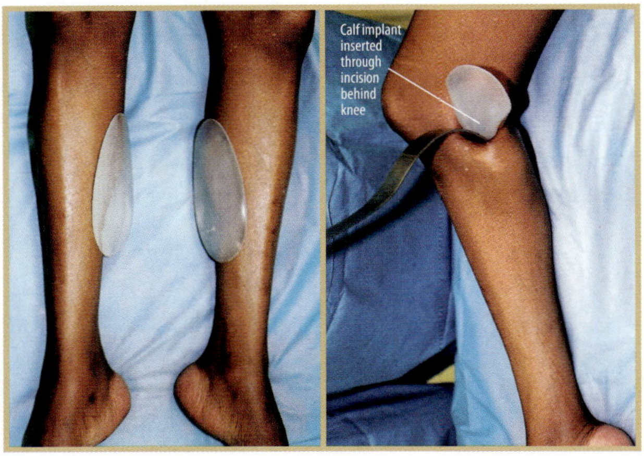

(*Left*) The implants are shown beside the legs of a woman with thin calves (See J.N., Patient Photographs). (*Right*) The implant may be folded on itself and then squeezed through an incision behind the knee. It slides into the space between the gastrocnemius muscle and the fascial (connective tissue) envelope that covers the muscle.

Patient Photographs

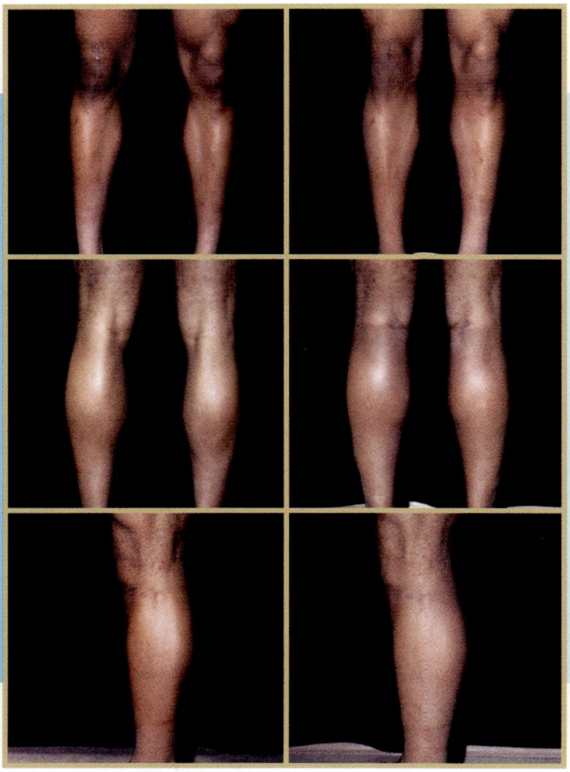

before ***10 days after***

Calf augmentation.

Comments: This 25-year-old bodybuilder was unable to develop his calves despite aggressive exercise. Ten days later he was walking without difficulty.

Height: 5'10"
Weight: 197 lbs.
A.A., age 25, hazardous materials technician

Calf augmentation with implants, and fat injection of lateral calves.

Comments: No amount of weight training had yielded results for this patient with hypoplastic calves. Calf implants were used in combination with fat injection to correct this disproportion. His calf circumference increased from 13½ inches to 15⅛ inches. The incisions are placed in the natural crease behind the knees, fade with time, and are well-concealed.

Height: 6'2"
Weight: 209 lbs.
J.J. age 39, director

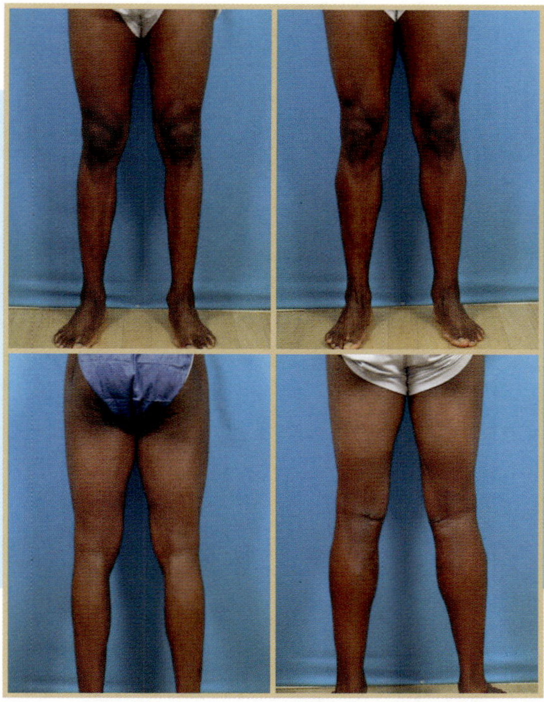

before *3 weeks after*

Calf augmentation with implants.

Comments: This patient would never show her "chicken legs." She would not wear shorts, even in the middle of summer. She returned to her office work two weeks after surgery. At first, she found heels more comfortable because it was hard to stretch out her legs completely. Her calf circumference increased from 11 inches to 12¾ inches. She was now comfortable showing off her legs. This had a major impact on her clothing options. Her intraoperative photographs are shown on the previous page.

Height: 5'2"
Weight: 111 lbs.
J.N., age 58, system analyst

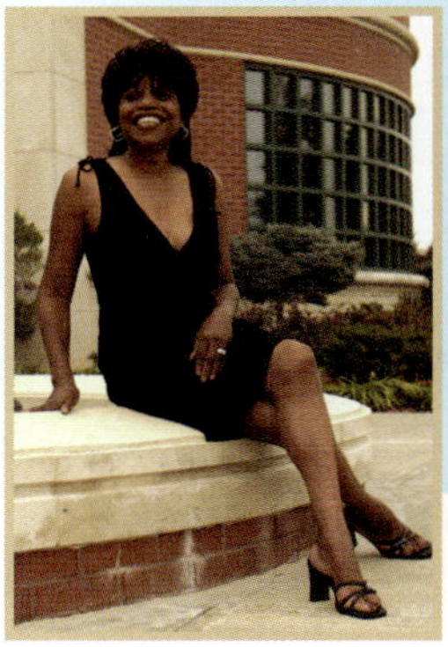

2 months after

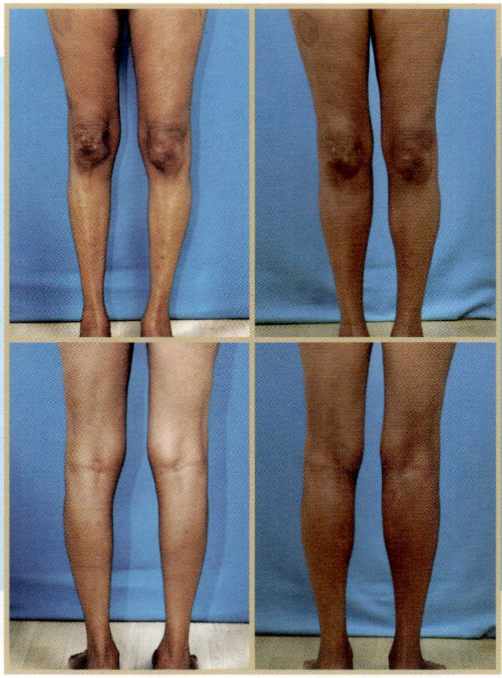

before *6 weeks after*

What to Expect after Surgery

The legs are wrapped with an Ace® wrap from the toes to the knees. The level of discomfort is usually tolerable. Patients are able to get up for short trips to the bathroom. When sitting, they need to keep their legs elevated on an ottoman.

I see patients the day after surgery in the office. I remove the dressing and examine the legs. The legs are then rewrapped with Kerlix® gauze and Ace® wrap. Patients may start bathing when they get home. The sutures dissolve on their own. I recommend that patients wait one month before resuming exercises and vigorous physical activity.

Complications

Infection

Similar to a breast augmentation, if an infection develops, the implant will probably need to be removed to clear the infection. The patient may return later to have a new implant inserted.

Hematoma

The surgical dissection is remarkably bloodless, so the risk of bleeding is low. A hematoma would cause excessive swelling and pain shortly after surgery, and would require a trip back to the operating room to release it.

Nerve Injury

A sensory nerve is at risk in this operation—the sural nerve, which supplies feeling to the foot. An injury to this nerve would cause numbness over the top of the foot, including possible permanent numbness. This nerve is often used as a donor nerve in reconstructive surgery because the consequences of such numbness are minimal. Nevertheless, care is taken to preserve this nerve and avoid this complication.

Malposition of the Implant

The implant may move after surgery and require repositioning.

A Larger Size

There is a limit to the size of implant that can be inserted, depending on the tension of the tissues. It may be necessary to come back later when the tissues have stretched to put in a larger implant, if desired.

Seroma

Any time a pocket is created under the skin, tissue fluid may accumulate, forming a seroma. This fluid is drained at regular intervals in the office until it stops forming.

Compartment Syndrome

If the pressure in the tissues is too great after insertion of an implant, this tension may cause a rare problem called compartment syndrome, which is signaled by excessive pain, due to lack of blood supply to the muscle tissue under the implant. This serious complication requires immediate surgical release of the tension by removing the implant.

Care after Surgery

- Minimize walking the first week after surgery.
- Wear Ace® wrap or compression stockings to reduce swelling.
- Keep your legs elevated when you are not walking.
- Most people take a week off work if their job is not physical.
- You can return to exercising one month after surgery.

Frequently Asked Questions

Q: What does the implant feel like?

A: It's a solid silicone material, made to be as soft as possible while preserving integrity. It typically feels quite natural, not unlike muscle.

Q: When can I start working out?

A: It is best to wait one month before resuming exercises.

Q: How much bigger can you make my calves?

A: The skin in this area is limited in how much it can expand at one operation. The surgeon typically adjusts the implant size to maximize the result, without making the skin too tight, which might increase the risk of complications. Fine-tuning is done by shaving the implant as necessary in surgery. The result is typically noticeable and flattering.

Q: One implant or two?

A: I use one implant on each side, but there are surgeons who place two.

Q: Is the implant solid or gel-filled?

A: Like most American surgeons, I use solid silicone implants. This is a hard form of silicone, not the gel form. Implant rupture is not a concern with this type of implant.

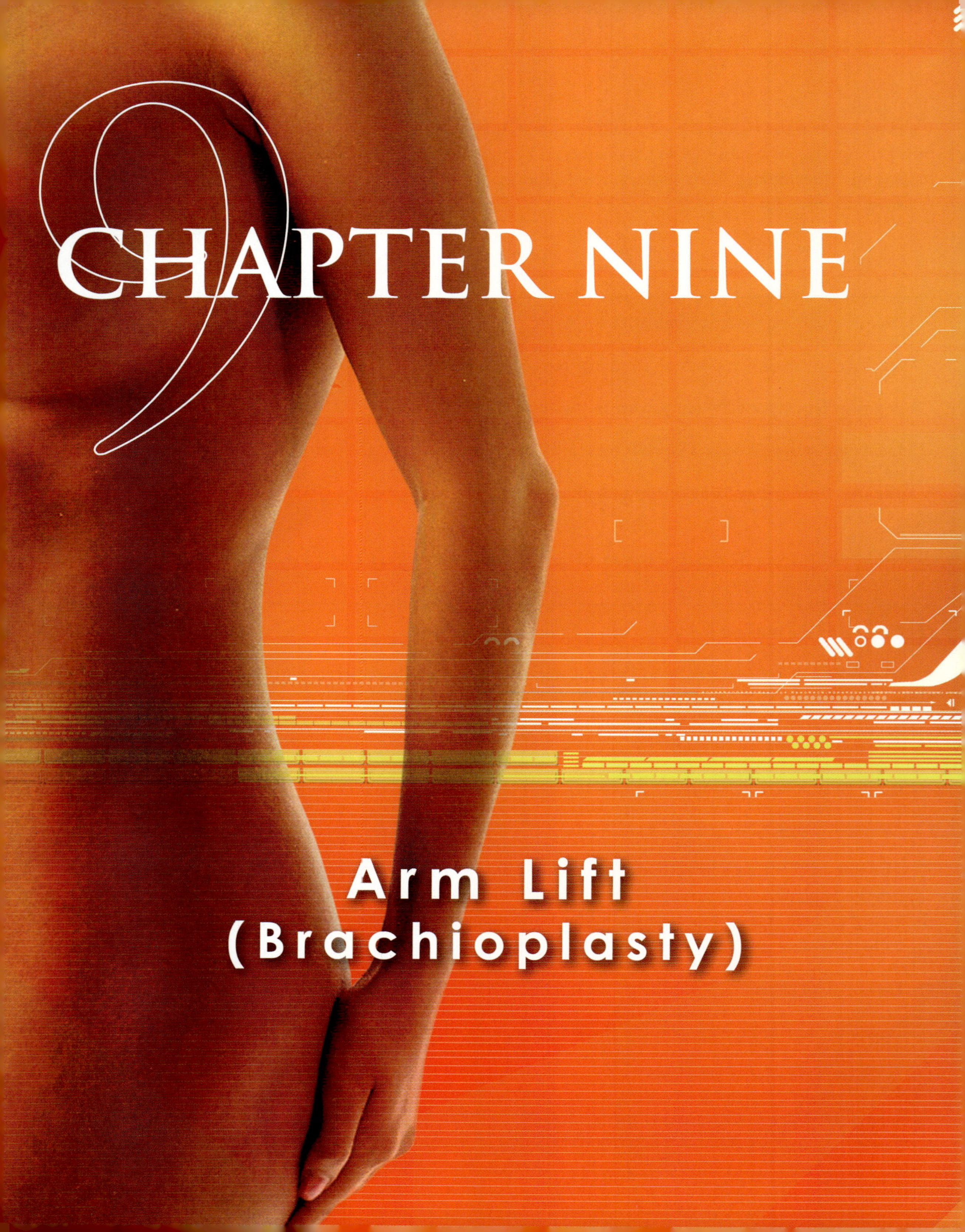

CHAPTER NINE

Arm Lift (Brachioplasty)

Introduction

Loose skin of the upper arms is a common problem and can be a source of embarrassment to women. They may not be able to go sleeveless, even during the summer. If the degree of skin laxity is mild, I recommend liposuction alone. However, if there is a lot of loose skin, it is best to proceed directly to a skin excisional procedure called brachioplasty.

Patients sometimes ask if it is possible to keep the incision contained up in the armpit (axilla). They may even show me by pinching the skin of the armpit area to demonstrate. The problem with this "minilift" is that the degree of improvement is limited to the uppermost part of the arm. For most women, this is not enough.

The skin problem is anatomically similar to excess skin of the inner thighs, which has traditionally been treated with the frequently disappointing inner thigh lift procedure, using an incision in the groin crease, but is now more effectively treated with a longitudinal excision running the full length of the inner thigh, much like the traditional brachioplasty incision on the arm.

An arm lift is usually done in conjunction with liposuction. An arm lift may be done on its own, but is more commonly performed at the same time as other body contouring procedures, especially in the treatment of deformities resulting from massive weight loss.

An arm lift may be done on its own, but is more commonly performed at the same time as other body contouring procedures, especially in the treatment of deformities resulting from massive weight loss.

How It's Done

Preoperative marking is performed. The arm is first treated with ultrasonic liposuction to remove extra fat and also develop a tissue plane to make skin removal easier and safer.

The Incision

An elliptical incision is used to cut out the extra loose skin. I prefer to position this ellipse over the back (posterior) margin of the upper arm. This way the scar is not conspicuous when the arm is in a resting position at the patient's side. The scar runs down the "inseam" of the arm from the armpit to a point just above the elbow.

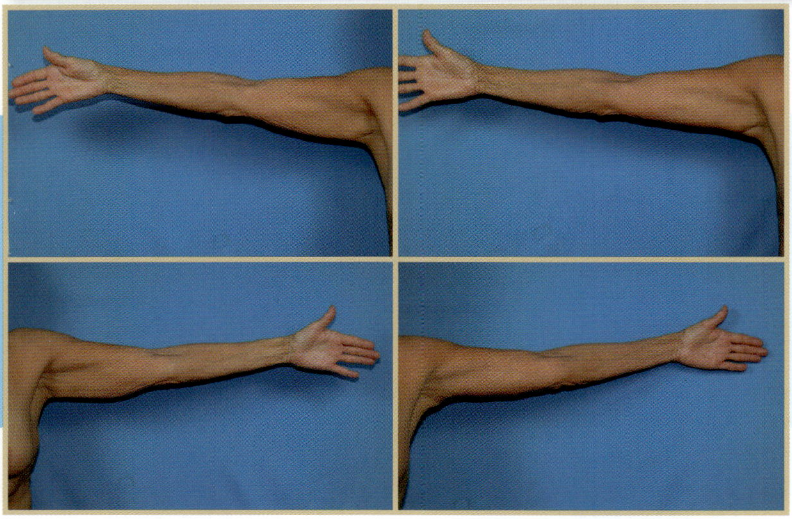

before 3 months after

Brachioplasties, breast lift, abdominoplasty, and inner thigh lifts.

Comments: This 65-year-old had loose skin of the arms. She underwent brachioplasties at the same time as an abdominoplasty and breast lift. The wrinkled appearance of her arms is eliminated.

Height: 5'4"
Weight: 132 lbs.
L.R., age 65, sales

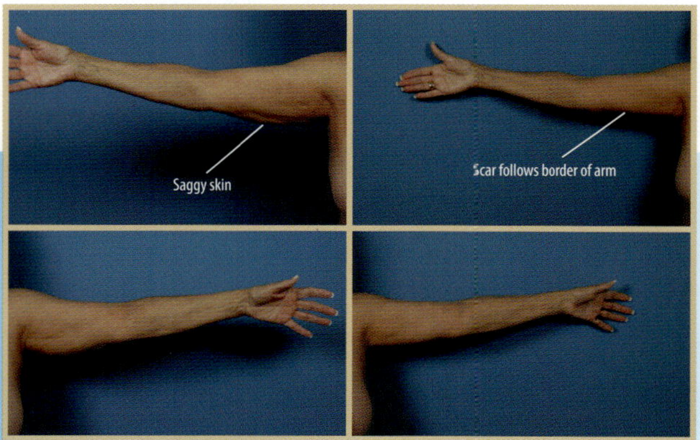

before 3 months after

Brachioplasties and ultrasonic liposuction of arms, axillae, and inner thighs.

Comments: This patient would not wear short sleeves during the summer because she was self-conscious about the flabby appearance of her arms. Her scars have healed well and are inconspicuous.

Height: 5' 3"
Weight: 143.5 lbs
R.J., age 70, retired

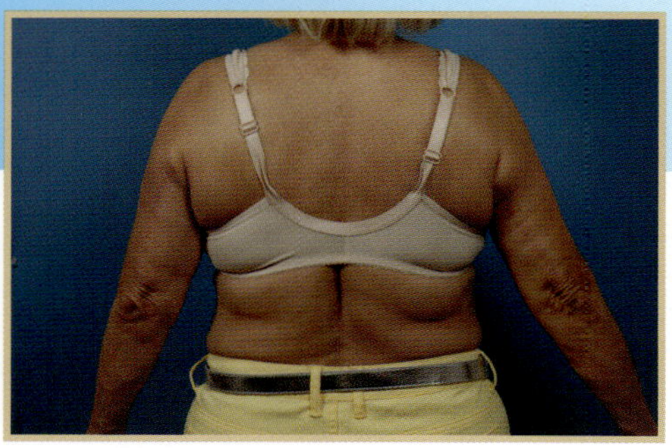

6 months after

What to Expect after Surgery

There is not much pain after this procedure. The dressings are removed the day after surgery. Steri-Strips™ are left on or replaced if they have become saturated. Bruising and swelling are to be expected, of course, but the improved tightness of the skin is already obvious.

Complications

Dog ear

I have occasionally treated a dog ear of either the upper ("proximal") or lower ("distal") end of the scar if the expected puckering does not settle down completely.

Excessive Scarring

Like all scars, sometimes the scar spreads. This scar widening may be improved by revising the scar at a later date, when there is less tension on the wound.

Numbness

An important sensory nerve (the "medial antebrachial cutaneous nerve") runs down the inside of the upper arm. It is important for the surgeon to avoid injuring this nerve, which might cause a painful neuroma. Typically, I resect the tissue more posteriorly, and anesthetic infiltration expands the subcutaneous plane, lifting the skin, and making nerve injury very unlikely.

Hematoma

Hematomas are unusual. The vessels are small and easily controlled with cautery. There is some compression from the tissue closure, which prevents a dead space. There is no need for a drain.

Seroma

With limited ultrasound times and the avoidance of cutting cautery, this complication can be avoided.

Care after Surgery

- The dressings come off when you return to the office the day after surgery.
- Bruising and swelling are normal. It is not unusual for the bruising to continue down the forearm.
- There is no garment that you need to wear. However, some patients prefer the gentle compression of tight-fitting long-sleeved athletic wear. One popular manufacturer is Under Armour®.
- Leave the Steri-Strips™ in place. They come off about a week after surgery.
- Start bathing normally again the day after surgery, after the dressings are removed.
- At first, there is some irregularity and gathering along the incision. This bumpiness smoothes out on its own.
- Vigorous physical activities should be deferred for about a month. Normal day-to-day activities may be resumed right away.
- Patients sometimes ask about swelling in the area of the elbow. In this area, liposuction is performed, but the skin incision has to end just above the elbow so as not to cross this joint level. Accordingly, there is less skin tightness and more room for swelling. This swelling gradually settles down.

Frequently Asked Questions

Q: Is it painful?

A: No.

Q: Can you keep the incision hidden in the armpit?

A: No. Unfortunately such a limited incision does not allow sufficient skin tightening.

Q: How visible is the scar?

A: It is exposed when you are sleeveless. However, it is kept close to the posterior border of the arm, where it is typically not obvious. Patients find the scar preferable to loose skin. If the skin is minimally saggy, liposuction is done instead.

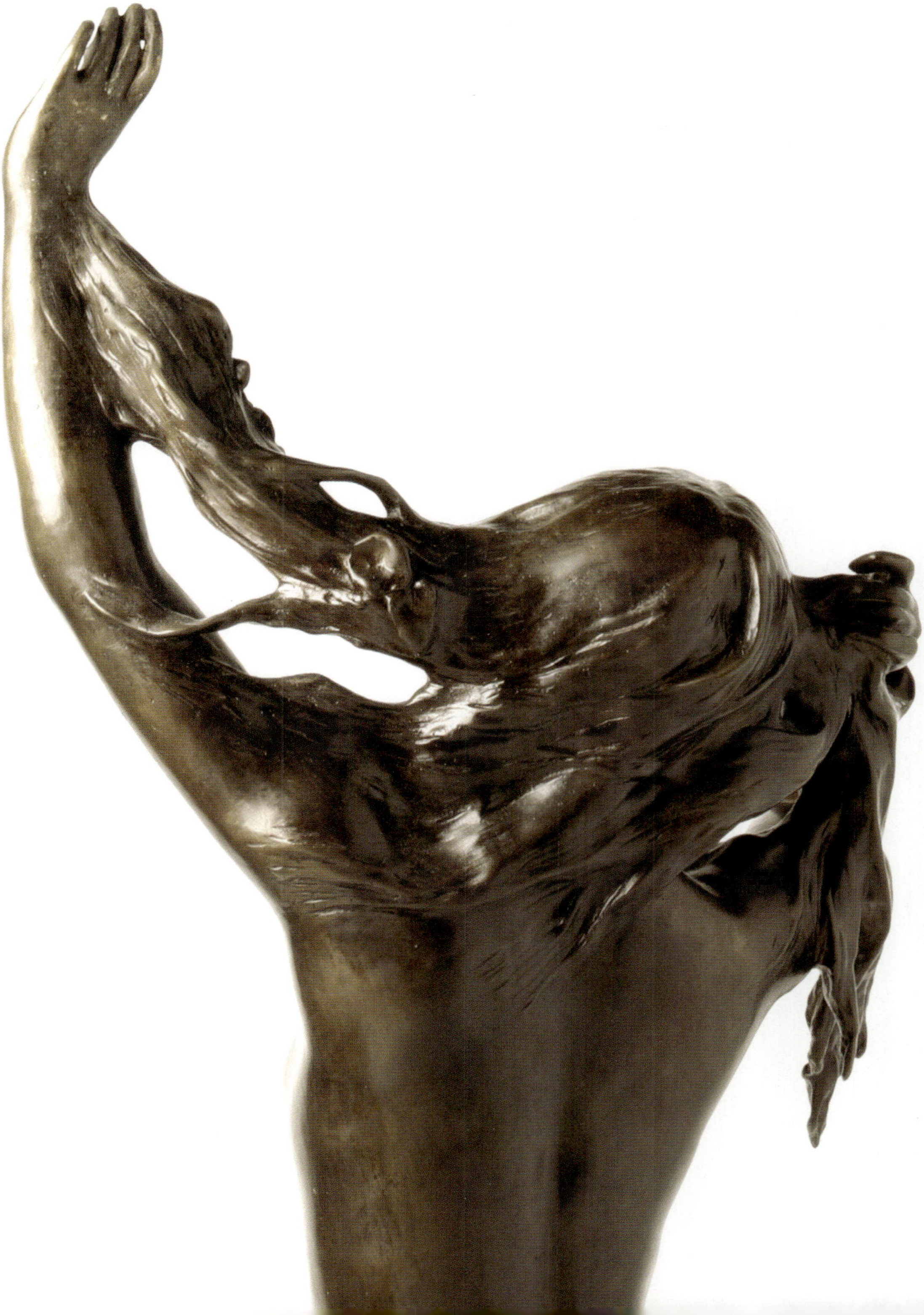

CHAPTER TEN

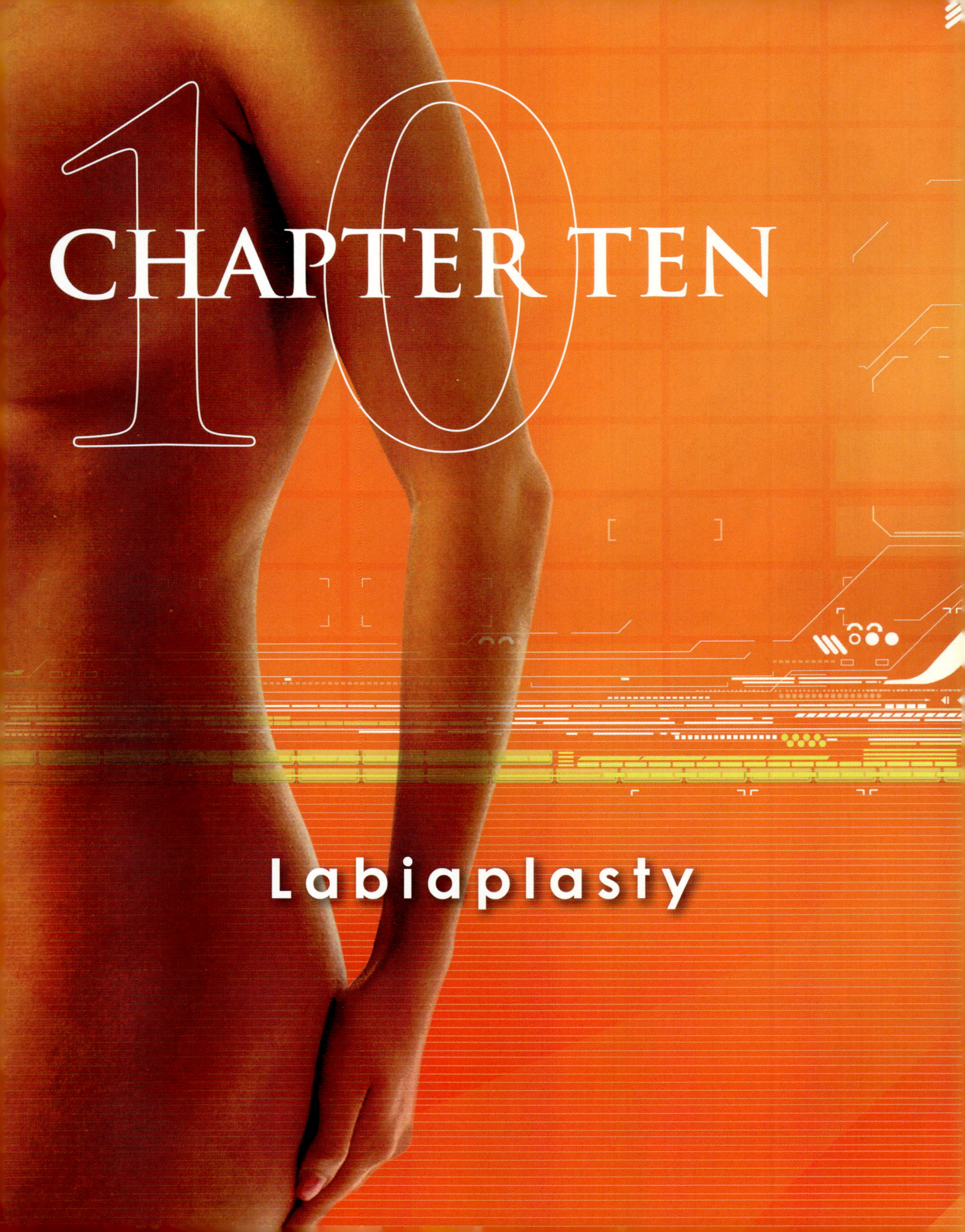

Labiaplasty

Introduction

This relatively new procedure reduces the size of the labia minora, which are the inner "lips" that border the vaginal opening. Like the lips of the face, they are composed of skin on the outside and mucosa on the inside.

The most common cause of enlarged labia is simply heredity. Women can be self-conscious about having excessive labial tissue. It can be embarrassing when they wear a bikini or tight-fitting clothing, or when they visit the gynecologist, not to mention intimate relationships. Women do not want to have any noticeable bump or irregularity in the genital area (which is also why I often perform liposuction of the pubic area). This can be a professional concern for models and actresses. Sometimes enlarged labia can chafe and cause pain when women engage in sports such as cycling and horseback riding. The labia can get in the way by folding in during intercourse.

Although this procedure may make women more comfortable in intimate relationships by making them less self-conscious and eliminate any problems caused by invagination of tissues, there is no suggestion that it otherwise enhances the sexual experience (See below).

Labiaplasty Is a Valid Procedure

Labiaplasty is a valid procedure, published in peer-reviewed plastic surgery journals. It successfully treats a real problem with predictable results and high levels of patient satisfaction. It is a relatively new tool in my armamentarium, and one that I find myself using more and more, often in conjunction with other body contouring procedures. Women should not feel embarrassed to ask about this procedure. With greater public and surgeon awareness, it will no doubt gain popularity.

"Vaginal Rejuvenation" – Buyer Beware

Labiaplasty is not to be confused with "vaginal rejuvenation" procedures, including Dr. David Matlock's patented "Laser Vaginal Rejuvenation," "Designer Laser Vaginoplasty," and "G-Shot Amplification," catchy labels (especially the last one) for techniques that are marketed to enhance sexual gratification in women. Dr. Matlock is a Los Angeles gynecologist, with an MBA, who found a niche in cosmetic surgery of the female genitalia, and has been featured on the popular *E! Entertainment* cable-television series *Dr. 90210*. The problem is an absence of scientific validation, with no published peer-reviewed studies. Dr. Matlock says that his patent attorneys told him not to publish his techniques so as to protect his intellectual property. He evidently does not subscribe to the time-honored Hippocratic oath, which calls for doctors to share their knowledge, as they were taught by others before them. Marketing 1, Hippocrates 0.

How It's Done

The excess labial tissue is resected as a triangle, removing the full thickness of the labia. The length of the free border is reduced. The edges are carefully sutured together. Asymmetry is common, so it is not unusual to remove more tissue on one side than the other. It is important to also repair the inner "stromal" layer of the labia, so as to maximize the strength of the repair.

This resection pattern does not place any important nerves at risk, so there is no diminished sensation. It preserves the normal anatomy of the free margin of the labia. Older techniques involved resection of the free margin of the labia, rather than a wedge, compromising the aesthetics of the labia. These women simply have too much of a desirable structure, so it makes sense just to remove the excess and preserve the rest in its anatomic condition.

Patient Photographs

Refer to Web site:
http://www.swansoncenter.com/content/ideal-body/procedures/labiaplasty/patient-photographs.asp

What to Expect after Surgery

There is typically minimal discomfort. In fact, if there is pain, the patient needs to be assessed. It could signal a hematoma. The sutures dissolve on their own in about two months. The suture ends are cut short to avoid irritation. Usually urination is not uncomfortable. It is recommended that women avoid intercourse for one month to ensure adequate healing before subjecting the labia to trauma that could cause a disruption of the wound.

The wound tends to heal extremely well, such that the surgical scar is almost invisible. The result is typically very natural, with no signs of surgery. Patient satisfaction is very high. A needless source of embarrassment is eliminated.

Complications

Wound Opening (Dehiscence)

The tissue can be fragile, which is why long-lasting sutures are used. The wound may come apart partially or fully. This problem is not painful, but requires surgical correction to avoid a V-shaped cleft in the labial margin.

Hematoma

The labia have an abundant blood supply. It is important for the surgeon to cauterize the vessels at surgery. Even doing so, it is possible for a clot to separate and a small collection of blood to develop within the labia. This is quite painful. Prompt surgical attention is needed to remove the clot and cauterize the vessel.

Infection

The perineal area is highly resistant to infection, so this is rarely a problem.

Under- or Overresection

As in most operations, underresection is preferable to overresection. It is easy to remove more labial tissue if needed, but impossible to restore it. With prudent but adequate resection, such problems can usually be avoided.

Care after Surgery

- Antibiotic ointment is applied to the incision lines twice a day.
- A gauze pad is used during the first 24 hours because there may be some oozing during this time.
- Most daily activities can be resumed right away. More vigorous activities that apply pressure to this area, such as cycling or horseback riding, should be avoided for at least 2 weeks.
- Avoid intercourse for one month.
- Usually the prescribed pain killers are not required after about 24 hours. If you have increased pain or swelling, or find that you have trouble walking because of discomfort, you should be assessed right away because these symptoms could signal a hematoma. A hematoma is unlikely to develop more than 24 hours after surgery.

Frequently Asked Questions

Q: Is it painful?

A: No. If there is pain, this may indicate a hematoma.

Q: When can I resume having intercourse?

A: It is best to wait a month to allow adequate healing.

Q: How bad are the scars?

A: The scars typically heal extremely well and are inconspicuous.

CHAPTER ELEVEN

Laser Hair Removal

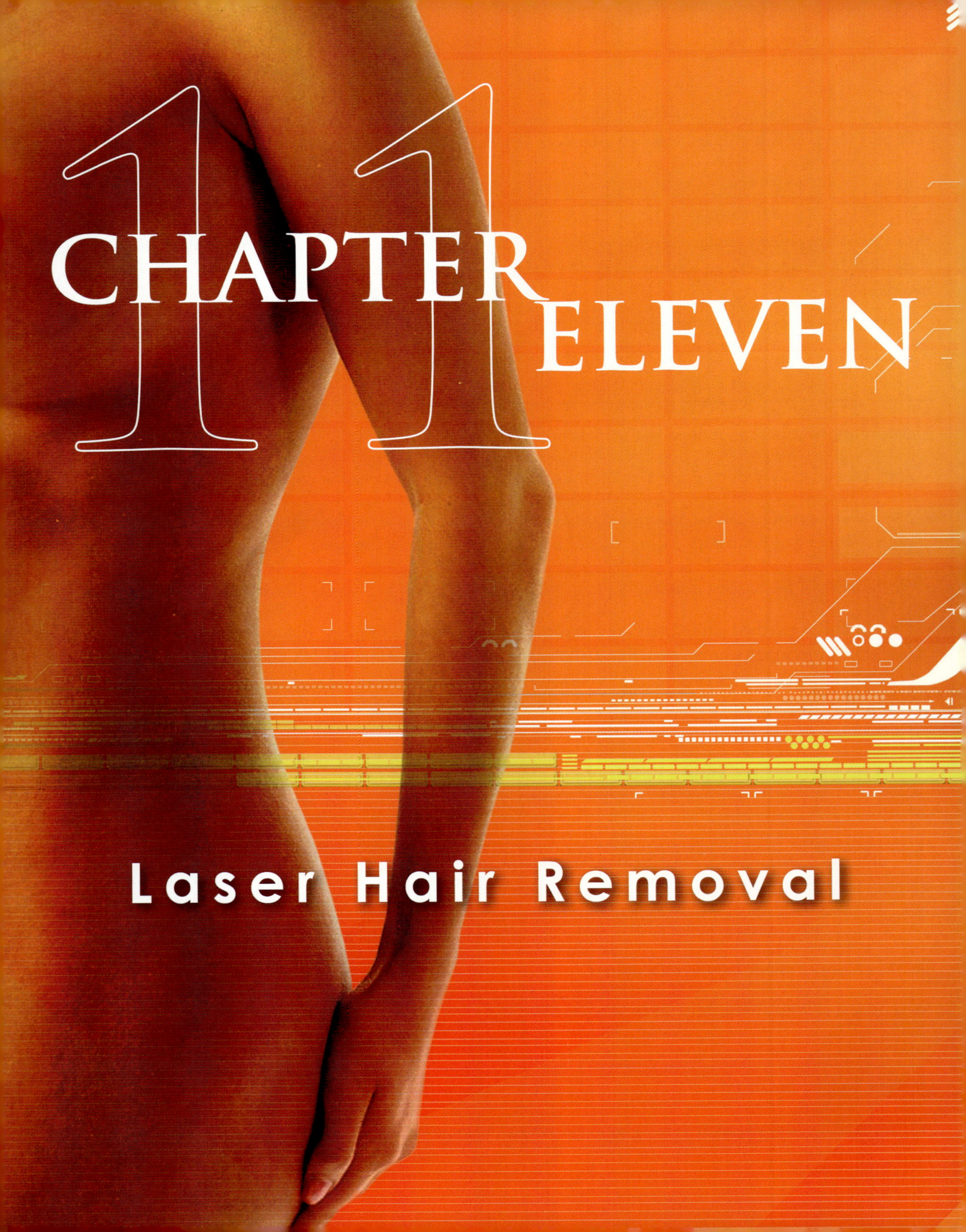

Introduction

Unwanted Body Hair

It is one of life's ironies that so many men lose hair where they want it and gain it where they don't. Facial hair on women can be socially debilitating. Any culture that uses cell phones disapproves of facial and body hair on women. Hirsutism is considered unfeminine, and indeed can signal, on a biological level, an androgynous hormonal imbalance. In North America, hairy underarms in women are undesirable, so much so that famous actresses sometimes find their photographs in tabloid magazines if they raise their arms and reveal body hair. At least such pictures are better than photographs of cellulite! Aversion to body hair is nothing new. Renaissance paintings by the masters rarely portray body hair on women, or men.

Shaving legs and underarms is part of the maintenance ritual of being an American woman. Most women shave their legs at least twice a week and would be embarrassed revealing hairy legs. Many women pluck facial hairs daily. Countless hours are wasted in this task that has no redeeming value. It is not quality time. Hair follicles may also be a nuisance when they become inflamed ("folliculitis") in the beard area in men and bikini area in women.

Supermodels are emblems of our society's physical ideals, even caricatures of them (it seems legs and necks cannot be too long.) After all, supermodels have one purpose—to sell their appearance. You don't find any body hair on supermodels. Their skin is as smooth as silk and unblemished.

Shaving legs and underarms is part of the maintenance ritual of being an American woman.

Hairy groins and inner thighs are completely unacceptable for women. Along with diets and tans, bikini waxes are part of the preparation before tropical holidays. A hair-free appearance does not stop at the bikini line. Today, women under 40 often shave their pubic areas, a "Brazilian," or they leave a small "Mohawk" strip.

Some unfortunate women have a syndrome characterized by polycystic ovaries and body hair—polycystic ovarian syndrome. Their hair growth is similar to a man's and they have had no option but to shave daily.

What about men? Some men shave twice daily to avoid the five o'clock shadow, or avoid taking off their shirt because of embarrassing body hair. Many men have told me they feel self-conscious about their body hair when they are shirtless on a beach or playing with their children. The Austin Powers look is decidedly out, along with crooked, yellow teeth, sideburns, and gold medallions. Among all the actors to play him, there has been only one hairy-chested Tarzan. None of the men on the cover of *Muscle and Fitness* magazine have hairy chests. George Carlin half-joked that when he sees a guy with hair on his back, he immediately relegates him to the animal kingdom. It's funny because you know there's an element of truth.

So what to do about it? Anyone who has seen Steve Carell's facial reactions in the movie *40-Year-Old Virgin* has some idea of the pain involved in body waxing. Fortunately, we have better options.

Temporary Treatments

Most treatments are of only a temporary nature, including plucking, waxing, and shaving. Depilatory creams are also of only temporary benefit and often irritate the skin. Plucking and waxing are especially painful and need to be repeated frequently. Why are these measures temporary? Because the hair is removed but the follicle is left intact, ready to produce a new hair. Many women believe that shaving accelerates hair growth and causes thickening of the hair, which is an old wives' tale (the hair follicle does not receive feedback as to whether the hair it produced is shaved or not). Shaving may cause skin irritation and folliculitis. Chemical applications may be complicated by dermatitis and burns.

Many women believe that shaving accelerates hair growth and causes thickening of the hair, which is an old wives' tale.

An improved method of hair removal, making use of laser technology, was long overdue. In the past, permanent hair removal for large areas such as the back (in men) and legs (in women) was not done simply because it was not possible.

Electrolysis

Everyone's heard of electrolysis, the only permanent technique for hair removal available before the advent of laser hair removal in the 1990s.

Electrolysis makes use of an electric current delivered by a needle directly into individual hair follicles. Each individual hair is grasped and an electric current is sent down the hair to heat and destroy the hair follicle. Because only one follicle is treated at a time, the technique is very tedious and time-consuming. The treatment is also painful. Many visits to the electrologist are needed to treat even areas the size of a postage stamp (which may include a few hundred hair follicles). There is a huge time investment. Patients may attend treatments weekly over periods of over a year. And the treatment is about 50% effective, meaning about half of the hairs survive treatment.

There are complications from this technique due to the effects of electrical current. Because some skin cells are burned along with the hair follicle, scarring and ingrown hairs may result. Nodules may form. Infection is possible because of the breakdown of the skin barrier function.

The technique is practical only for small areas such as the upper lip and chin. It is completely out of the question for large areas such as the back or legs. Although it was introduced in the mid-20th century, the technology is from the 19th century. It is an antiquated treatment.

The Hair Follicle

The hair follicles are specialized structures in the skin that produce hairs. They are like tiny tulip bulbs, "planted" deeply in the skin. In fact, they stick out of the underside of the skin and are easily visible in surgery when the skin is lifted. They are well-protected in this location. Any treatment to remove the hairs without damaging the skin must be selective. The puzzle has always been how to destroy the hair follicle without damaging the surrounding skin.

Lasers that nonselectively remove the top layers of the skin are ineffective because of the deep location of the hair follicles. Sometimes patients ask if resurfacing lasers such as the erbium:YAG laser and the CO_2 laser can also get rid of their facial hair. These lasers can vaporize surface hair (which is why hair-free or shaved areas are treated, so that the laser energy is not wasted), but because they do not penetrate deeply into the dermis, the hair follicle is unaffected. A new hair simply grows out to replace the vaporized one.

However, lasers that produce wavelengths that penetrate more deeply into the skin are ideally suited for this purpose. All that remained was a suitable target that could absorb the laser energy and deliver it to the hair follicle.

Targeting Melanin

For years, lasers have been used to treat a variety of skin conditions, such as port wine stains, benign pigment conditions, and tattoos. In 1983, the concept of "selective photothermolysis" was introduced, describing the use of medical lasers of the appropriate wavelength and energy settings to act on targets in the skin, without causing damage to the surrounding tissue.

It's hard to imagine now, but there was no such thing as "laser hair removal" before the 1990s. Like so many important discoveries (microwaves, for example), the use of a laser for hair removal was discovered by accident. Doctors noticed that when they treated tattoos with a ruby laser, fewer hairs grew back in the treated area. They recognized a new application of the laser to the old problem of hair removal. The laser target was the pigment in the skin—melanin.

Doctors noticed that when they treated tattoos with a ruby laser, fewer hairs grew back in the treated area.

Fortunately, you don't need to have a tattoo for the treatment to work. Pigment cells containing melanin are concentrated around hair follicles. Melanin is a naturally-occurring pigment in the skin that may be targeted by a laser using a wavelength that is well absorbed by melanin. By absorbing and then releasing the laser energy next to the hair follicle, the follicle may be disabled. The energy is concentrated in a very short pulse (milliseconds), so that the heat does not build up sufficiently to cause damage to the surrounding skin cells. Hair follicles may be safely deactivated with minimal risk of scarring.

Lasers For Hair Removal

In 1991 the use of the ruby laser for hair removal was patented. Several clinical studies were performed and, in 1997, the FDA approved three types of ruby lasers for hair removal, including the EpiTouch and EpiLaser. The FDA-approved alexandrite and diode lasers, with similar specificity for melanin, were introduced shortly afterward. Our facility has considerable experience with the long-pulsed alexandrite Apogee® laser (Cynosure Inc., Westford, Ma.).

The ruby (694 nm), alexandrite (755 nm), and diode (800 nm) lasers all have wavelengths that are appropriate for hair removal. Shorter wavelengths are better absorbed by melanin, but do not penetrate as deeply into the skin. Longer wavelengths penetrate better, but are not absorbed as well by melanin. The alexandrite laser provides a favorable balance of penetration and melanin absorption (See Illustration).

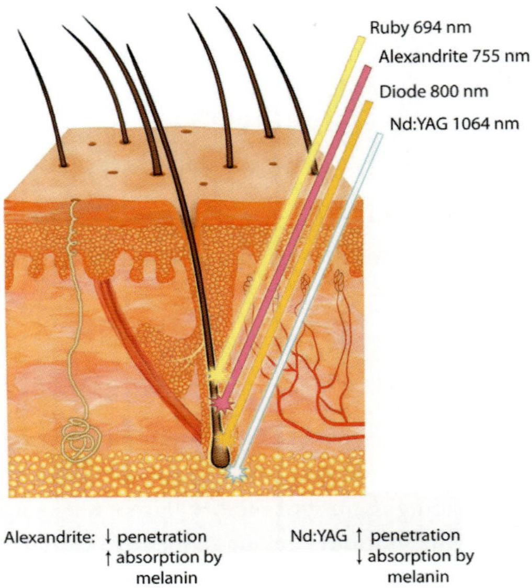

Lasers for Hair Removal

The Nd:YAG laser has a wavelength of 1064 nm. This laser penetrates more deeply into the skin, but at the price of much reduced melanin absorption. To compensate for this decreased absorption, early investigators rubbed a black carbon-mineral oil preparation into the skin to act as a target for the laser energy. This concept was used in the first laser system marketed for hair removal (Softlight, manufactured by Thermolase). Patients needed to be waxed first to remove the hairs from the follicles and let the lotion penetrate the hair follicles. The need for waxing and a rubbed-in ointment were obvious disadvantages and this system is no longer used. However, the Nd:YAG laser is used today to treat patients with dark skin types (Fitzpatrick V and VI), whose skin contains too much melanin to be safely treated with the alexandrite laser, but the reduced melanin absorption also compromises its effectiveness.

The alexandrite laser offered advantages–a larger spot size and a faster repetition rate.

Our center first used the ruby laser before switching to the long-pulsed alexandrite laser. The alexandrite laser offered advantages—a larger spot size and a faster repetition rate, reducing treatment times and making them less expensive. Also, the longer "pulse duration" offered an advantage in spreading out the energy delivery, particularly for patients with darker skin types or dense hair. Although the evidence is anecdotal, our patients seem to require fewer treatments with the long-pulsed alexandrite laser than other laser systems. A cooling unit that blows refrigerated air over the skin provides sufficient cooling, reducing discomfort. Topical anesthetic cream such as EMLA is not required.

Treatment Areas

Most areas of the face and body may be treated. Women often wish to have the upper lip, chin, lower face, and neck treated. These are common areas of unwanted hair, usually an inherited tendency. The bikini area and underarms are also frequently treated. Treatment times are usually 20 minutes or less. Of course, the arms and legs are larger areas and take longer to treat.

Men may experience overgrowth of hair in the beard area causing the five o'clock shadow. The lower face and neck may be treated to reduce growth in these areas. Laser hair removal may also be used to treat troublesome ingrown hairs, which can cause folliculitis. The male beard has dense, coarse hair and requires more treatments than other areas. The back of the neck, shoulders, and back are the most common areas treated in men.

The Hair Cycle

While laser treatment is a huge step forward, making possible what was previously impossible, it is not perfect. Hair follicles are not all vulnerable to the laser treatment at one time, so it's not possible to eliminate them all in one laser treatment. Hair follicles cycle from a dormant resting stage of invulnerability ("telogen") to the growth phase ("anagen"), then to a brief breakdown phase ("catagen"), and then back to the telogen phase again. The cycle length is different, depending on the anatomic location. For most areas of the body, it's between four and 10 months long and about half this time is spent in the anagen phase. The scalp has a much longer anagen phase, accounting for the longer length of scalp hairs.

Of course, hairs are not all in the same phase of their cycle at one time. They only seem to be vulnerable to laser treatment in their growth phase, perhaps owing to the presence of a hair shaft in the follicle to absorb laser energy (the reason to avoid plucking before laser hair removal). Furthermore, even hair follicles that are in anagen may not be permanently deactivated with a single laser treatment. A significant percentage survive, although the hair they produce may be less coarse and lighter. Consequently, laser hair removal cannot remove all the hair growth in one treatment. Treatments are spaced out at least a month apart, to treat hair follicles just emerging from their "hibernation," as I like to think of it. Over the course of treatments, few hair follicles will escape exposure to the laser energy.

Alternative Light-Based Systems

There are alternative Intense Pulsed Light (IPL™) systems (such as Epilight™) that use a flashlamp and then a filter to narrow the range of wavelengths. These light-based systems are sometimes confused with lasers. The advantage of *laser* treatment is specificity. All of the energy is delivered on the desired wavelength so that there is less wasted energy.

How It's Done

Avoid Plucking

The treated area is shaved prior to treatment. This removes the portion of the hair above the surface of the skin and leaves a small piece of the hair still in the hair follicle. This way the laser energy is not wasted by singeing the hair on the outside, but used where it is needed, heating the melanin contained in the cells at the base of the hair follicle and in the piece of the hair which remains in the hair follicle. This is also the reason that we recommend that patients do not pluck their hairs before treatment. Not only is plucking painful and unnecessary, but leaving the small piece of hair in the follicle may improve results by absorbing more laser energy.

Eye protection is worn. The laser emits pulses of light that are slightly uncomfortable. A unit that blows cool air on the skin helps. In our facility, a nurse or an aesthetician typically performs the procedure.

Skin Types

The most favorable combination for treatment is dark hair and light skin. Such patients have maximum contrast between pigment concentration in the hair follicle and the skin, so that there is minimal skin absorption of laser energy, making the treatments safe and not overly uncomfortable. High energy settings may be safely used, targeting the laser energy where we want it—on the melanin lining the hair follicles.

Patients with darker skin types have more melanin in their skin, so there is a higher risk of "hypopigmentation," or lightening of the skin in the area of treatment. Blisters or even burns are possible. For this reason, darkly-complected African-Americans (Fitzpatrick skin type VI) are not good candidates for laser hair removal.

Patients with white, grey, or very blond, wispy ("villous") hairs do not respond well either, because there is minimal melanin present around the hair follicle or in the hair shaft itself.

Many patients with darker skin types may still be treated, but with lower energy settings to avoid burning the skin. This includes most Asian, Hispanic, southern Mediterranean, middle Eastern, and East Indian skin types (Fitzpatrick skin types IV and V). Lightly-complected blacks may also be treated. There is less contrast between skin color and hair color, so lower energy settings and a longer pulse duration are used. I tell these patients they should expect to have more treatments.

It does seem unfair that people with darker skin types are less ideal candidates, but this is simply a reality of the physics of the treatment. Lightly-complected patients with light hair are not good candidates either.

Avoid Tanning before Treatments

It is best to avoid tanning prior to treatments. Tanning increases the melanin content in the skin, so the skin absorbs more of the laser energy, making treatments more uncomfortable. Also, lower energy settings must be used in tanned patients, compromising effectiveness.

Minimal Discomfort

Unlike other techniques such as waxing, there is no need to grow out the hair before treatment. It can be helpful to have a few days' growth of hair to help demonstrate the area to be treated.

Treatments vary in length from just a few minutes to treat a small area (for example, the upper lip) to over an hour for very large areas (the shoulders and back, or both legs). Patients are quite comfortable and tolerate the laser treatment well. The feeling is similar to the snap of a rubber band on the skin. No anesthetic is required. We have treated many teenagers and even some 11- and 12-year-old girls.

Spacing of Treatments

The number of treatments depends on the individual and the area treated. Facial hair cycles quickly, so that the second treatment may be performed four weeks after the first. This spacing of treatments allows hair follicles in their resting phase time to cycle into their growth phase, so they are susceptible to treatment. Each additional treatment provides greater clearance of hair. My advice is that patients schedule their first two treatments four weeks apart to provide an effective one-two combination and ensure that few hair follicles escape treatment. Additional treatments are at the patient's discretion. Patients who wish to be on the fast track can return as frequently as monthly until they are satisfied.

Treatment Photograph

A patient's back is treated with the alexandrite laser.

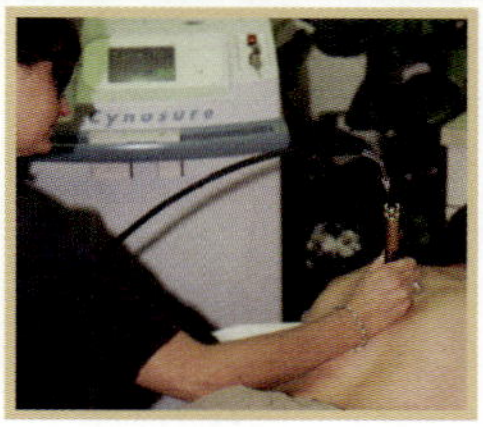

Patient Photographs

Laser treatment of chin and neck.

Comments: This 30-year-old woman had unwanted hair on her chin and neck, and her skin became irritated and inflamed. Past treatments had been unhelpful. She noticed an improvement after her first alexandrite laser treatment. She is seen after one treatment, and again two-and-a-half years later, after six treatments.

T.W., age 30/32, manager

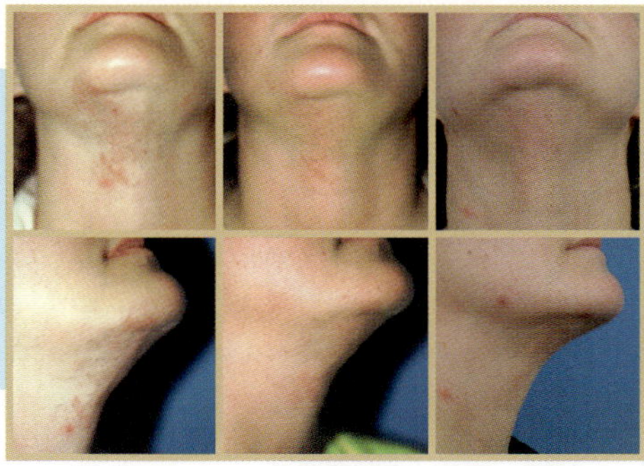

before *1 month after* *2½ years later*

Laser treatment of back and shoulders.

Comments: This 50-year-old man had always been self-conscious about his body hair. His neck had been shaved in the "before" picture. He is seen six weeks after his third treatment (15 months after his first treatment). His back and neck were not shaved in the after picture.

E.D., age 50

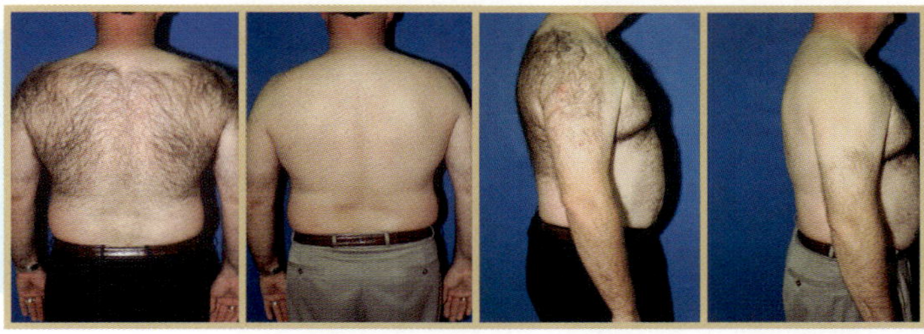

before *15 months after* *before* *15 months after*

What to Expect after Treatment

The skin is typically red immediately after the procedure, like a sunburn. There are tiny areas of swelling that cause little bumps around the hair follicles ("follicular edema"). Hydrocortisone cream, 1%, is applied to reduce inflammation. Usually the redness fades over a period of hours. The patient may see hair fragments fall out over the next week or two. There may be a hair-free period of a few weeks (longer with additional treatments), followed by a less dense growth of new hair.

Each Treatment Reduces Hair Density

Patients need to know that repeated treatments are needed. The exact number is unknown and varies from patient to patient depending upon the area treated, treatment response (related to hair color, skin color, and hair density), and patient expectations.

I explain to patients that each treatment reduces the hair density by a certain percentage, for example 20%. The first treatment or two may not produce a conspicuous difference, but the reduction becomes more obvious with more treatments. It takes about a 50% reduction to produce a noticeable difference, so if the patient can see a difference they likely have already reached this milestone. Most patients are satisfied with a reduction of about 80%. This level may be reached after three to six treatments in patients with favorably dark hair and light skin. At this point, they may be shaving infrequently enough that their hair no longer constitutes a nuisance. Of course, they can always return in the future for additional treatments, if desired. On the other hand, there are patients who have two or three treatments, are pleased with the result, and do not return for more.

There is a small subset of patients who really want to *eliminate* the unwanted hair. These patients typically return every month and may have 10 treatments or more. Each treatment is less uncomfortable than the preceding one because there are fewer hairs to absorb the laser energy. You might think that such patients would be dissatisfied, returning for so many treatments. On the contrary, they are happy to have a safe, effective treatment that has helped tremendously with a problem that has caused them social embarrassment. They simply want more of a good thing.

Because of this variation between individual responses and expectations, it is impossible to predict exactly how many treatments will be needed. Therefore, laser hair removal is priced by the treatment, not for a package of treatments.

Are the Results Permanent?

When we first started doing laser hair removal, we did not know whether the effects were permanent, although early studies were encouraging. With greater experience, researchers found that the disabled hair follicles did not regain function; the effect appears to be permanent.

Patient satisfaction is remarkably high. Since 1997, our center has successfully treated thousands of patients, mostly women, but also a large number of men who typically have their backs treated.

Complications

Infection

Because the laser does not produce a break in the surface of the skin, the risk of infection is minimal.

Hyperpigmentation

Hyperpigmentation can occur after treatment, particularly in patients with darker skin types. Hyperpigmentation is both prevented and treated by strict avoidance of ultraviolet exposure, sunblock, and a bleaching cream. It can take several months to fade.

Hypopigmentation

There is a risk of lightening of the skin, particularly in patients with darker complexions. This is rarely an issue of practical importance for patients, who may not mind some skin lightening in the treatment areas anyway.

Blistering

Blistering is more likely in tanned patients or those with darker skin types because more energy is absorbed by the skin. When they do rarely occur, these blisters are superficial and unlikely to leave scars.

Scarring

The risk of scarring is minimized by the use of appropriate energy settings, taking into account the skin pigmentation.

Care after Treatment

A moisturizer may be used after treatment. For persistent redness or a prickly sunburn sensation, a mild steroid cream such as hydrocortisone, 1%, may be applied to the affected areas. This is an over-the-counter medication. It is wise to avoid sun exposure for at least a few days after treatment, or longer if another treatment is contemplated.

Frequently Asked Questions

Q: Is there any cream that works to remove hair?

A: There is a product called Vaniqa® that is marketed for hair removal. I have prescribed it on occasion to patients that request it. Tellingly, no one has asked for a renewal of the prescription. It appears to have minimal effectiveness.

Q: Are there any restrictions after the laser treatment?

A: Avoidance of ultraviolet light (i.e., sun exposure) for a period of at least several days (longer in some cases) after treatment is recommended to avoid hyperpigmentation (skin darkening) due to temporary melanocyte hypersensitivity.

Avoid the sun and tanning *before* treatments to reduce the amount of melanin in the skin that would otherwise absorb the laser energy, causing more discomfort and making it necessary to reduce the energy setting on the laser.

Q: Is the hair removal permanent?

A: Studies show that the hair follicles that are disabled by the laser treatment do not tend to recover, so that, yes, the effect is permanent. But, of course, not all hair follicles are deactivated with each treatment. Each treatment reduces the hair count (density).

Q: What results should I expect after my first treatment?

A: I use the analogy of cutting trees in a forest. If an enthusiastic woodsman were to cut down every fifth tree in a forest, the forest would still resemble a forest. It may take three or more such tree-cutting sessions, cutting down 20% each time, before the forest starts to look thinned out. Once about half the trees are eliminated, the results are noticeable. So you should not expect too much from just one or two treatments. Be patient and after your third or fourth treatment you should notice a difference. For my more mathematically-inclined patients, an exponential curve is a useful reference. In the midportion of the curve, there is a rapid decline, but then the curve flattens out, approaching but never actually reaching zero hairs.

Q: Is it painful?

A: Yes, there is some discomfort, similar to a rubber band snapping on the skin. After awhile it does not seem to hurt as much. However, there are areas of the face and body, such as the upper lip and flanks, which seem to be more sensitive. The cooling unit helps to make the procedure more comfortable. The energy setting is adjusted to strike the right balance between comfort and effectiveness. A clue to effectiveness is the redness of the skin. Excessive redness may be an indication the power setting is a little too high, but a little redness is to be expected and confirms energy delivery. Almost everyone can tolerate these treatments. We've even treated 12-year-old girls on occasion.

Q: How many treatments will I need?

A: The number of treatments depends on your skin type, hair color and density, area of the body, and your expectations. If you have dark hair and light skin, you have the ideal combination and should have a favorable result. If your hair is very dense, or if you have more pigment in your skin, you will need more treatments. Most patients are satisfied with a hair reduction of about 80%. This result may reduce the need for shaving from a daily ritual to perhaps weekly or less often.

The average patient has between three and six treatments. However, many patients report a satisfying reduction after as few as two treatments. On the other hand, some patients, who are intent on removing as much hair as possible, have returned for 10 or more treatments over a period of a few years.

The male beard area is notoriously dense. Men having this area treated should expect to have more treatments.

Q: I have a big problem with ingrown hairs. Will this help?

A: Yes. Ingrown hairs can be a nuisance, causing chronic inflammation. The hair is difficult to extract because it is buried by the skin. Laser hair removal can effectively treat buried hair follicles that tend to become painfully inflamed.

Q: Should I let the hair grow out before my laser treatment?

A: It can be helpful to have the slightest amount of hair growth at the time of treatment, just enough to show the affected area. But any more than this is unnecessary. Accordingly, you should stop shaving the day before your treatment or perhaps the morning of your treatment if your hair comes in quickly.

Q: I heard that shaving is to be avoided because this makes the problem worse. Is this true?

A: No. This is an old wives' tale. Shaving is to be encouraged, not discouraged. Women can shave too and should not be embarrassed about doing so. Shaving is much faster and less painful than plucking or tweezing. The new hair that erupts from the surface of the skin does seem to be coarser than the old one but this is simply because it is short. It has not yet grown out enough to be flexible. If anything, shaving can be healthy for skin, providing a little exfoliation. Women should not regard shaving as unfeminine. With laser hair removal treatments, it is not necessary to shave as often.

Q: Do the hairs just fall out?

A: Yes. You may see hair fragments that get pushed out of the hair follicles during the week or two after treatment.

CHAPTER TWELVE

Tattoo Removal

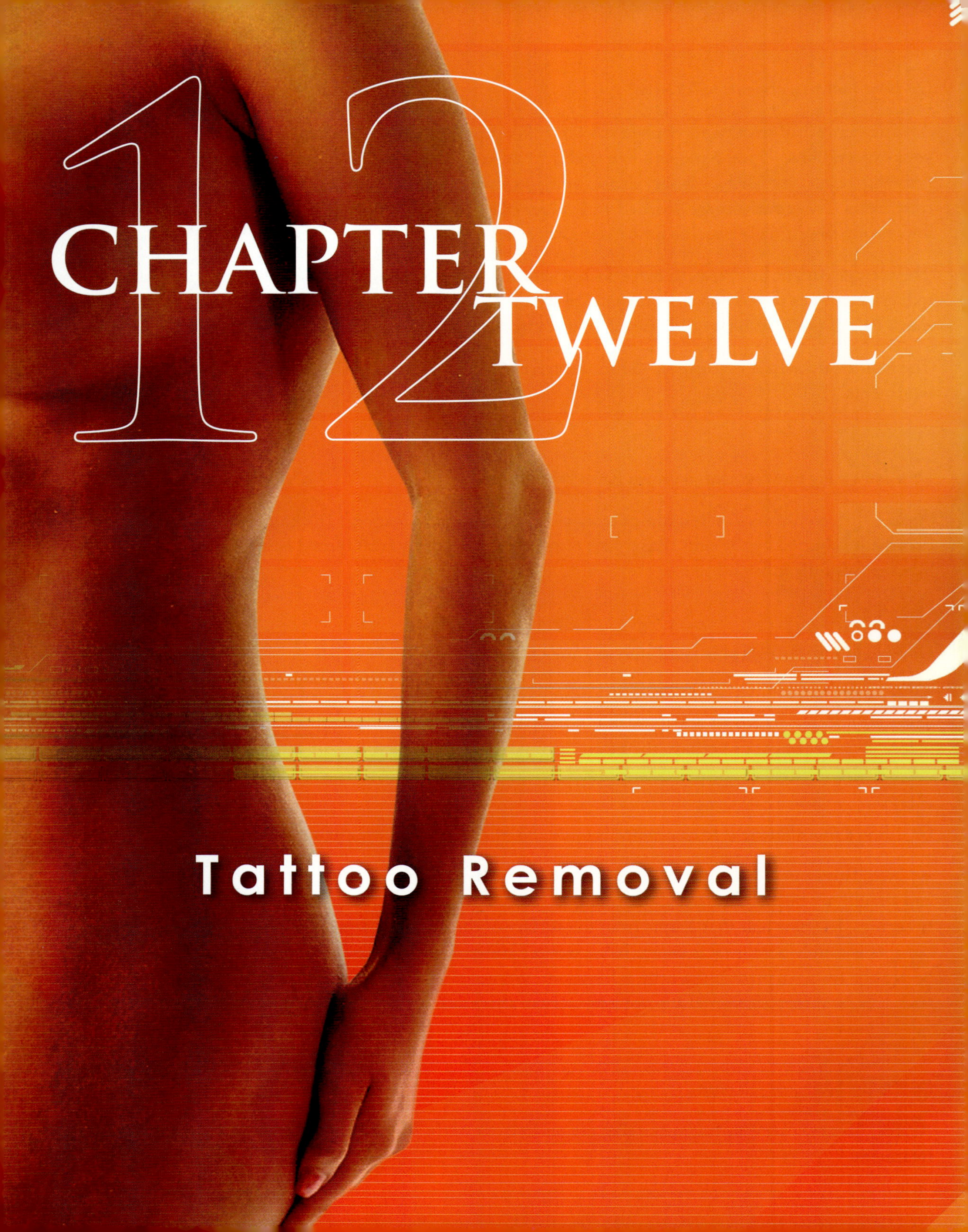

Introduction

Today, almost as many women (13%) as men (15%) have tattoos. A 2004 telephone survey among young adults, ages 18-29, found 36% had tattoos. Despite their popularity, a large percentage of people with tattoos eventually regret having them.

How It's Done

Like life in general, it's always easier to get into trouble than out of it. Removing a tattoo is more difficult and costly than getting one. Tattoo removal presents a number of challenges. Often, multiple colored dyes are used by the tattoo artist, and the pigment is typically injected deep into the dermis.

Laser Treatment

Laser treatment uses light energy delivered on a specific wavelength that is absorbed by a pigment in the skin. One laser cannot treat all colors. Dark ink tattoos (black and blue) are most successfully treated with the laser.

The "Q-switched" Nd:YAG and ruby lasers work well on black and blue dyes, but not as well on green pigment (the Q-switched alexandrite laser works better for this), and not at all on red or yellow colors (a pulsed dye laser is needed for these). Ironically, the tattoo pigment may even be made darker by laser treatments, particularly flesh-toned pigments.

Multiple treatments are needed, as many as 10, at monthly intervals. Some colors are difficult or impossible to remove, and there is always a blemish that remains. Patients are invariably disappointed to hear about these limitations of laser treatment of tattoos, the expense, and the time investment.

Patients are invariably disappointed to hear about these limitations of laser treatment of tattoos, the expense, and the time investment.

However, there may be no alternative treatment. Laser treatment is the only option for large tattoos or tattoos that are placed in areas where surgical excision is not feasible. Examples are a large tattoo on the back or a circumferential arm tattoo.

A new tattoo ink, composed of tiny plastic beads that contain bioremovable dyes ("Infinitink" manufactured by Freedom2Ink) has been developed that is more susceptible to laser treatment and can be removed in fewer sessions. The laser energy ruptures the microscopic beads, allowing the ink to be absorbed by the body. This innovation appears to be a step in the right direction. If all tattoo ink colors could be manufactured using such a process (currently, just black ink is available), and proved acceptable to tattoo artists, this would be a huge advantage for patients, and possibly for the tattoo industry as well.

Surgical Removal

It is usually preferable to have small tattoos surgically removed, although this does leave a scar and may necessitate staging (repeated excisions) if the tattoo is too large to be removed in one treatment (See M.R., Patient Photographs). Most patients are willing to trade their tattoo for a scar, particularly if the tattoo has negative psychological connotations or creates a limitation in the workplace.

A common example of a tattoo that lends itself to surgical removal is a dolphin tattoo on an ankle. Although such a tattoo may be small, the skin is tight, with little room to stretch, so that two or three excisions may be needed. A more ideal placement is the lower abdomen, where there is plenty of loose skin and the scar from tattoo removal can be placed inconspicuously along the bikini line. It is usually possible to remove a small or intermediate-sized tattoo in one stage in this location.

Patient Photographs

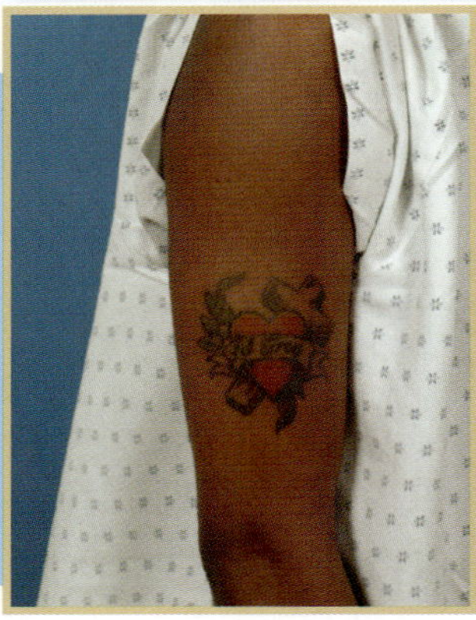

before

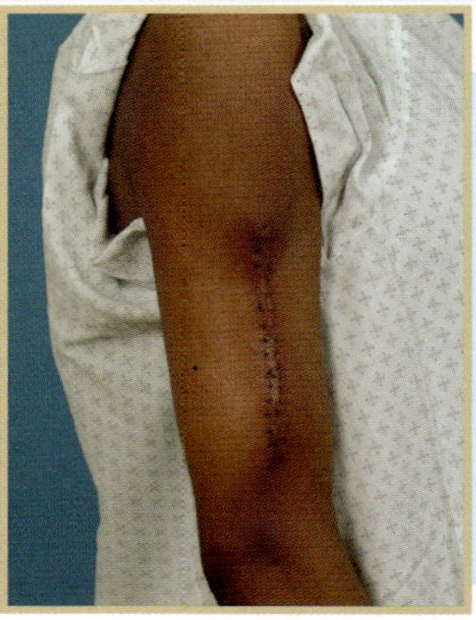

2 weeks after 3rd procedure

Staged tatto removal.

Comments: This patient wished to have a tattoo removed from her right upper arm. Her after photograph was taken on the day her sutures were removed, two weeks after her third-stage excision. The suture tracks are still conspicuous. She has some early puckering at each end (dog ears) that flattened out over the next few months. Because of the large size of her tattoo, three procedures were needed, all done in the office under local anesthesia.

M.R., age 32, office worker

What to Expect after Surgery

Depending on the size of the tattoo and the location, one or more procedures are needed. The scar is longer than the diameter of the tattoo. There may be puckering at the ends of the incision. These gradually settle down.

Complications

Laser Treatment

Complications include scarring, hypopigmentation, darkening of flesh-toned tattoo colors, and inadequate clearance of the tattoo, especially multicolored tattoos.

Surgical Removal

Complications are the same as for any surgical scar—scarring, infection, wound dehiscence, and hematoma (rarely). The scar is the trade-off for removal of the tattoo. If the scar is under excessive tension, due to removal of a large tattoo, it is likely to spread more and may require a revision later on. This tendency for scars to widen under tension is the reason it is often better to remove a sizable tattoo in stages rather than trying to do too much in one operation.

Care after Surgery

The wound should be kept clean. Resume bathing right away. Apply topical antibiotic ointment twice a day. Depending on the location of the tattoo and the skin tension, the sutures come out in 10-14 days.

Frequently Asked Questions

Q: Does laser treatment work?

A: Laser treatment does lighten tattoos, but there are limitations depending on the number of colors used in the tattoo. Complete elimination is usually not possible; a blemish remains on the skin.

Q: If I have it removed surgically, how big is the scar?

A: The scar needs to be longer than the diameter of the tattoo.

Q: How many treatments will I need?

A: This depends of course on the site and size of the tattoo. The number of anticipated treatments is discussed with your surgeon at your consultation.

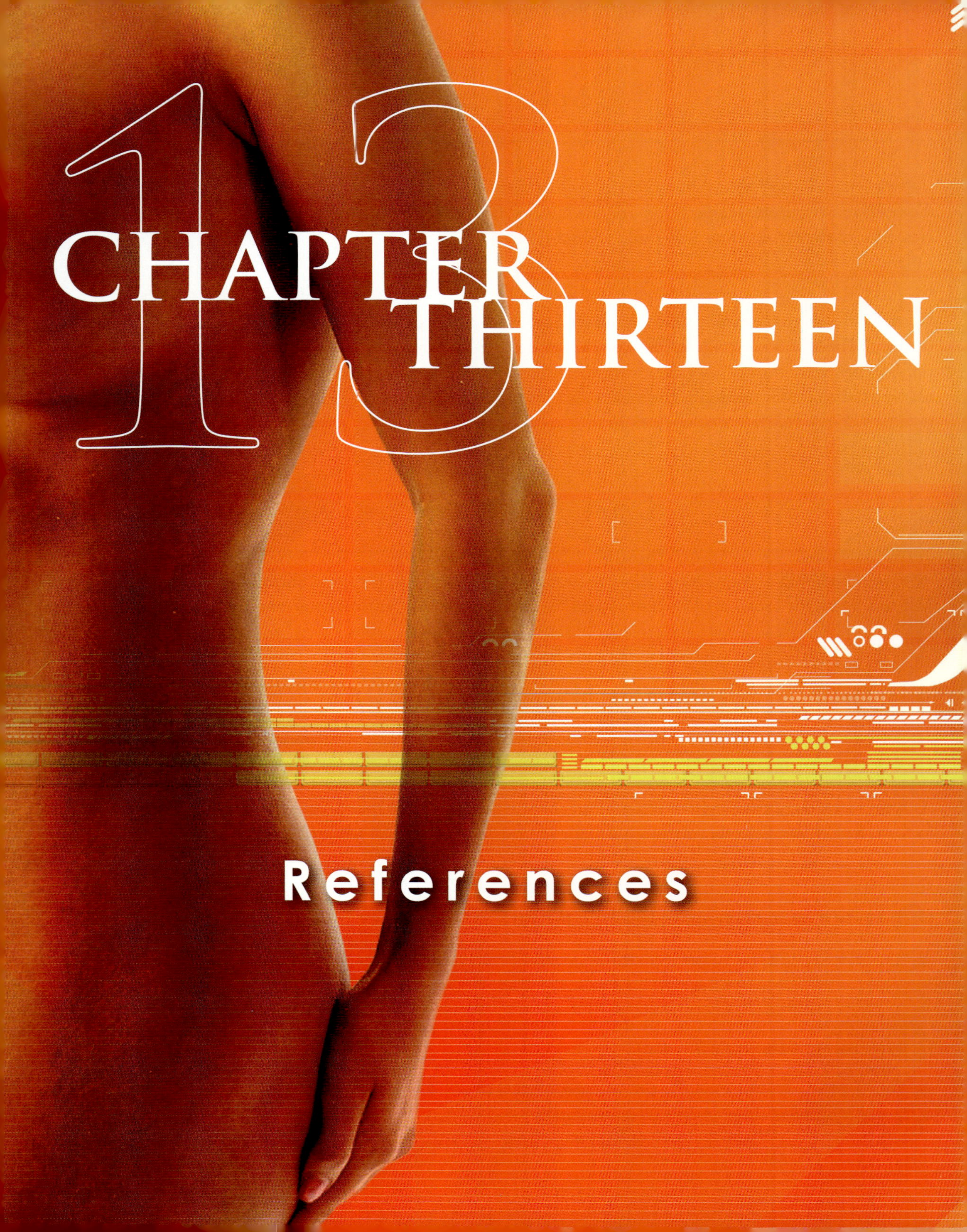

13 CHAPTER THIRTEEN

References

Foreword – Science and the Ideal Body

Page 9

"Obesity is a huge problem today in the United States, with one third of adults obese and another third in the overweight category."

American Obesity Association. Web site available at http://www.obesity.org. Accessed September 2008.

"In France, only 9% of adults are obese; in Japan, only 3%."

http://www.aneki.com/obesity.html. Accessed June 11, 2009.

Page 11

"'VelaShape™', an upgrade of the VelaSmooth™ System, (Syneron Inc., Irvine, Ca.) is a machine that uses a combination of four modalities—radiofrequency energy, infrared light, rollers, and suction …to smooth cellulite. The manufacturer also claims this can reduce the circumference of the abdomen, buttocks, and thighs."

http://www.velashape.com/how-velashape-works. Accessed July 11, 2009.

"Liposuction has been subjected to scientific study by pioneers in the field of ultrasonic liposuction."

Rohrich, R.J., Beran, S.J., and Kenkel, J.M. *Ultrasonic-assisted Liposuction*. St. Louis: Quality Medical Publishing, 1998.

Kenkel, J.M., Lipschitz, A.H., Shepherd, G., Armstrong, V.W., Streit, F., Oellerich, M., Luby, M., Rohrich, R.J., and Brown, S.A. Pharmacokinetics and safety of lidocaine and monoethylglycinexylidide in liposuction: a microdialysis study. *Plast. Reconstr. Surg.* 114: 16, 2004.

Brown, S.A., Lipschitz, A.H., Kenkel, J.M., Sorokin, E., Shepherd, G., Grebe, S., Oliver, L.K., Luby, M. and Rohrich, R.J. Pharmacokinetics and safety of epinephrine use in liposuction. *Plast. Reconstr. Surg.* 114: 756, 2004.

Liposuction

Page 13

"Healthy premenopausal women have waist-to-hip ratios of 0.67 to 0.80. This means that their waist circumference is seven- to eight-tenths as large as their hips. A healthy man's waist-to-hip ratio is between 0.85 and 0.95."

Singh, D. Adaptive significance of female physical attractiveness: role of waist-to-hip ratio. *Journal of Personality and Social Psychology*. 65: 293, 1993.

"Men have an innate preference for female bodies with narrow waists and full hips, which signal high fertility, high estrogen, and low testosterone."

Ibid.

"this preference for feminine waist-to-hip ratios is not limited to Caucasian males, but is true for women and other cultures and races as well."

Singh, D. Body fat distribution and perception of desirable female body shape by young black men and women. *International Journal of Eating Disorders*. 16: 289, 1994.

Singh, D. and Luis, S. Ethnic and gender consensus for the effect of waist-to-hip ratio on judgment of women's attractiveness. *Human Nature*. 6: 51, 1995.

"The 1950s bombshell and early *Playboy* centerfold, Jayne Mansfield, reportedly had measurements of 40-21-35, for a waist-to-hip ratio of 0.60. (She also said her IQ was 163, but the public was more interested in her other measurements.)"

http://en.wikipedia.org/wiki/Jayne_Mansfield. Accessed July 19, 2009.

"Barbie™ (1959-) has measurements of 36-18-33, with a 0.54 waist-to-hip ratio."

Etcoff, N. *Survival of the Prettiest. The Science of Beauty*. New York: Anchor Books, 2000. Page 192.

"at least before 'breaking up' with Ken in 2004"

http://www.foxnews.com/story/0,2933,111234,00.html. Accessed August 9, 2009.

"During the 20th century, Miss Americas (1923-87) and *Playboy* centerfolds (1955-65, 1976-90) alike had waist-to-hip ratios that ranged from 0.68 to 0.72. The average Miss America measurements in 1940 were 34-24.5-35; in 1987, they were a slightly bustier and trimmer 35-23.5-34.5."

Singh, D. Adaptive significance of female physical attractiveness: role of waist-to-hip ratio. *Journal of Personality and Social Psychology*. 65: 293, 1993.

Page 14

"By the end of the 20th century, the average fashion model was four inches taller than the average woman, but maintained an hourglass 0.70 waist-to-hip ratio, combining a tall, lean body with curves."

Tovee, M.J., Mason, S.M., Emery, J.L., McClusky, S.E., and Cohen-Tovee, E.M. Supermodels: stick insects or hour-glasses? *Lancet* 350: 1474, 1997.

"The Miss Americas of the 1960s averaged five feet six inches tall and weighed 120 pounds. Twenty years later they had gained two inches in height but remained the same weight. *Playboy* playmates also gained an inch in height and dropped several pounds in weight during the same period."

Mazur, A. U.S. trends in feminine beauty and overadaptation. *Journal of Sex Research*, 22: 281, 1986.

"Even the Columbia Pictures logo, the torch-bearing woman, was slimmed down in 1992."

Etcoff, N. *Survival of the Prettiest. The Science of Beauty*. New York: Anchor Books, 2000. Page 201.

"Today, 64% of American adults are overweight, defined as having a body mass index of 25 or greater, and 31% are obese, having a body mass of 30 or greater."

American Obesity Association. Web site available at http://www.obesity.org. Accessed September 2008.

"Only one state, Colorado, can claim less than a 20% obesity rate…six states have rates higher than 30%."

http://www.cdc.gov/obesity/data/trends.html. Accessed July 19, 2009.

"The proportion of overweight children (ages 6-19) has jumped from about 5% to 17% in the last 30 years."

http://www.cdc.gov/obesity/childhood/prevalence.html. Accessed July 19, 2009.

"An excellent resource on this topic of interest to almost everyone is Robert Pool's scholarly review, *Fat. Fighting the Obesity Epidemic.*"

Pool, R. *Fat: Fighting the Obesity Epidemic*. Oxfordshire: Oxford University Press, 2001.

"Nonobese people form fat cells only up to age two, and then again from age 10 to 18...obese children continue to form fat cells up to the age of 24"

Knittle, J.L., Timmers, K., and Ginsverg-Fellner, F. The growth of adipose tissue in children and adolescents. *Journal of Clinical Investigation*. 63: 239, 1979.

"An adult female who weighs 160 pounds has about 40 pounds of fat. Her lean body mass is 120 pounds. At 200 pounds, she has about 70 pounds of fat, but her lean body mass increases only about 10 pounds (accounting for the extra weight of connective tissue, muscle and blood vessels to support the fat)…this additional fatty tissue adds little to the body's energy requirements."

Pool, R. *Fat: Fighting the Obesity Epidemic*. Oxfordshire: Oxford University Press, 2001. Page 247.

"Research showed that, as a person's weight increases from ideal body weight to obesity, the number of fat cells remains the same. Each fat cell swells to accommodate more fat-storing triglycerides. But this cellular expansion has a limit. A fat cell can expand to about four times its original size before it needs to divide to store more fat."

Hirsch, J., Knittle, J.L., and Salans, L.B. Cell lipid content and cell number in obese and non-obese human adipose tissue. *Journal of Clinical Investigation*. 45: 1023, 1966.

"This works out to about a 60 pound weight gain in the average adult, corresponding to a body mass index well over 30. So within a range of about 60 pounds over ideal weight, fat cell numbers stay the same. Any changes are purely due to an increase or decrease in the size of individual fat cells."

Bulfer, J.M. and Allen, C.E. Fat cells and obesity. *Bioscience*. 29: 736, 1979.

Page 15

"An average fat cell is about one-tenth of a millimeter in diameter, about the width of a human hair. In obese people the fat cell may be twice as big, and in lean people half as big."

Pool, R. *Fat: Fighting the Obesity Epidemic.* Oxfordshire: Oxford University Press, 2001. Page 63.

"Body Mass Index"

http://apps.who.int/bmi/index.jsp?introPage=intro_3.html. Accessed July 19, 2009.

"Researchers found that in extremely obese patients who underwent successful bariatric surgery, lost massive amounts of weight, and maintained the weight loss, fat cell size dropped sharply. However, reduction in cell *number* was not as impressive; only about a sixth of the fat cells seemed to disappear."

Naslun, I., Hallgren, P., and Sjöström, L. Fat-cell weight and number before and after gastric surgery for morbid obesity in women. *International Journal of Obesity*. 12: 191, 1988.

"The primary problem in obese people is a change in homeostasis—the "set point" for their weight. The set point is the weight that the body considers normal. In obesity, this equilibrium may become reset at a much higher weight than normal. If their weight creeps up *above* this point, their metabolic rate increases to burn calories, they tend to lose their hunger, and their weight drifts back to this set point. If their weight drops *below* this set point, their brain gets receives hunger signals, their metabolic rate drops to conserve energy."

Pool, R. *Fat: Fighting the Obesity Epidemic.* Oxfordshire: Oxford University Press, 2001. Page 72.

Page 16

"In the obese person whose weight drops below this elevated set point, the body wrongly reacts as if it is starving and needs to conserve fuel"

Leibel, R.L., Rosenbaum, M., and Hirsch, J. Changes in energy expenditure resulting from altered body weight. *N. Engl. J. Med.* 332: 621, 1995.

"People born without the gene for this hormone, an exceedingly rare condition, always feel hungry and become severely obese (and may be successfully treated with injections of this hormone)."

Pool, R. *Fat: Fighting the Obesity Epidemic.* Oxfordshire: Oxford University Press, 2001. Page 3.

"The problem is that obese people already have high levels of circulating leptin, so this strategy would not work for them."

Ibid. Page 132.

"In nonobese people, this homeostatic mechanism is normally very finely tuned, so that normally our weight changes little in the course of a year, despite large swings in the number of calories in and calories out. However, there is a general trend upward, with the average American man or woman gaining about 20 pounds between the age of 25 and 55."

Rosenbaum, M., Leibel, R.L., and Hirsch, J. Obesity. *N. Engl. J. Med.* 337: 396, 1997.

"Studies in volunteers have shown that nonobese people who gain weight intentionally tend to lose it quickly, and the weight gain is entirely due to fat cell expansion."

Pool, R. *Fat: Fighting the Obesity Epidemic.* Oxfordshire: Oxford University Press, 2001. Pages 70, 85.

"This fact explains why the people who have successfully dropped hundreds of pounds without surgery are so few and far between, and almost maniacal in their efforts to stay thin. They must exert tremendous willpower to stay thin because they often feel hungry. They may have even developed some obsessive behavior in an effort to keep the weight off, such as jogging six miles a day."

Ibid. Page 84.

Page 17

"There are rare cases of genetic mutations causing obesity (Prader-Willi syndrome), but in these patients the obesity is extreme, and there are other obvious physical abnormalities."

Ibid. Page 3.

Rosenbaum, M., Leibel, R.L., and Hirsch, J. Obesity. *N. Engl. J. Med.* 337: 396, 1997.

"A review of increasing obesity rates in the United States."

http://www.cdc.gov/obesity/data/trends.html. Accessed July 19, 2009.

"22% of American adults exercise regularly."

http://news.msu.edu/story/31/. Accessed July 19, 2009.

"Recent studies suggest that proper diet is much more important because the calories burned by exercise are so modest in comparison to the calories consumed in a single serving of french fries, for example, or a muffin. Furthermore, exercise tends to increase hunger."

Church, T.S., Martin, C.K., Thompson, A.M., Earnest, C.P., Mikus, C.R., and Blair, S.N. Changes in weight, waist circumference and compensatory responses with different doses of exercise among sedentary, overweight postmenopausal women. *PLoS ONE.* 4(2): e4515. http://www.plosone.org/article/info:doi/10.1371/journal.pone.0004515. Accessed August 10, 2009.

"One study found that 75% of children who were obese at age 10-14 were obese at age 25."

Whitaker, R.C., Wright, J.A., Pepe, M.S., Seidel, K.D., and Dietz, W.H. Predicting obesity in young adulthood from childhood and parental obesity. *N. Engl. J. Med.* 337: 869, 1997.

"Body Shape is Hereditary"

Rosenbaum, M., Leibel, R.L., and Hirsch, J. "Obesity." *N. Engl. J. Med.* 337: 396, 1997.

"When we gain weight, our existing fat cells swell and when we lose weight, they shrink. *But their number and distribution remain the same.*"

Kreider, J.W., Hughes, K.C., Smeal, D., Hirai, T., and Manders, E.K. Obesity. *Clin. Plast. Surg.* 23: 671, 1996.

Spalding, K.L., Arner, E., Westermark, P.O., Bernard, S., Buchholz, B.A., Bergmann, O., Blomqvist, L., Hoffstedt, J., Näslund, E., Britton, T., Concha, H., Hassan, M., Rydén, M., Frisén, J. and Arner, P. Dynamics of fat cell turnover in humans. *Nature.* 453: 783, 2008.

Page 19

"Our studies showed that three months after liposuction, patients lost an average of 2.2 pounds overall. Patients with liposuction volumes over 3,000 cc lost an average of 5.2 pounds."

Swanson, E. Unpublished data. Swanson Center, 2009.

Page 20

"We know from our studies that liposuction can lower circulating triglycerides. This effect is particularly pronounced in patients with liposuction volumes over three liters."

Ibid.

"Using the 'tumescent' technique, fluids are injected into the tissues before liposuction is performed."

Klein, J.A. Tumescent technique for regional anesthesia permits lidocaine dose of 35 mg/kg for liposuction. *J.Dermatol Surg. Oncol.* 16: 248, 1990.

"The 'superwet' technique is a modified form of tumescent liposuction, in which fluids are infused in approximately a 1:1 ratio with the volume suctioned off by liposuction (the 'aspirate')."

Rohrich, R.J., Beran, S.J., Fodor, P.B. The role of subcutaneous infiltration in suction-assisted lipoplasty: A review. *Plast. Reconstr. Surg.* 99: 514, 1997.

Page 23

"A long time coming, liposuction was a huge step forward in body contouring surgery when the technique burst on the scene after a presentation by Dr. Illouz in 1982."

Illouz, Y.G. Body contouring by lipolysis: a 5-year experience with over 3,000 cases. *Plast. Reconstr. Surg.* 72: 591, 1983.

"In 1990 an American dermatologist, Dr. Jeffrey Klein, described the tumescent technique."

Klein, J.A. tumescent technique for regional anesthesia permits lidocaine dose of 35 mg/kg for liposuction, *J.Dermatol Surg. Oncol.* 16: 248, 1990.

Page 24

"Ultrasonic liposuction, also called ultrasonic-assisted liposuction, was developed by an Italian plastic surgeon, Dr. Michele Zocchi, in 1988."

Zocchi, M. Ultrasonic liposculpting. *Aesthetic Plast. Surg.* 16: 287, 1992.

"It improves results in fibrous areas that are difficult to treat with traditional liposuction—the upper abdomen, flanks, back, and male breasts. The fat is liquefied before its removal, so that the resulting contours are smooth. Because ultrasonic energy is used to break up the fat cells, less physical force may be required from the plastic surgeon."

Rohrich, R.J., Ha, R.Y., Kenkel, J.M., and Adams, W.P. Classification and management of gynecomastia: defining the role of ultrasound-assisted liposuction. *Plast. Reconstr. Surg.* 111: 909, 2003.

"An added advantage of ultrasonic liposuction may be improved skin tone and appearance, due to improved preservation of the underlying connective tissue. With selective defatting under the skin, the skin's capacity to contract is optimized."

Ibid.

Zocchi, M.L. Ultrasound assisted lipoplasty: technical refinements and clinical evaluations. *Clin. Plast. Surg.* 23: 575, 1996.

Page 25

"Another favorable observation has been the rarity of infection after ultrasonic liposuction. Dr. Zocchi attributes this finding to the conversion of some of the water molecules into peroxide molecules as they are exposed to ultrasonic energy."

Ibid.

"In the past, surgeons have relied on physical energy alone to dislodge fat cells. The surgeon literally pummeled the fat with a blunt instrument (cannula). The flimsy fat cells were dislodged from their attachments and suctioned away. This technique is effective, but nonselective. Other tissues were traumatized too."

Gupta, S.C., Khiabani, K.T., Stephenson, L.L., and Zamboni, W.A. Effect of liposuction on skin perfusion. *Plast. Reconstr. Surg.* 110: 1748, 2002.

"If a fat cell is exposed to high frequency sound waves, microbubbles are generated from pressure changes, called cavitation. The fragile cell membrane cannot contain these bubbles, and gives way, releasing its liquid fat contents ('emulsification'), which are then suctioned out of the body."

Zocchi, M.L. Ultrasound assisted lipoplasty: technical refinements and clinical evaluations. *Clin. Plast. Surg.* 23: 575, 1996.

"No question, these tissues have been traumatized, but not as much as they would have been without the benefit of ultrasound."

Kenkel, J.M., Robinson, J.B., Beran, S.J., Tan, J., Howard, B.K., Zocchi, M.L., and Rohrich, R.J. The tissue effects of ultrasound-assisted lipoplasty. *Plast. Reconstr. Surg.* 102: 213, 1998.

Page 26

"Surgeons have noticed improved skin contraction after ultrasonic treatment."

Rohrich, R.J., Beran, S.J., Kenkel, J.M., Adams, W.P. Jr., and DiSpaltro, F. Extending the role of liposuction in body contouring with ultrasound-assisted liposuction. *Plast. Reconstr. Surg.* 101: 1090, 1998.

Page 27

"One plastic surgeon is fond of reminding surgeons at meetings, 'Remember, we enjoy surgery much more than our patients.'"

Paul, M. Presentation at the meeting of the Kansas City Plastic Surgery Society, December 2008.

Page 30

"Laser systems are costly and add a price increment to surgery because a nonreusable tip is needed for each patient. Importantly, laser use in liposuction does not selectively target fat cells, which is the principle advantage of ultrasonic assistance. Studies have failed to show a definite advantage for liposuction devices that incorporate a laser. Investigators found greater cellular damage to the fat cells and greater release of triglycerides from laser treatments (versus liposuction without laser pretreatment) and no improvement in skin retraction. The word 'laser' has marketing appeal in medicine, and investigators caution against 'putting commerce before research.'"

Prado, A., Andrades, P., Danilla, S. et al. A prospective, randomized, double-blind, controlled clinical trial comparing laser-assisted lipoplasty with suction-assisted lipoplasty. *Plast. Reconstr. Surg.* 118: 1032, 2006.

"Studies have failed to show a definite advantage for liposuction devices that incorporate a laser."

Fodor, P.B. Progress report on multicenter study of laser-assisted liposuction. *Aesthetic Plast. Surg.* 19: 379, 1995.

Apfelberg, D. Results of a multicenter study of laser-assisted liposuction. *Clin. Plast. Surg.* 23: 713, 1996.

"The latest marketing scheme is external laser treatment that is being sold as a noninvasive way to lose fat 'without the dangers of surgery'"

http://www.myzerona.com. Accessed October 20, 2009.

Page 31

"According to Dr. Rod Rohrich, the editor of the *Journal of Plastic and Reconstructive Surgery*, 'it is mind-boggling to think that a physician would inject patients—or that patients would allow physicians to inject them—with unknown, unproved substances based on hearsay and unsubstantiated clinical findings.' And that it is 'inconceivable' that plastic surgeons would embrace such a treatment."

Rohrich, R.J. Mesotherapy: What is it? Does It Work? *Plast. Reconstr. Surg.* 115: 1425, 2005.

"Dr. Alan Matarasso, a New York plastic surgeon and expert in body contouring surgery, cautions: 'To ensure some level of safety before using phosphatidylcholine in mesotherapy, it would be prudent to know the products of dissolution, whether or not free fatty acids are released into the patient's bloodstream, whether the injected chemical is absorbed into the bloodstream, the effects on the liver and other organs, the appropriate dose, and so on.'"

Mesotherapy for body contouring. *Plast. Reconstr. Surg.* 115: 1420, 2005.

Page 32

"Such devices have been tried since ultrasound was first used internally to assist liposuction. However, the results have been underwhelming."

Teitelbaum, S.A., Burns, J.L., Kubota, J., Matsuda, H., Otto, M.J., Shirakabe, Y., Suzuki, Y., and Brown, S.A. Noninvasive body contouring by focused ultrasound: safety and efficacy of the Contour I device in a multicenter, controlled, clinical study. *Plast. Reconstr. Surg.* 120: 779, 2007.

Page 35

"Muscle relaxants, such as succinylcholine, reduce the sympathetic tone to the leg veins, possibly setting the stage for blood clots."

Kryger, Z.B., Fine, N.A., and Mustoe, T.A. The outcome of abdominoplasty performed under conscious sedation: six-year experience in 153 consecutive cases. *Plast. Reconstr. Surg.* 113: 1807, 2004.

Ersek, R.A. Fatal pulmonary embolism, letter to editor, *Plast. Reconstr. Surg.* 113: 1868, 2004.

"trigger malignant hyperthermia"

Friedberg, B.L. Lethal pulmonary embolisms are avoidable. *Plast Reconstr. Surg.* 123: 768, 2009.

Page 38

"Avoidance of a general anesthetic likely reduces the risk of a pulmonary embolus."

Ersek, R.A. Fatal pulmonary embolism, letter to editor, *Plast. Reconstr. Surg.* 113: 1868, 2004.

Witt, P.D. Reply. *Plast. Reconstr. Surg.* 113: 1868, 2004.

Mustoe, T.A. Discussion. Abdominoplasty: a comparison of outpatient and inpatient procedures shows that it is a safe and effective procedure for outpatients in an office-based surgery clinic. *Plast. Reconstr. Surg.* 118: 523, 2006.

"Surgeons who avoid general anesthesia report low incidences of this dangerous complication."

Kryger, Z.B., Fine, N.A., and Mustoe, T.A. The outcome of abdominoplasty performed under conscious sedation: six-year experience in 153 consecutive cases. *Plast. Reconstr. Surg.* 113: 1807, 2004.

Friedberg, B.L. Lethal pulmonary embolisms are avoidable. *Plast Reconstr. Surg.* 123: 768, 2009.

"Some surgeons have recommended the use of blood-thinners such as heparin"

Hatef, D.A., Kenkel, J.M., Nguyen, M.Q., Farkas, J.P., Abtahi, F., Rohrich, R.J., and Brown, S.A. Thromboembolic risk assessment and the efficacy of enoxaparin prophylaxis in excisional body contouring surgery. *Plast. Reconstr. Surg.* 122: 269, 2008.

Page 67

"Our Survey Says"

Unpublished data. Swanson Center, 2009.

Page 68

"To better answer these questions, our center undertook a study using MRIs."

Ibid.

Page 72

"Our study found a modest, but statistically significant ($p < 0.05$), average weight loss of 2.2 pounds three months after surgery for all liposuction patients. Patients with liposuction volumes of 3,000 cc or more experienced a greater average weight loss, dropping 5.2 pounds three months after surgery. Most notably, there was a highly significant drop in the fasting triglyceride level ($p<0.001$) after liposuction. Triglyceride levels dropped from an average of 152 mg/dL to 113 mg/dL for all liposuction patients. The decrease was even more impressive for patients with liposuction volumes over 3,000 cc, whose average fasting triglyceride level dropped from 186 before surgery to 118 after! There was no significant change in total cholesterol, LDL (the 'bad' cholesterol), or HDL (the 'good' cholesterol). Also, there were no significant changes in control patients tested at the same time intervals, confirming that these changes are caused by liposuction."

Ibid.

"The American Heart Association classifies triglyceride levels below 150 mg/dL normal and above 150 borderline-high risk. Patients with triglyceride levels over 150 are more likely to develop metabolic syndrome, increasing the risk of atherosclerosis."

http://www.americanheart.org/presenter.jhtml?identifier=183#Triglyceride. Accessed July 15, 2009.

Page 73

"Plaque buildup in arterial walls can lead to coronary artery disease, stroke and peripheral vascular disease. Metabolic syndrome also raises the risk of Type II insulin-resistant diabetes."

http://www.americanheart.org/presenter.jhtml?identifier=4756. Accessed July 15, 2009.

"Our study showed a drop in hemoglobin (the oxygen-carrying molecule contained in our red blood cells) level immediately after surgery, as expected. Three months after surgery, hemoglobin levels were back to normal."

Unpublished data. Swanson Center, 2009.

"Our study showed that levels of circulating anesthetic agents given in the anesthetic solution, lidocaine and bupivicaine (used for abdominoplasty patients), remain below toxic levels. There are no significant changes in liver enzymes or blood sugar."

Ibid.

Page 74

"Also, limiting the duration of ultrasonic treatment to a few minutes per area helps prevent complications, such as burns or seromas."

Fodor, P.B. Personal experience with ultrasound-assisted lipoplasty: a pilot study comparing ultrasound-assisted lipoplasty with traditional lipoplasty. *Plast. Reconstr. Surg.* 113: 1852, 2004.

Page 76

"Normally, some fat is released into the bloodstream during liposuction and travels to the lungs."

Kenkel, J.M., Brown, S.A., Love, E.J., Waddle, J.P., Krueger, J.E., Noble, D., Robinson, J.B., and Rohrich, R.J. Hemodynamics, electrolytes, and organ histology of larger-volume liposuction in a porcine model. *Plast. Reconstr. Surg.* 113: 1391, 2004.

El-Ali, K.M. and Gourlay, T. Assessment of the risk of systemic fat mobilization as a consequence of liposuction: ex vivo study. *Plast. Reconstr. Surg.* 117: 2269, 2006.

"Evaluation of circulating triglyceride levels after ultrasonic liposuction shows that these levels actually decrease after ultrasonic liposuction, an important safety consideration."

Zocchi, M.L. Ultrasound assisted lipoplasty: technical refinements and clinical evaluations. *Clin. Plast. Surg.* 23: 575, 1996.

Unpublished data. Swanson Center, 2009.

Ideal Buttocks

Page 81

"In fact, surveys suggest that men rate the attractiveness of the female buttocks on par with their breasts."

Mazur, A. U.S. trends in feminine beauty and overadaptation. *Journal of Sex Research*, 22: 281, 1986.

"'high and hard,' as Joan Rivers puts it."

Rivers, J. *Men are Stupid…and They Like Big Boobs*. New York: Pocket Books, 2009. Page 3.

Page 85

"We estimate about 50%"

Kaufman, M.R., Bradley, J.P., Dickinson, B., Heller, J.B., Wasson, K., O'Hara, C., Huang, C., Gabbay, J., Ghadjar, K., and Miller, T. Autologous Fat Transfer National Consensus Survey, Trends in techniques for harvest, preparation, and application, and perception of short- and long-term results. *Plast. Reconstr. Surg.* 119: 323, 2007.

Abdominoplasty

Page 87

"Surveys indicate that 57-71 percent of women are dissatisfied with their midtorso!"

Bolton, M.A., Pruzinsky, T., Cash, T.F., and Persing, J.A. Measuring outcomes in plastic surgery: Body image and quality of life in abdominoplasty patients. *Plast. Reconstr. Surg.* 112: 619, 2003.

Page 90

"When endoscopic procedures were introduced in the 1990s, plastic surgeons tried this approach on the abdomen, to determine whether an effective abdominoplasty could be performed used smaller incisions, with endoscopic tightening of the muscles."

Eaves, F.F., Nahai, F., and Bostwick, J. Endoscopic abdominoplasty and endoscopically assisted miniabdominoplasty. *Clin. Plast. Surg.* 23: 599, 1996.

"However, this approach did not prove practical because the skin remained stretched out. The skin did not contract sufficiently. It was clear that removal of excess skin was needed in most patients. Unlike the forehead lift… abdominoplasty did not prove to be a worthwhile application of endoscopy."

Nahai, F. Discussion. Circumferential suction lipectomy of the trunk with anterior rectus fascia plication through a periumbilical incision: an alternative to conventional abdominoplasty. *Plast. Reconstr. Surg.* 113: 733, 2004.

Page 108

"Our Survey Says"

Unpublished data. Swanson Center, 2009.

Page 111

"It takes months for the feeling to gradually return, starting with the sides of the tummy. The last area to recover feeling is the area below the umbilicus, which can take up to two years."

Farah, A.B., Nahas, F.X., Ferreira, L.M., Mendes, J.A., and Juliano, Y. Sensibility of the abdomen after abdominoplasty. *Plast. Reconstr. Surg.* 114: 577, 2004.

"Dog ears occur after abdominoplasties with some regularity."

Matarasso, A. Discussion. Geometric incision designing for abdominoplasty. *Plast. Reconstr. Surg.* 109: 2537, 2002.

Page 112

"A small, oval umbilicus with a skin fold over the top part is the goal."

Craig, S.B., Faller, M.S., and Puckett, C.L. In search of the ideal female umbilicus. *Plast. Reconstr. Surg.* 105: 389, 2000.

Page 117

"Cessation of smoking greatly reduces the risk of this complication."

Manassa, E.H., Hertl, C.H., and Olbrisch, R.R. Wound healing problems in smokers and nonsmokers after 132 abdominoplasties. *Plast. Reconstr. Surg.* 111: 2082, 2003.

Page 120

"Presently, acetaminophen toxicity is the leading cause of acute liver failure in the United States."

Larson, A.M., Polson, J., Fontana, R.J., Davern, T.J., Lalani, E., Hynan, L.S., Reisch, J.S., Schiødt, F.V., Ostapowicz, G., Shakil, A.O., and Lee, W.M. Acetaminophen-induced acute liver failure: results of a United States multicenter prospective study. *Hepatology* 42: 1364, 2005.

"at the time of this writing, an FDA advisory panel is recommending reducing the maximum daily dose from 4000 mg to 2600 mg and limiting the amount in a pill to 325 mg (so that 500 mg extra-strength Tylenol® would no longer be available)."

http://www.fda.gov/ForConsumers/ConsumerUpdates/ucm168830.htm. Accessed July 10, 2009.

Page 121

"However, a study showed similar pain scores and use of prescription pain killers in patients with and without these pumps after abdominoplasty. Possible reasons for its ineffectiveness are a lack of penetration of the muscle fascia, and a compromised distribution in the wound due to gravity and suction drains used after surgery that may drain off the local anesthetic solution."

Bray, D.A., Nguyen, J., Craig, J., and Cohen, B.E. Efficacy of a local anesthetic pain pump in abdominoplasty. *Plast. Reconstr. Surg.* 119: 1054, 2007.

Thigh and Buttock Lifts

Page 129

"Seromas are relatively common (about one-third of patients) because large areas may be undermined, particularly when thigh lifts are done in combination with an abdominoplasty."

Aly, A.S., Cram, A.E., Chao, M., Pang, J., and McKeon, M. Belt lipectomy for circumferential truncal excess: the University of Iowa experience. *Plast. Reconstr. Surg.* 111: 398, 2003.

Leahy, P.J., Shorten, S.M., and Lawrence, W.T. Maximizing the aesthetic result in panniculectomy after massive weight loss. *Plast. Reconstr. Surg.* 122: 1214, 2008.

Body Contouring after Massive Weight Loss

Page 133-134

"Patients who undergo Lap-Band® surgery do not tend to have nutritional deficiencies because the absorptive capability of the digestive tract is preserved. The digestive tract remains intact. It is a purely restrictive procedure. A small gastric pouch and outlet are created, so that patients feel satisfied earlier. Absorption is preserved, and nutritional deficiency is unlikely. This is the most common bariatric procedure performed today and the safest.

By contrast, gastric bypass surgery, most commonly the Roux-en-Y procedure, not only reduces the stomach size, but also interferes with absorption of nutrients ('malabsorption'), by literally bypassing portions of the digestive tract. These patients are often anemic, as a result of reduced absorption of iron, vitamin B12, and folate, and need to supplement their diets accordingly. One-third of gastric bypass patients may remain iron-deficient, even with oral supplementation. Their hemoglobin levels are often below normal or borderline. In addition, they may be deficient in protein, vitamin A and C, selenium and zinc—all important nutrients for wound healing and immune function. These patients may have a more dramatic weight reduction than Lap-Band patients, but their nutrition is jeopardized."

Agha-Mohammadi, S., and Hurwitz, D.J. Nutritional deficiency of post-bariatric surgery body contouring patients: what every plastic surgeon should know. *Plast. Reconstr. Surg.* 122: 604, 2008.

Page 134

"Combination procedures can increase surgical blood loss because of greater tissue resections. This needs to be considered in surgical planning. Patients also need to be aware of the possible need for a blood transfusion."

Leahy, P.J., Shorten, S.M., and Lawrence, W.T. Maximizing the aesthetic result in panniculectomy after massive weight loss. *Plast. Reconstr. Surg.* 122: 1214, 2008.

"It is more common today to use a longitudinal incision down the inseam of the inner thigh, rather than an incision in the groin crease, to remove the greatest amount of excess skin and provide maximum circumferential tightening of the thigh."

Kenkel, J.M., and Eaves, F.F. Medial thigh lift. *Plast. Reconstr. Surg.* 122: 621, 2008.

"flaps raised at the time of the outer thigh lift may be transposed to help fill out the buttocks."

Pascal, J.G., and Le Louarn, C. Remodeling body lift with high lateral tension. *Aesthetic Plast. Surg.* 26: 223, 2002.

Page 138

"Deep venous thrombosis can occur after any long procedure, and the risk may be as high as 9% in patients undergoing body contouring surgery after massive weight loss, occurring almost exclusively in patients who remain obese (BMI>35)."

Shermak, M.A., Chang, D.C., and Heller, J. Factors impacting thromboembolism after bariatric body contouring surgery. *Plast. Reconstr. Surg.* 119: 1590, 2007.

Breast Reduction in Men

Page 141

"It is a common condition, affecting about one-third of males overall, and an even larger percentages of adolescent boys and men over 65."

Rohrich, R.J., Ha, R.Y., Kenkel, J.M., and Adams, W.P. Classification and management of gynecomastia: defining the role of ultrasound-assisted liposuction. *Plast. Reconstr. Surg.* 111: 909, 2003.

"Most of the time, there is no known cause."

Ibid.

"Sometimes gynecomastia may be caused by a specific drug or medical problem. Chronic alcoholics and men who use anabolic steroids as part of a bodybuilding program are more likely to develop this condition. Certain hormonal abnormalities, inherited or acquired, usually involving either a deficiency of testosterone or excess of estrogen, can cause breast enlargement. Hyperthyroidism can cause it too. Marijuana and cancer chemotherapeutic agents can bring it on. Gynecomastia can also be a side effect of a number of heart and blood pressure medications. In rare cases it may be associated with an estrogen-producing testicular tumor."

Ibid.

Page 142

"This breast tissue can be quite fibrous, and ultrasound helps to break down the fat component, facilitating its removal. *Liposuction is not very effective in removing breast tissue itself.*"

Hammond, D.C., Arnold, J.F., Simon, A.M., and Capraro, P.A. Combined use of ultrasonic liposuction with the pull-through technique for the treatment of gynecomastia. *Plast. Reconstr. Surg.* 112: 891, 2003.

Page 148

"It is important to leave a cushion of breast tissue under the nipple to avoid a saucer-like depression, which can be difficult to correct."

Ibid.

Hand Rejuvenation

Page 153

"Hands can be a giveaway for aging."

Bains et al. Hand aging: Patients' opinions. *Plast. Reconstr. Surg.* 117: 2212, 2006.

"Fat injection can help by providing a layer of cushioning between the skin and the underlying tendons and veins, making them less conspicuous."

Coleman, S.R. Hand rejuvenation with structural fat grafting. *Plast. Reconstr. Surg.* 110: 1731, 2002.

Arm Lift (Brachioplasty)

Page 165

"An arm lift may be done on its own, but is more commonly performed at the same time as other body contouring procedures, especially in the treatment of deformities resulting from massive weight loss."

Gusenoff, J.A., Coon, D., and Rubin, J.P. Brachioplasty and concomitant procedures after massive weight loss: a statistical analysis from a prospective registry. *Plast. Reconstr. Surg.* 122: 595, 2008.

Page 167

"An important sensory nerve (the 'medial antebrachial cutaneous nerve') runs down the inside of the upper arm. It is important for the surgeon to avoid injuring this nerve, which might cause a painful neuroma."

Knoetgen, J. and Moran, S.L. Long-term outcomes and complications associated with brachioplasty: a retrospective review and cadaveric study. *Plast. Reconstr. Surg.* 117: 2219, 2006.

Labiaplasty

Page 171

"The most common cause of enlarged labia ('labia minora') is simply heredity."

Giraldo, F., Gonzalez, C., and de Haro, F. Central wedge nymphectomy with a 90-degree Z-plasty for aesthetic reduction of the labia minora. *Plast. Reconstr. Surg.* 113: 1820, 2004.

"Labiaplasty is a valid procedure, published in peer-reviewed plastic surgery journals. It successfully treats a real problem, with predictable results and high levels of patient satisfaction."

Alter, G. A new technique for aesthetic labia minor reduction. *Ann. Plast. Surg.* 40: 287, 1998.

Girlado, G., Gonzalez, C., and de Haro, F. Central wedge nymphectomy with a 90-degree Z-plasty for aesthetic reduction of the labia minora. *Plast. Reconstr. Surg.* 113: 1820, 2004.

"Dr. Matlock says that his patent attorneys told him not to publish his techniques so as to protect his intellectual property."

Valenza, T. Cosmetic surgery's G-man. *Plastic Surgery Practice.* May 2009. Page 10.

Laser Hair Removal

Page 175

"Renaissance paintings by the masters rarely portray body hair on women, or men."

Bresc-Bautier, G. and Morvan, F. (eds.) *The Louvre Collections*. 1999. Paris: Réunion des musées nationaux. 1999.

"Among all the actors to play him, there has been only one hairy-chested Tarzan."

Etcoff, N. *Survival of the Prettiest. The Science of Beauty*. New York: Anchor Books, 2000. Page 98.

"George Carlin half-joked that when he sees a guy with hair on his back, he immediately relegates him to the animal kingdom."

Carlin, G. *Napalm & Silly Putty*. New York: Hyperion, 2001. Page 30.

Page 176

"And the treatment is about 50% effective, meaning about half of the hairs survive treatment. There are complications from this technique due to the effects of electrical current. Because some skin cells are burned along with the hair follicle, scarring and ingrown hairs may result. Nodules may form. Infection is possible because of the breakdown of the skin barrier function."

Chana, J.S. and Grobbelaar, A.O. The long-term results of ruby laser depilation in a consecutive series of 346 patients. *Plast. Reconstr. Surg.* 110: 254, 2002.

Page 177

"In 1983, the concept of 'selective photothermolysis' was introduced."

Anderson, R.R. and Parrish, J.A. Selective photothermolysis: precise microsurgery by selective absorption of pulsed radiation. *Science* 220: 524, 1983.

"Doctors noticed that when they treated tattoos with a ruby laser, fewer hairs grew back in the treated area. They recognized a new application of the laser to the old problem of hair removal."

Alster, T.S. *Manual of cutaneous laser techniques*. Second ed. Philadelphia: Lippincott Williams & Wilkins, 2000. Page 110.

Page 178

"Also, the longer 'pulse duration' offered an advantage in spreading out the energy delivery, particularly for patients with darker skin types or dense hair."

Finkel, B., Eliezri, Y.D., Waldman, A., and Slatkine, M. Pulsed alexandrite laser technology for noninvasive hair removal. *J. Clin. Laser Med. Surg.* 15: 225, 1997.

Page 179

"The cycle length is different, depending on the anatomic location. For most areas of the body, it's between four and 10 months long and about half this time is spent in the anagen phase."

Chana, J.S. and Grobbelaar, A.O. The long-term results of ruby laser depilation in a consecutive series of 346 patients. *Plast. Reconstr. Surg.* 110: 254, 2002.

"They only seem to be vulnerable to laser treatment in their growth phase, perhaps owing to the presence of a hair shaft in the follicle to absorb laser energy."

Ibid.

Page 180

"The most favorable combination for treatment is dark hair and light skin."

Ibid.

Page 182

"With greater experience, researchers found that the disabled hair follicles did not regain function; the effect appears to be permanent."

Dierickx, C.C., Grossman, M.C., Farinelli, W.A., and Anderson, R.R. Permanent hair removal by normal-mode ruby laser. *Arch. Dermatol.* 134: 837, 1998.

Tattoo Removal

Page 187

"Today, almost as many women (13%) as men (15%) have tattoos."

http://www.harrisinteractive.com/harris_poll/index.asp?PID=868. Accessed March 4, 2009.

"A 2004 telephone survey among young adults, aged 18-29, found 36% had tattoos."

http://www.aad.org/media/background/factsheets/fact_tattoos.html. Accessed March 4, 2009.

"Despite their popularity, a large percentage of people with tattoos eventually regret having them."

http://emedicine.medscape.com/article/1121212-overview Accessed March 4, 2009.

ARTISTIC CREDITS

Page 79	Vanni Saltarelli. "Piccolo scherso."
Page 131	Jean-Baptiste Carpeaux. "La toilette de Venus." 1855.
Page 139	Wayland Bartlett. "Torso of a seated woman." 1895. Musée d'Orsay, Paris.
Page 151	Ancient Greek statue. Male torso, Louvre Museum.
Page 157	Kirsten Kokkin. "Flight to Infinity." 1991.
Page 169	French Bronze, circa 1910-1920.

INDEX

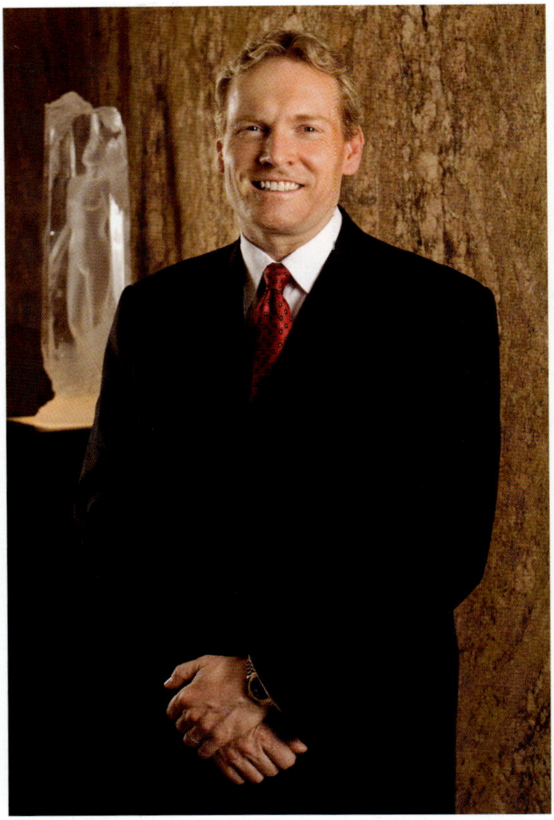

Dr. Swanson completed medical school at the University of Toronto, where he received his M.D. at the age of 22. In 1988, he completed a residency in plastic and reconstructive surgery at the University of Toronto, followed by a fellowship in cosmetic surgery. Dr. Swanson moved to Kansas City in 1989, where he started practice. From 1991 to 1995, he served as Director of the Cleft Palate and Craniofacial Clinic at Children's Mercy Hospital. He also served as Director of the Residency in Plastic Surgery at the University of Missouri-Kansas City from 1991 to 1993. Dr. Swanson was a visiting surgeon, performing cleft lip and palate surgery on children in the Dominican Republic, during three missionary excursions in 1991-1993.

In 1998, Dr. Swanson opened the Swanson Center for Cosmetic & Laser Surgery and Leawood Surgery Center, Kansas City's first licensed ambulatory surgery center specializing in cosmetic surgery.

In 2002, the Swanson Center embarked on a multipart clinical investigation of cosmetic surgery, including outcome studies, prospective clinical studies, and measurements using specialized computer imaging and MRIs. In 2008, Dr. Swanson presented the original findings at the meeting of the American Society of Plastic Surgeons, followed by another presentation at the 2009 meeting of the American Society for Aesthetic Plastic Surgery.

In 2009, Dr. Swanson completed his landmark four-part *Ideal Look* series, subtitled *The New Science of Cosmetic Surgery*, the product of a large body of clinical experience and studies. Dr. Swanson is an outspoken advocate for the application of the scientific method to cosmetic surgery, an approach known as evidence-based medicine.

Dr. Swanson is certified in plastic surgery by the Royal College of Surgeons of Canada, a member of the American Society of Plastic Surgeons, a Fellow of the American College of Surgeons, and a Fellow of the Royal College of Surgeons of Canada. He has practiced in Kansas City since 1989 and specializes exclusively in cosmetic surgery.